D0845884

Training for Sport and Activity

Training for Sport and Activity
The Physiological Basis
of the Conditioning Process

Second Edition

Jack H. Wilmore
University of Arizona

ALLYN AND BACON, INC.
Boston   London   Sydney   Toronto

Library of Congress Cataloging in Publication Data

Wilmore, Jack H., 1938–
   Training for sport and activity.

   Rev. ed. of: Athletic training and physical fitness.
   Bibliography: p.
   Includes index.
   1. Exercise—Physiological aspects. 2. Physical
fitness—Physiological aspects. 3. Physical education
and training. I. Title.
QP301.W675 1982   612'.044   81-17605
ISBN 0-205-07761-7   AACR2

Managing Editor: Hiram Howard

Printed in the United States of America

10 9 8 7 6 5 4 3 2 1   87 86 85 84 83 82

This book is dedicated to those who have made the greatest impact on my life: to Dottie, my lovely wife, and our three beautiful daughters, Wendy, Kristy, and Melissa, for their patience and love; to Mom and Dad, for their love, direction, and encouragement; and to my Lord, Jesus Christ, who is always there providing for every one of my needs.

Contents

Preface

Like the previous edition, this book is designed to provide the sport practitioner—the coach, the athlete, the team trainer, and the team physician—with a basic understanding of the physiological principles underlying the physical conditioning process that is so important to athletic performance and physical fitness. This book is also written for the undergraduate major in physical education with the intent of providing a clear understanding of the fundamental principles of exercise physiology as applied to sport and physical activity.

Over the years, research in the exercise and sport sciences has provided the practitioner with relatively little information of practical value. In addition, the information that has been provided has been poorly utilized. Unfortunately, there is a large chasm between the researcher in the laboratory and the practitioner in the gym, beside the pool, or on the field. They live in two different worlds, neither completely understanding the language, complexity of the situation, or problems of the other. On the positive side, however, during the past few years research has taken a turn toward problems of a more practical nature, and a wealth of information is now available to the practitioner. To achieve maximum utilization of this information, one must have or acquire a basic understanding of the foundations of exercise and sport.

It has been less than five years since the publication of the first edition of this book. Knowledge and understanding in the exercise and sport sciences have advanced rapidly during this intervening period of time. This has necessitated rather major revisions in the original material, and the inclusion of two new chapters. Almost all of the original artwork has been redrawn, with the intent of simplifying basic concepts and complementing the revisions in the text. Again, I must extend my thanks to all of those whose encouragement and assistance made this book a reality.

J. H. W.

SECTION A

Physiological Foundations

The present book is designed to provide the reader with a fundamental understanding of the physiological principles underlying the body's responses and adaptations to acute and chronic exercise. This section deals first with a brief review of the foundational areas of anatomy and physiology. The emphasis then shifts to an explanation of the physiological alterations that result from an acute or single bout of exercise. Those changes that typically result from chronic exercise, i.e., a long-term program of physical training, will then be discussed. This section should give the reader the basic language that he or she will need to more fully understand the subsequent sections of this book.

1

Basic Anatomical and Physiological Considerations

INTRODUCTION

The human body is an amazing creation. In the resting state, countless events are occurring simultaneously, in perfect coordination, allowing complex functions such as hearing, seeing, smelling, tasting, breathing, and thinking to continue without conscious effort. The transition from rest to exercise is accompanied by substantial alterations in a number of the body's functions, which allow the body to successfully adapt to this additional stress. As the body is subjected to repeated bouts of exercise, such as in a physical conditioning program, long-term adaptations in bodily function occur which allow higher levels of exercise to be tolerated without fatigue, as well as provide the body with a feeling or sense of well-being.

People have been able to achieve rather remarkable physical feats in the realm of sport. They can sprint 100 meters in less than ten seconds, run a sub-four-minute mile, and complete a 26.2-mile marathon in less than two hours and ten minutes. They can jump over 29 feet horizontally, and over 7 feet vertically. They can swim for both speed and distance, and perform many other tasks which require high levels of skill and dexterity.

Such feats can be accomplished only through a series of complex interactions within the body involving nearly all of the body's systems. The bones provide the basic skeletal framework through which the muscles can perform. The heart and blood vessels deliver nutrients via blood to the various cells of the body, and, with the help of the lungs, provide oxygen to and remove carbon dioxide from these same cells. The nervous and endocrine systems integrate all of this activity into a meaningful performance. Practically no cell, tissue, or organ escapes involvement in even the simplest movement. At the level of the cell, various enzymes are activated and energy is generated to enable muscles to contract. The skin plays a vital role in maintaining body temperature through its various avenues of heat loss, as body heat would tend to accumulate with prolonged exercise. Also, the kidneys assist in maintaining fluid balance. This chapter will focus on the basic anatomical structures, and the physiological function of the various body systems that enable the individual to successfully adapt to short-term, prolonged, and repeated bouts of exercise.

The science of *anatomy* deals with the structure of the body and the interrelationship of its parts. The science of *physiology* deals with the mechanisms through which the body functions, or more simply, understanding how the various systems of the body work. The systems that will be reviewed in this chapter will include the skeletal, muscular, nervous, cardiovascular, respiratory, metabolic, and endocrine systems. Since it is difficult to separate structure and function, the anatomical and physiological aspects of each system will be discussed concurrently.

SKELETAL SYSTEM

The skeletal system is composed of all of the bones in the body, and, for purposes of discussion in this chapter, will include the articulations of these bones, which are referred to as joints, and the cartilage and ligamentous tissue that supports the structure of the joints. The bones, joints, cartilage, and ligaments form the supporting framework for the body, and the bones specifically serve as the basis of attachment for the muscles, provide protection for delicate structures in certain parts of the body, act as a reserve for calcium stores in the body, and are involved in the formation of red blood cells.

Bone Development

Bone develops from fibrous membranes and hyaline cartilage starting at approximately the eighth week of embryonic life. Flat bones, such as those of the face and skull, develop from fibrous membranes, while the remaining bones, which include most of the bones of the body, develop from hyaline cartilage. *Hyaline cartilage* is a special form of cartilage that covers the surface of bones within joints, and forms the rib cartilages and many of the other cartilages found in the body. As the body is being formed and the bones continue to grow, both during fetal development as well as during the initial fourteen to twenty-two years of life, the membrane and cartilage are transformed into bone through the process of *ossification*.

Since most bones originate from hyaline cartilage, particularly the long bones which are of greatest interest to the present discussion, the ossification process from hyaline cartilage to the fully mature bone will be discussed briefly. This is a particularly important concept to understand, for athletic injuries to immature bone, i.e., not fully developed, can have serious long-term consequences, including complete cessation of growth of the involved bone or bones.

The ossification process involves the conversion of cartilage to bone, a process which may not be complete in all of the bones in the body until about the twenty-fifth year of life. First, the general contour of the cartilage in the early embryonic stages resembles the future shape of the mature bone. The central shaft of the long bone is referred to as the *diaphysis*, or the primary center of ossification. The

ends of the long bone are referred to as the *epiphyses*. Bone formation, or the transformation of cartilage to bone, begins at the diaphysis. The *periosteum*, which is the external or outer covering of bone, is first to develop, and forms a ring or collar of bone around the central shaft or diaphysis. At the same time, the cartilage cells in the area of the diaphysis undergo a series of complex changes which eventually result in the formation of bone. The cartilage continues to grow in length and thickness, and the periosteum and the bone formation from the center of the diaphysis continues toward the ends of the bone, or the epiphysis. Eventually, the periosteum reaches the epiphysis and establishes secondary centers of ossification in each epiphysis, thus allowing bone formation from cartilage to begin at the ends of the long bones. Once this occurs, there are plates of cartilage that lie between the diaphysis and the epiphyses which persist for periods of time until full maturation, allowing for growth in the length of the bone. These plates of cartilage are known as *epiphyseal cartilage*. Cartilage continues to grow on the epiphyseal border of these plates, and cartilage is replaced on the diaphyseal border, so that the plates or discs of cartilage remain approximately the same thickness. Ossification is complete and bone growth ceases when the cells of cartilage cease to grow and the entire discs are replaced by bone. This results in the uniting of the diaphysis with each epiphysis, and growth in length is no longer possible. The ossification process is illustrated in Figure 1–1. In the tibia, ossification is completed in the distal epiphysis (epiphysis farthest from the center of the body) by the age of seventeen years, and in the proximal epiphysis by the age of twenty years, although the exact age will vary considerably from one individual to the next.

The structure of the mature long bone is surprisingly complex. Bones must have a blood supply, for they are metabolically active, requiring essential nutrients. In addition, the center of the long bone is hollow and is referred to as the *medullary cavity*. It is in the medullary cavity and in the spaces of spongy bone that one finds the *bone marrow*. Bone marrow aids in the nutrition of the bone as well as serving as a center for red blood cell production and limited white blood cell production. Bone tissue consists of cells that are distributed throughout a matrix or lattice-type of arrangement. Bone tissue

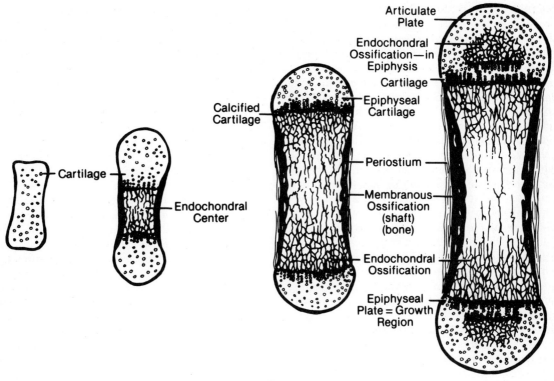

Figure 1–1 Illustration of the growth of a long bone from total cartilage in the embryonic stages to an almost mature bone.

is dense and hard due to deposits of lime salts, mainly calcium phosphate and calcium carbonate. Calcium is therefore an essential nutrient, particularly during periods of bone growth, and in the latter years of life when bone tends to become brittle with aging.

Articulations

The bones of the skeletal system join together to form the supporting framework of the body. Whenever two or more bones meet, articulations or joints are formed. The articulation of the femur with the tibia forms the knee joint. The humerus articulates with the radius and ulna to form the elbow joint. And the three phalanges of each finger articulate to form several joints for each finger. Several types of joints exist in the body. Essentially there are three primary classifications of joints: fibrous, cartilaginous, and synovial. *Fibrous joints*

are those joints where bones are joined together by fibrous-like elastic connective tissue, allowing little or no movement. The bones of the cranium or skull cap are joined together in this fashion. *Cartilaginous joints* are similar in characteristic, there being no space or joint cavity between bones, and there is only limited motion. The bodies of the vertebrae are joined in this manner. *Synovial joints* are of the greatest importance for purposes of discussion in this book. Synovial joints are formed by the articulating bones, a thin layer of cartilage on the ends of the bones and a fibrous capsule that encloses the joint. All the joints of the extremities are synovial joints. The fibrous joint capsule is lined on the inside with a membrane which has a rich capillary network of blood vessels. This membrane is referred to as the *synovial membrane*, and it produces a viscous or relatively thick fluid, *synovial fluid*, which provides a natural lubrication for all joint movement. The smooth hyaline cartilage on the ends of those bones involved in the articulation provides a surface that has a greatly reduced friction, which, when combined with the synovial fluid, provides a relatively free motion within the joint. Figure 1–2 illustrates a synovial joint.

A disc of fibrous cartilage is present in some joints, dividing the joint cavity and providing a smoother surface for joint action. The knee joint has several of these discs or menisci which allow for a better articulation of the femur with the tibia. Frequently, when the knee is injured in athletics, the meniscus is damaged and must be removed through surgery. However, loss of one or both menisci in a single knee joint does not greatly limit joint movement, although the articulation is not as smooth. Joint swelling and pain are often the result, with the possibility of arthritis in the later years.

Ligaments are cords or bands of fibrous tissue which cross the joint, attaching one bone to another, providing strength to the joint capsule so it won't be pulled apart or disrupted in any fashion. Ligaments typically lie outside the joint capsule, but are also found within the joint capsule for certain joints, e.g., cruciate ligaments inside the knee joint. *Tendons* are formed of connective tissue and provide the means by which muscles are attached to bones. Tendons cross joints and thus provide additional support for that specific joint. *Bursae* are small sacs that are filled with synovial fluid and are present in the area of joints where tendons are likely to rub against bone, ligaments, or other tendons, or at locations where skin moves over a bony prominence. They function to reduce friction at these points of movement.

MUSCULAR SYSTEM

There are basically three kinds of muscle tissue: smooth, cardiac, and skeletal. *Smooth muscle* is also referred to as involuntary muscle as it is not usually under the conscious control of the individual; its contractions being controlled automatically through the autonomic nervous system. Smooth muscle is found in the walls of the internal or visceral organs, e.g., blood vessels, stomach, and intestines. *Cardiac muscle* is found only in the heart. It has characteristics similar to skeletal muscle, but, like smooth muscle, is not under direct voluntary control. *Skeletal muscles*, also referred to

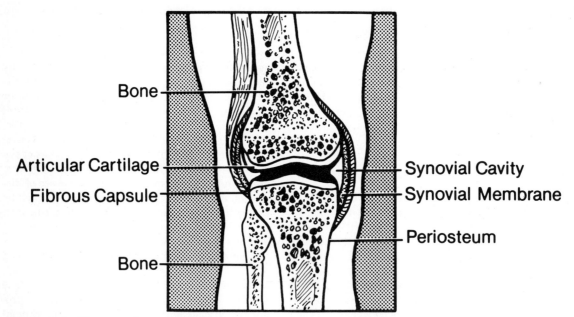

Figure 1–2 Diagram of a synovial joint, illustrating the articular cartilage, synovial membrane, articular capsule, and ligamentous support.

as voluntary muscles, are those muscles we are consciously aware of and are able to control, which attach to and cause movement of the skeleton. The remainder of this section will concentrate entirely on a discussion of the characteristics of skeletal muscle.

Skeletal muscle, in combination with the bones and joints, is responsible for all human movement. Obviously, any one single muscle does not work by itself, contracting at will, independently of the other muscles in the body. All skeletal muscles are coordinated simultaneously by a master network of nerve cells, both inside and outside the brain. The nervous system's control of muscular movement will be discussed in more detail in the next section of this chapter.

Structure and Function of Skeletal Muscle

Figure 1–3 illustrates the basic structure of muscle. A single muscle is composed of a number of individual muscle fibers. The individual *muscle fiber* is a single cell with many nuclei and is the structural unit of muscle. The number of muscle fibers per whole muscle will vary considerably, depending on the size and function of the muscle. Within a given muscle, the individual muscle fibers are grouped into bundles of fibers which are termed *fasciculi*. The *endomysium* is connective tissue that surrounds individual fibers and binds them together to form the fasciculi. The *perimysium* is white fibrous connective tissue that binds adjacent fasciculi together. The *epimysium* is the external connective tissue that surrounds the entire muscle, binding all of the fasciculi together into the whole muscle. Each muscle fiber has a protective covering or membrane which surrounds it, the *sarcolemma*. Inside each muscle fiber are numerous *myofibrils* which are comparable to numerous wires comprising a large cable (fiber). The *sarcoplasm* is a gelatin-like substance that surrounds the myofibrils within each fiber and serves as the protoplasm of the muscle cell or fiber. The *mitochondria* are the small rod-shaped bodies in the sarcoplasm that serve as the powerhouses of the cell, and are involved in providing energy for muscular contraction.

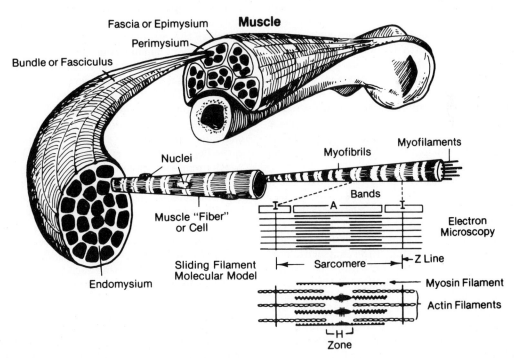

Figure 1–3 Structure of human skeletal muscle.

The myofibrils have distinct markings and the individual myofibrils are lined up in register with the adjacent myofibrils. A closer look at these markings indicates a definite repetitive pattern. These markings are referred to as *striations*, and skeletal muscle has been referred to as striated muscle, although this is a characteristic shared in common with cardiac muscle. The repetitive pattern defines the *contractile unit* of muscle, the *sarcomere*. In Figure 1–3, the sarcomere is bound on each end by a *Z-line*. Between each pair of Z-lines are, in sequence, a light or isotropic zone referred to as the *I-band*; a dark, or anisotrophic zone, referred to as the *A-band*; an *H-zone* of slightly lighter contrast which lies in the middle of the A-band; and a second I-band. Each myofibril is composed of numerous sarcomeres which are joined end-to-end at the Z-line.

These variations in light and dark patterns are thought to be the result of the alignment of individual *myofilaments* which comprise the myofibrils. Looking through an electron microscope, it is possible to differentiate two small protein filaments, *actin* and *myosin*. The thinner of the two filaments is the protein actin, while the protein myosin forms the thicker filament. The I-band reflects that region of the sarcomere where there are only thin, or actin filaments; the A-band reflects that region where there are both thick, or myosin, as well as thin, or actin, filaments; and the H-zone is that central portion of the A-band occupied only by the thick filaments when the sarcomere is in a resting state. The H-zone will disappear when the muscle contracts, for the thin filaments will extend into this zone—as will be defined in the next paragraph.

When a muscle fiber contracts, the individual sarcomeres of each myofibril actually shorten, i.e., the Z-lines move closer together. How does a muscle or the individual sarcomeres contract? With the use of an electron microscope it is possible to begin to obtain an understanding of the contractile process. An electron microscope allows maximum magnification of the tissue sample and is required for muscle analysis since myosin filaments are only 160 angstrom units in diameter, and actin filaments are only 50 to 70 angstrom units in diameter. To relate this to a more familiar standard of comparison, there are 10,000 angstrom units in a micron, and 1,000 microns in a millimeter. Since there are 25.4 millimeters in an inch, there would be a total of 254,000,000 or 2.54×10^8 angstroms per inch! The most widely accepted theory of how muscle contraction occurs at the level of the sarcomere is illustrated in Figure 1–4. The contraction or shortening of the sarcomere appears to be the result of the thin actin filaments sliding past the thick myosin filaments, a theory which has been referred to as the *sliding filament theory*. This conclusion was reached when it was observed that during contraction, there is a decrease in the length of the I-band, while the A-band remains essentially unchanged and the H-zone disappears. Small projections, referred to as *cross bridges*, have been identified on the thick myosin filaments and these appear to make contact with the thin actin filaments. It is postulated that those cross bridges move in a ratchet-like fashion when energy is available, pulling the thin filaments toward the center of the sarcomere, shortening the distance between the Z-lines. Apparently, neither the actin or myosin filaments alter their length, but simply alter the extent of their overlap.

The actual contraction process is quite complex. A nerve impulse from the specific nerve serving that muscle fiber travels along the *sarcolemma*, which is the cell membrane or outer cover of the muscle fiber, depolarizing this outer membrane along its length. A series of tubules enter this individual muscle fiber through pores in the sarcolemma. These tubules are referred to as *T-tubules*, and they conduct the impulse toward the center of the fiber, connecting with the *sarcoplasmic reticulum* a system of channels that spread out over the surface of the myofibrils. The nerve impulse is spread along the sarcolemma and down the T-tubules to the sarcoplasmic reticulum. Calcium ions are stored within the sarcoplasmic reticulum and are released once the nerve impulse reaches the sarcoplasmic reticulum. It is the release of these calcium ions that allows the process of contraction to begin. There are two *regulatory* proteins that are a part of the actin filament which serve to keep the actin and myosin filaments from interacting with one another, resulting in contraction or shortening of the myofibril. These proteins, *troponin* and *tropomyosin*, work in an intricate fashion along with the calcium ions to maintain relaxation or initiate contraction. Once calcium ions are released from the sarcoplasmic reticulum,

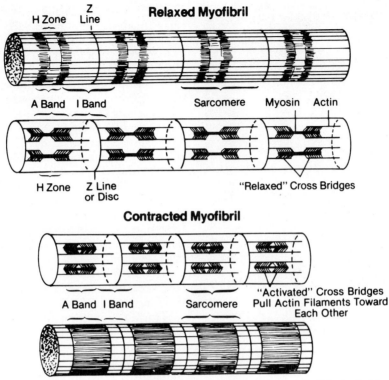

Figure 1–4 The proposed mechanism of muscular contraction at the level of the individual sarcomere unit.

they bind troponin, which in turn blocks the function of tropomyosin, which is to keep the actin and myosin filaments from interacting. The enzyme *ATPase*, located on the head of the cross bridge of the myosin filament, is then freed to act on *ATP* (adenosine triphosphate), causing it to break down to *ADP* (adenosine diphosphate), phosphate and energy for contraction. ATP is the chemical molecule in the body most available for energy release, and is the primary source of energy for muscular contraction. When ATP breaks down to ADP, releasing energy for contraction, there is an interaction between the myosin filament and the actin filament, involving the specific action of the cross bridges. The details of the mechanism of cross bridge involvement are not clear at this time, but are undergoing investigation by a number of scientists. The extent of contraction of the individual sarcomere units appears to be limited by the myosin filaments and the Z-lines, i.e., the contraction will be complete when the myosin filaments reach the Z-lines. Schematic representations of this discussion are illustrated in Figures 1–5 and 1–6.

Muscle Fiber Types

Are all muscle fibers identical? Recent research over the past ten years has identified the fact that there are different types of muscle fibers; this has definite implications relative to successful athletic performance. Muscle fiber type is dictated by the characteristics of the *motor unit* to which that particular muscle fiber belongs. A motor unit is composed of a nerve fiber or *neuron* which transmits the nervous impulse from the spinal cord to the muscle fiber, and is referred to as a *motor fiber* or *motorneuron*, and the muscle fibers that are controlled or innervated by that motorneuron. Each muscle fiber is innervated by only one motorneuron, but each motorneuron innervates from several fibers to several hundred fibers, depending on the function of that particular muscle. Muscles that

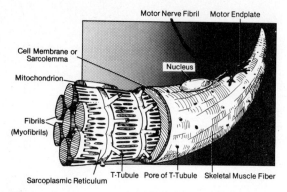

Figure 1–5 Nerve impulse transmission from the sarcolemma to the sacroplasmic reticulum.

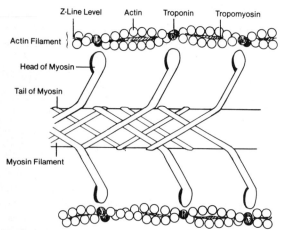

Figure 1–6 The molecular structure of the actin and myosin filaments and their related interaction in contraction.

exert control over fine movements, such as those muscles that control movements of the eyes, are characterized by a small number of muscle fibers for each motorneuron. Those muscles that have more general functions, such as the gluteal muscles that form the buttocks, have a very high number of muscle fibers for each motorneuron. Motor units are characterized on the basis of speed, force, and endurance, the latter term being defined as the length of time a muscle fiber can contract without loss of tension.

With respect to speed, there are two basic classifications into which all motor units fall: fast and slow. There are three classifications into which all motor units fall with respect to force: high, medium, and low. Finally, there are two classifications into which all motor units fall with respect to endurance: fatigue-resistant and fatigable. Looking at all motor units with respect to the characteristics of speed, force, and endurance, three basic fiber types can be identified: slow-twitch, oxidative; fast-twitch, high-oxidative, and glycolytic; and fast-twitch, glycolytic. For most purposes, the latter two types are combined and referred to as *fast-twitch fibers*, providing a simple two-component system of classification, i.e., fast-twitch and slow-twitch. Slow-twitch oxidative fibers are characterized as being slow in speed of contraction, low force-producing, and high endurance or fatigue-resistance. The fast-twitch, high oxidative and glycolytic fibers are characterized as being fast in speed of contraction, moderate in force-producing, and high in endurance or fatigue-resistance. The fast-twitch glycolytic fibers are characterized as being fast in speed of contraction, high force-producing, and low in endurance or fatigable. The terms *oxidative* and *glycolytic* refer to the primary energy source for muscular contraction.

How does all of this relate to athletic performance potential? Over the past few years, researchers have started looking at fiber types in athletes representing various sports, or positions, or events in specific sports. This is accomplished through a muscle biopsy, which involves removing a very small piece of muscle from the belly of a muscle for subsequent analysis. The area where the biopsy is to be taken is deadened with a local anesthetic. Once anesthetized, a scalpel is used to make a small, approximately one-inch, incision through the skin and outer connective tissue. A biopsy needle is then inserted into this incision and is pushed through the belly of the muscle to the appropriate depth. A small plunger is pushed through the center of the needle, snipping off a very small sample of the muscle. The sample is removed immediately and quickly frozen in liquid nitrogen. It is then sliced thinly, stained, and examined under a microscope. Figure 1–7 illustrates the biopsy technique, and Figure 1–8 illustrates a micrograph of a sectioned muscle, illustrat-

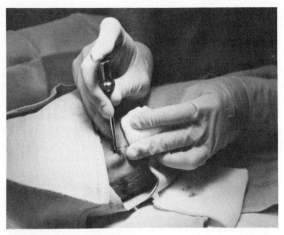

Figure 1–7 Illustration of a muscle biopsy of the lateral gastrocnemius.

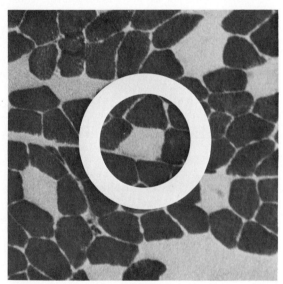

Figure 1–8 Illustration of fast-twitch (dark stained) and slow-twitch (light stained) muscle fibers from a cross-section of the gastrocnemius muscle.

ing the basic differences in fibers, stained to differentiate between fast- and slow-twitch fibers.

When biopsies are taken from athletes in various sports, or positions, or events in specific sports, an interesting pattern develops. Athletes who compete in sports or events that require speed have a high percentage of fast-twitch fibers. Those who are in sports or events that require endurance have a high percentage of slow-twitch fibers. As an example, track and field sprinters will typically have a fiber composition of 60 to 90 percent fast-twitch and 10 to 40 percent slow-twitch fibers, while the marathon runner will have 60 to 90 percent slow-twitch and 10 to 40 percent fast-twitch fibers. To date, it appears that fiber composition characteristics are determined hereditarily, although longitudinal studies starting early in life have not been conducted. Several studies have trained subjects in an attempt to develop either endurance or speed, and have found that fiber composition remains unchanged even though the subjects demonstrate improved speed or endurance. It does appear, however, that the fast-twitch glycolytic fiber can change to a fast-twitch, high oxidative and glycolytic fiber with endurance training. While it does not make the actual transition from a fast-twitch to slow-twitch fiber, it does develop endurance or fatigue-resistant qualities.

Since fiber type is essentially determined hereditarily, and doesn't change with training, it has been suggested that fiber composition could be determined at an early age, and then young athletes could be advised as to those sports for which they would be best suited. In the age of test-tube babies and proposed cloning procedures, this would seem to be a natural course to follow. Fortunately, for those who would argue for maintaining purity in sport, the fiber composition pattern of athletes in specific sports or events is not as absolute as was once thought. As an example, while the majority of world class marathon runners have a very high percentage of slow-twitch fibers, approximately 80 percent slow-twitch compared to 60 percent slow-twitch for middle-distance runners, one of the top five finishers at the 1976 Olympic Games held in Montreal, Quebec, had only 55 percent of his total fiber population as slow-twitch fibers. Thus, while the trend is toward a very high population percentage of slow-twitch fibers, there are always notable exceptions, and it is the exception that would make the selection of athletes solely on the basis of fiber type an undesirable practice.

NERVOUS SYSTEM

The muscular system provides the force that causes movement of the skeletal system. The nervous system acts to initiate this movement. Just as the skeleton is motionless without muscle, the muscle is motionless without the nervous system's control. The nervous system is probably the most complex of the body's systems. The master control center is located in the brain, although simple movement patterns which originate from reflexes, such as the "knee-jerk" reflex, do not depend on the brain for initiating or controlling the resulting movement. In addition to the brain, intricate networks of nerve cells go out to all parts of the body from the brain and spinal cord, while others originate in such areas as vessels, organs, muscle, and skin, and end in the spinal cord or brain. In an attempt to simplify the discussion of the nervous system, the total system is subdivided into the following classification:

A. Central Nervous System
   1. Anatomical Classification
      a. brain
      b. spinal cord
      c. peripheral nerves
   2. Functional Classification
      a. sensory division
      b. motor division
      c. integrative division
B. Autonomic Nervous System
   1. Sympathetic Division
   2. Parasympathetic Division

Anatomically, the nervous system has a central and peripheral component. The central nervous system is comprised of the brain, the spinal cord, and the peripheral nerves which have their cell bodies in the spinal cord. The brain serves as the master control center of the human body, functioning in much the same way as a computer. The brain and its various functional areas are illustrated in Figure 1–9. Information coming into the brain from various regions of the body is transmitted by the *sensory division* of the nervous system. The sensory division conducts impulses from the various sensory organs or receptor areas to the brain by *sensory nerves*. Vision, hearing, touch, smell, pressure, and pain illustrate a few of the various sources of sensory information, which allow the brain to be aware of its immediate surrounding environment. The brain transmits information out to various regions of the body through the *motor division* of the nervous system.

Once the brain has processed the information it receives through the sensory division, a decision is made, and the action is initiated by impulses traveling from the brain to that area of the body where movement is to occur. The motor division controls the contraction of skeletal muscle, the contraction of smooth muscle in the internal organs, and the secretion of the exocrine and endocrine glands. Skeletal muscles are controlled by impulses conducted by *motor nerves* originating from any one of three levels: the motor area of the cerebral cortex, the basal regions of the brain, and the spinal cord. As the level of control moves from the spinal cord to the *motor cortex*, the degree of movement complexity increases from simple reflex control to complicated movements requiring basic thought processes. The *integrative division* of the nervous system is where all information processing occurs. Numerous centers are located immediately adjacent to all sensory and motor centers in both the brain and the spinal cord. Some of these areas store information, a process more commonly referred to as *memory*, while others are involved in abstract thinking, and still others are involved with the evaluation of incoming information and then making decisions on the basis of that information, relative to all aspects of body movement and general physiological function.

The basic functional unit of the nervous system is the *neuron* or nerve cell. It has been estimated that there are approximately 12 billion neurons in the

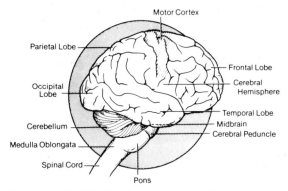

Figure 1–9   The brain and its functional areas.

brain and spinal cord, with approximately 75 percent of these located in the cerebral cortex, the center for thinking and memory storage. A typical neuron is composed of three parts: the *soma* or cell body of the neuron, the *dendrites*, and the *axon*. A nerve impulse can be transmitted only in one direction. It proceeds from the dendrite to the cell body and then out along the axon to either the end organ, such as the muscle, or to another neuron. Each neuron contains many dendrites which function to transmit impulses from adjacent neurons to the cell body of that neuron. There is, however, only one axon for each neuron, and the impulses travel from the cell body along the length of the axon to the

point where it branches into many terminal fibrils. Figure 1–10 illustrates the basic neuron.

The small terminal fibrils from a single neuron either connect to a muscle fiber, forming the *neuromuscular junction*, or to adjacent neurons forming a *synapse*. The neuromuscular junction is composed of the terminal fibrils of the neuron which end in sole feet, and the muscle fiber, which is invaginated at that point forming a cavity to accommodate the sole feet of the terminal fibrils. The cavity is referred to as the *synaptic gutter*, and the small space between the sole feet and the muscle fiber is referred to as the *synaptic cleft*. When one neuron connects with an adjacent neuron

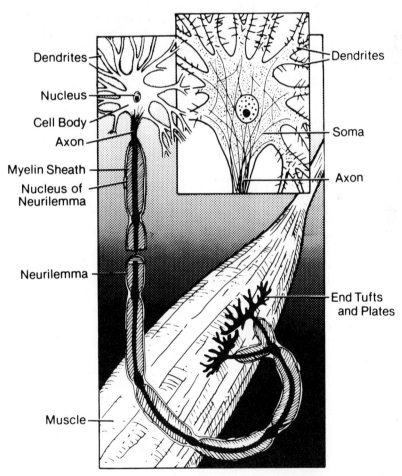

Figure 1–10 The neuron and its connection with muscle and adjacent neurons.

to form a synapse, the terminal fibrils end in synaptic knobs, which lie on the surface of the cell body and the dendrites of the adjacent neuron. The synapse is the actual junction between each synaptic knob and the dendrite or soma. Branches on terminal fibrils from many different axons of other neurons can all converge on the dendrites and cell body of a single neuron.

The transmission of impulses from one neuron to another, from one neuron to a single muscle fiber, and even from the dendrite of a neuron to the terminal fibrils of the same axon, is a complex act. Once a single neuron is stimulated, the impulse is transmitted the length of that neuron to the terminal fibrils through the process of depolarization. The neuron cell membrane has a resting electrical membrane potential which is disrupted by the incoming impulse, causing the membrane potential to be altered from a negative charge to a positive charge for a fraction of a second (depolarization) before returning to its normal resting potential (repolarization). This depolarization typically begins in the dendrites or cell body and progresses down the length of the axon in a wave-like action. Once the impulse reaches the neuromuscular junction, a chemical, *acetylcholine*, is released from the nerve terminals, and this chemical substance transmits the impulse from the sole feet, across the synaptic cleft to the muscle fiber, which in turn starts depolarization in the muscle fiber. Acetylcholine is referred to as a *transmitter substance*, and is immediately destroyed following stimulation of the muscle fiber by another chemical substance called *cholinesterase*. With respect to the synapse, the impulse is transmitted from the synaptic knobs across the synapse to the dendrites or soma of an adjacent neuron in much the same way as it is transmitted across the neuromuscular junction, i.e., via a transmitter substance. Unlike the neuromuscular junction, however, the transmitter substance at the synapse can be inhibitory as well as excitatory. Thus, some terminal fibrils excite the adjacent neuron while others inhibit the adjacent neuron. The concept of excitatory and inhibitory transmitter substances is very important when discussing the physiological basis for gaining strength.

Sensory Division

The sensory division of the nervous system receives information from the body from four primary sources: exteroceptive sensation, *proprioceptive sensation*, *visceral sensation*, and the *special senses*. Exteroceptive sensations are those that arise from the skin, including touch, pressure, heat, cold, and pain. Proprioceptive sensations arise from special sensory organs that sense muscle tension, tendon tension, joint angle, and deep pressure from the bottom of the feet. Visceral sensations are received from the internal organs, and include the sensations of pain, fullness, and heat. The special senses include vision, hearing, taste, and smell.

Sensations are detected by special nerve endings in the skin, muscles, tendons, or deeper areas of the body. The impulses are transmitted via the sensory nerves to the spinal cord, at which point the nerve either ends, forming a local reflex at that level of the spinal cord, or travels up to the upper regions of the spinal cord and brain. Sensory pathways to the brain terminate either in the sensory areas of the brain stem, the cerebellum, the thalamus, or the cerebral cortex. Impulses that terminate in the spinal cord initiate cord reflexes. This would be exemplified by the individual who touches a hot stove, and pulls back one's hand quickly to avoid further pain and discomfort. The sensory impulses from heat and pain travel to the spinal cord, terminate at that level of entry, connect with a motor nerve, which then activates the muscles necessary to withdraw the hand. Sensory signals that terminate in the lower brain stem result in subconscious motor reactions of a higher and more complex nature than those resulting in simple spinal cord reflexes. Postural control would be an example of this level of sensory input. Sensory signals that terminate at the level of the cerebellum also result in subconscious control of movement. This appears to be the center of coordination, smoothing out movements by coordinating the actions of the various muscle groups that are contracting to perform the desired movement. Both fine and gross motor movements appear to be coordinated through the cerebellum. Without the control exerted by the cerebellum, all movement would be uncontrolled and obviously uncoordinated. Sensory signals that terminate at the thalamus begin to enter the level of consciousness, and one begins to distinguish between the various types of sensation. Only when the sensory signals enter the cortex is one able to discreetly localize the nature of the signal.

Sensory receptors are basically of two types: *free nerve endings* and *special end-organs*. Free nerve endings detect the sensations of crude touch, pressure, pain, heat, and cold. Special end-organs are of several types and have several different functions. Each type of end-organ is sensitive to a specific sensation. The end-organs of most significance to human movement are the proprioceptive receptors. The joint *kinesthetic receptor* is located in the joint capsule, and is sensitive to joint angles and rates of change in joint angles. *Muscle spindles* and *Golgi tendon organs* are specialized receptors which provide information on the status of muscle. Muscle spindles provide information regarding the degree to which a muscle is stretched, and Golgi tendon organs detect the resulting tension applied to the tendon, providing information relative to the strength of muscle contraction.

Motor Division

Once a sensory impulse is received, this typically evokes a response through a *motorneuron*, irrespective of the level at which the sensory impulse stops. In a simple reflex, such as the example used earlier of touching a hot stove, the sensory receptor detects heat and pain, and transmits this information by impulses to the spinal cord through sensory nerve fibers. At this point, the impulses continue to the brain, informing the brain of what has transpired, but, more importantly, the impulses are transmitted by an interneuron at that same level in the spinal cord to a motorneuron, which then activates the appropriate muscle group to withdraw the hand. As reflexes or conscious movements become more complex, the sensory impulses travel further up the spinal cord, with the most complex terminating in the brain. The motor response to the more complex movement patterns typically originate in the motor cortex of the brain.

Skeletal muscle function is finely controlled by a complex series of events that transpire within the muscle, and between the muscle and its sensory and motor activation. Muscle spindles and Golgi tendon organs, previously described, play a vital role in controlling muscle contraction and the resulting tension developed by the muscle. Between the normal muscle fibers, which are referred to as *extrafusal fibers,* lie the muscle spindles, which are composed of several small specialized muscle fibers called *intrafusal fibers*, and nerve endings attached to these fibers. The endings of the intrafusal fibers are attached to the sheaths of the surrounding skeletal muscle fibers. These specialized muscle fibers, i.e., the intrafusal fibers, are controlled by a specialized motor nerve fiber, which is referred to as a *gamma motorneuron*, while normal or extrafusal muscle fibers are controlled by motorneurons referred to as *alpha motorneurons*. The middle portion of the intrafusal fiber does not have the ability to contract, thus when the ends of these fibers contract they stretch or elongate the central portion. Sensory nerve endings are wrapped around this middle portion of the intrafusal fibers and transmit information back to the central nervous system, informing the higher centers of the state of contraction or relaxation of that portion of the muscle. The muscle spindle is illustrated in Figure 1–11.

When a muscle is suddenly stretched, such as when a heavy weight is placed in the palm of an extended arm, this stretches or elongates the middle of the muscle spindle, which sends impulses to the spinal cord, which then excites the alpha motorneurons, causing the muscle to contract, overcoming the stretch. The gamma motorneurons function to excite the intrafusal fibers, placing them into a slightly prestretched position, making the central portion of the fiber more sensitive to even small degrees of stretch. The muscle spindle also assists in normal muscle contraction. It appears that when the alpha motorneurons are stimulated to excite contraction of the extrafusal muscle fibers, the gamma system is activated at the same time, causing contraction of the ends of the intrafusal fibers. This elongates the middle portion of

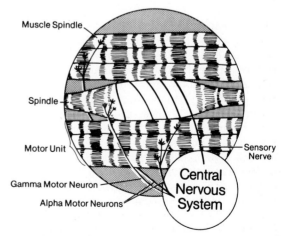

Figure 1–11 The muscle spindle.

the muscle spindle which stimulates impulses to travel back through the sensory nerves to the spinal cord and immediately back to the muscle to facilitate the original impulses. Thus, the contraction and final force or tension development is a result of both direct stimulation through the alpha motorneuron and indirect stimulation through the muscle spindle.

There are a number of reflexes that enable the body to function under a variety of conditions. Each of these reflex patterns has an intricate control system. The reader is referred to current texts in physiology or neurophysiology for additional information, since further discussion in this area falls outside the scope of this book.

Most movements involved in sport activities involve control and coordination through the higher brain centers, specifically the motor cortex, the basal ganglia, and the cerebellum. The motor cortex is a part of the cerebral cortex in the higher brain centers, and is responsible for the control of fine and discreet muscle movements. The basal ganglia are located deep in the cerebral hemispheres, and are composed of separate large pools of neurons that control complex, semi-voluntary movements such as walking and running. The cerebellum is located behind the lower brain stem, and it assists both the motor cortex and the basal ganglia in the performance of their functions. It facilitates movement patterns by smoothing out the movement, which would normally be jerky and uncontrolled in the absence of the cerebellum.

Autonomic Nervous System

The preceding discussion of neural control was based solely on the sensory and motor aspects of body movement. The *autonomic nervous system* controls the internal functions of the body typically not subject to voluntary control. Blood pressure, heart rate, and respiration are among those involuntary activities that fall under the control of the autonomic nervous system. The autonomic nervous system has two major divisions: the *sympathetic nervous system* and the *parasympathetic nervous system*. The two divisions originate from different sections of the spinal cord or the base of the brain, the effects of the two systems are often antagonistic to one another, and the two systems usually secrete different transmitter substances. The sympathetic division originates from the thoracic and upper lumbar regions of the spinal cord, while the parasympathetic division originates from the cranial nerves and the sacral region of the spinal cord. Approximately 90 percent of the parasympathetic fibers originate from the tenth cranial nerve, which is referred to as the *vagus nerve*.

As was stated, the transmitter substance secreted by these two divisions is essentially different. The sympathetic division secretes *norepinephrine* or noradrenalin, and the neurons are referred to as *adrenergic*, while the parasympathetic division secretes *acetylcholine*, thus the neurons are referred to as *cholinergic*. A few of the fibers originating from the sympathetic division secrete acetylcholine. Acetylcholine and norepinephrine both have the ability to excite some end-organs and inhibit others, although they usually act in opposition.

The functions of the two divisions are typically different. As an example, sympathetic stimulation of the heart increases heart rate, while parasympathetic stimulation decreases heart rate. In controlling the blood vessels, the sympathetic nervous system is responsible for constriction of most of the blood vessels, providing control over blood pressure and the volume of blood pumped by the heart each minute, referred to as the cardiac output. Sympathetic stimulation results in dilation of the coronary blood vessels which supply the heart muscle. Thus, during exercise, sympathetic stimulation is very important since it results in an increase in heart rate which increases the work of the heart, a dilation of the coronary blood vessels which allows more blood to perfuse the heart muscle to provide the necessary nutrients and remove the waste products associated with an increased rate of work, and, finally, to maintain and even elevate the blood pressure to allow sufficient blood to return to the heart to maintain an adequate cardiac output. If all of the blood vessels in the body were to dilate simultaneously, there would be no return of blood to the heart since the capacity of the blood vessels far exceeds the total volume of blood in the body. This is essentially what happens when one goes into the state of shock referred to as *neurogenic shock*. There is a sudden cessation of sympathetic impulses, the blood vessels dilate, the blood pressure drops, and blood pools in the veins, thus greatly reducing the return of blood to the heart. This is the typical series of events when one faints following an acute emotional stress. The parasympathetic nervous system plays a very minor role in controlling the systemic blood vessels.

Closely related to the example of sympathetic nervous system control during exercise, the sympathetic nervous centers in the brain, when excited, produce a mass discharge throughout the body, preparing the body for action. A sudden loud noise, a life-threatening situation, or the athlete waiting those last few seconds prior to the start of a race or game, are examples of times when one would experience this mass sympathetic discharge. Heart rate and blood pressure increase, the rate of metabolism increases, the degree of mental activity is increased and facilitated, glucose is released into the blood from the liver as an energy source, kidney function decreases, and sweating is initiated. These basic alterations in body function facilitate action, thus the sympathetic nervous system is essential for proper responses to these types of acute situations or stresses.

CARDIOVASCULAR SYSTEM

The cardiovascular system is responsible for numerous functions in the body that are essential for survival. The body depends on the cardiovascular system to provide nutrients to and remove waste products from every cell in the body; to provide a means of cooling the body when it is overheated as a result of exercise or environmental temperature; to control the degree of acidity and alkalinity of the body; and to promote resistance to invasion by disease organisms. The cardiovascular system also provides other important functions which will not be discussed at this time.

Any system of circulation requires three essential components: a pump, a system of channels or vessels, and a fluid medium. The heart, blood vessels, and blood, respectively, comprise the essential components of the cardiovascular system. Each of these will be discussed individually.

Heart

The heart is a four-chambered organ that serves as the primary pump for circulating blood throughout the entire cardiovascular system. In reality, the heart is really two separate pumps, one pumping blood through the *pulmonary circulation* to the lungs, and the other pumping blood through the *systemic circulation* to the rest of the body. Figure 1–12 schematically illustrates the heart and the pulmonary and systemic circulation systems. Blood enters the right side of the heart, from the great veins, into the *right atrium*. From the right atrium, the blood is pumped through the *tricuspid valve* into the *right ventricle*, where the right ventricle pumps the blood through the *pulmonary valve* into the *pulmonary artery* which transports the blood directly into the lungs. The blood exits the lungs through the pulmonary vein into the left atrium. From the left atrium, the blood is pumped into the left ventricle through the mitral valve. The left ventricle is the most powerful of the four chambers, since it must then pump the blood through the aortic valve, into the aorta, and out through the total systemic circulation. The blood travels through the major arteries to minor arteries, and then to the arterioles before it reaches the capillary bed. From the capillaries, the blood returns via venules to the lesser veins, and then to the greater veins back to the right atrium. The circulation from the right ventricle through the lungs and back to the left atrium is referred to as the lesser or *pulmonary circulation*, while circulation from the left ventricle through the remainder of the body and back to the right atrium is referred to as the *systemic circulation*.

The heart is essentially a muscle, which is distinctly different from both skeletal and smooth muscle. The heart muscle is called the *myocardium*. The inner lining is referred to as the *endocardium*, and the outer lining is the *epicardium*. The thickness of the myocardium varies in direct relationship to the stress placed on the walls of a specific chamber. The left ventricle, therefore, has the thickest walls since it pumps blood against a much greater resistance than any of the other three chambers.

Heart muscle is striated like skeletal muscle, but has the unique feature of being able to contract rhythmically on its own in the absence of nervous stimulation. As was discussed in the preceding section, however, the heart rate is controlled by both the sympathetic (increases rate) and parasympathetic (decreases rate) nervous systems. The resting heart rate, or the number of heart contractions

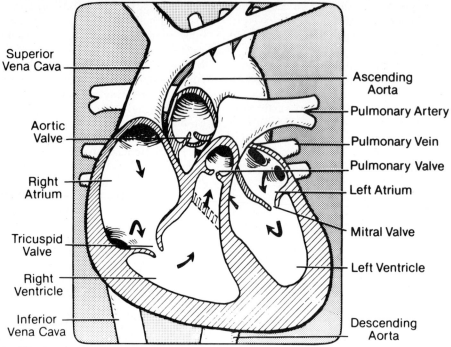

Figure 1–12   The heart, illustrating the pulmonary and systemic circulation systems.

or beats per minute, typically varies between sixty and eighty-five beats per minute. With extended periods, i.e., months to years, of physical conditioning or training of a cardiovascular endurance nature, the resting heart rate can decrease to thirty-five beats per minute or lower. It is postulated that these lower resting rates are the result of increased parasympathetic stimulation through the vagus nerve.

As was stated earlier, the myocardium has its own rate of contraction independent of nervous stimulation. In fact, various areas within the myocardium have their own rates of contraction. The sinoatrial or *S-A node* is a small group of cardiac muscle fibers located on the posterior wall of the right atrium. Without nervous stimulation, it will contract at approximately seventy-two times per minute. Similarly, the atrium and the ventricle will contract at sixty and twenty times per minute respectively. Since the S-A node has the faster rate of rhythm compared to other parts of the heart, the impulses generated by the S-A node spread into the atria and ventricles at a rate that exceed their natural slower rhythm. Thus, the S-A node sets or

establishes the rhythm for the entire heart, and for this reason it is referred to as the *pacemaker* of the heart. Occasionally, chronic problems develop within the S-A node which create problems of maintaining the appropriate rhythm. In such cases it is becoming quite common to surgically install an artificial pacemaker.

Once the impulse is initiated at the S-A node, it spreads by special pathways to the atrioventricular or *A-V node*, which is located toward the center of the heart on the right atrial wall. From the A-V node, the impulse spreads rapidly through the *A-V bundle* out of the atria and into the ventricles. The A-V bundle is composed of small bundles of specialized fibers called *Purkinje fibers*, which transmit the impulse at a velocity approximately six times faster than normal heart muscle. The A-V bundle divides into a left and right bundle branch shortly after entering the ventricles. On reaching the walls of the ventricles, each branch divides into many small Purkinje fiber branches which make direct contact with the cardiac muscle. The speed of conduction of the impulses along the Purkinje fibers is an important aspect of ventricular contraction, allowing all parts of the total ventricle to contract in unison, and not one section at a time.

The sequence of contraction is as follows: First, the impulse travels relatively slowly from the S-A node to the A-V node, where the A-V node delays the impulse before sending it on to the ventricles. Since the impulse travels through the atria on its way from the S-A node to the A-V node, contraction of the atria occurs at this time. The delay of the impulse at the A-V node allows the atria to complete their contraction, in which blood is pumped into the ventricles, before the ventricles initiate their contraction. Occasionally, disturbances occur in this normal sequence of events which lead to an irregular heart rhythm. These vary in the degree of seriousness from premature ventricular contractions, which result in the feeling of either skipped beats or extra beats, and result from an impulse outside the S-A node; atrial flutter or atrial fibrillation, where the atria contract at rates of 200 to 400 times per minute, but pump little or no blood; and ventricular fibrillation, in which the ventricles contract continuously without pumping any blood, and this rapidly leads to death.

The electrical activity of the heart, as just described, can be recorded for purposes of diagnosing potential cardiac problems. Electrodes are placed in specific locations on the arms, legs, and multiple locations on the chest, and a permanent recording of the electrical activity between any two or more electrodes is made using an *electrocardiograph*. The resulting tracing is referred to as an *electrocardiogram*. Heart defects, disease, and electrical conduction abnormalities can be identified from a detailed interpretation of the electrocardiogram.

The contraction phase for either the atria or ventricles is referred to as the period of *systole*; while the relaxation phase, during which time the atrium or ventricle fills with blood, is referred to as the period of *diastole*. At a heart rate of seventy-four beats per minute, diastole accounts for 0.50 second and systole for 0.31 second, for a total of 0.81 second for the entire cardiac cycle. As the heart rate increases, these absolute time intervals are proportionally shortened. During systole, a certain volume is ejected from the left ventricle, which is called the *stroke volume* (SV) of the heart, or the volume of blood pumped per stroke. As was defined earlier, cardiac output ($\dot{Q}$) is the volume of blood pumped per minute, or simply the product of the heart rate

(HR) and the stroke volume (SV); hence, ($\dot{Q}$ = HR $\cdot$ SV). The stroke volume at rest in the standing position will average between 60 and 100 milliliters in an average sized adult. Thus, at a resting heart rate of eighty beats per minute, the resting cardiac output will vary between 4,800 and 8,000 milliliters per minute or 4.8 to 8.0 liters per minute.

Vascular System

The vascular system is composed of a series of vessels that transport the blood from the heart to the tissues and back to the heart. In addition, the heart, as an active muscle, has its own vascular system to provide it with its necessary nutrients and to rid it of its waste products. With respect to systemic circulation, blood is pumped from the powerful left ventricle through the aorta into the arteries and from the arteries into the arterioles. From the arterioles, the blood goes directly to the capillaries where oxygen and nutrients are released, and carbon dioxide and additional metabolic waste products are collected. The blood is then returned to the right atrium of the heart via the venules and veins to the inferior and superior vena cava. In the pulmonary circulation, blood is pumped from the right ventricle to and from the lungs via the pulmonary arteries and pulmonary veins, respectively.

Since people spend so much time in the upright position, either sitting or standing, it is necessary to provide assistance in returning the blood from the lower extremities back up to the heart. This is accomplished by a series of valves located in the veins which allow blood to flow in only one direction, i.e., back to the heart. Thus backward flow is prevented. Each time the surrounding muscles contract, the veins in the immediate vicinity are compressed and the blood is pushed up towards the heart. When the individual stands for an extended period of time with minimal contraction of the muscles of the leg, there will be a pooling of blood in the leg veins as they become distended three to five times their normal size. When the valves undergo progressive destruction, the same problem develops, even in the presence of muscle contractions, and this leads to the medical condition of *varicose veins*.

Blood flow to all parts of the body is controlled largely by the autonomic nervous system. At rest, under normal conditions, the total blood flow is distributed as follows: brain, 14 percent; heart, 4 percent; kidneys, 22 percent; liver, 27 percent; muscle, 15 percent; bone, 5 percent; skin, 6 percent; and other tissues, 7 percent. Under the stress of exercise, following a big meal, or after exposure to a very cold environment, there is a general redistribution of blood flow, redirecting or shunting blood to those areas where it is needed most. With heavy endurance exercise, as an example, this shunting is rather remarkable in that the muscles receive up to 70 to 75 percent of the available blood. All arteries, arterioles, and veins of the systemic circulation are supplied by nerves from the sympathetic nervous system. Sympathetic stimulation results in a constriction of these vessels. Under normal conditions, the sympathetic nerves transmit impulses continuously to the blood vessels, which maintain the vessels in a continuous state of moderate constriction. This is referred to as *vasomotor tone*. Increasing the intensity of stimulation further constricts blood vessels in a certain area, while decreasing this base level of stimulation to low levels allows the vessels in that immediate area to dilate.

When it becomes necessary to redistribute blood to areas where there is a greater need, e.g., the muscles during exercise, this is accomplished by sympathetic stimulation of those areas from which blood flow is to be reduced, since constriction of those vessels will divert the flow of blood away from those areas. In contrast, to those areas needing an increased blood supply, the sympathetic stimulation is reduced, the local vessels dilate, and additional blood is supplied. Regulation of body temperature is controlled in much the same way. During heavy exercise or in a hot environment, blood is shunted to the skin through reduced sympathetic stimulation leading to dilation of the superficial vessels supplying the skin. This promotes heat loss and allows the maintenance of a constant body temperature. When faced with a cold environment, body heat is conserved by increasing sympathetic stimulation and thus constriction of the superficial vessels diverting blood away from the surface of the skin. The bright red color of the skin in the heat, and the white color of the skin in the cold provides visual evidence of the effective shunting of blood.

The rate of blood flow through the various areas or regions of the body is controlled primarily by the arterioles. This is the direct result of the fact that: (1) approximately 50 percent of the total resistance to blood flow in the systemic circulation is in the arterioles; (2) the arterioles have a strong muscular wall that allows the diameter of the vessel to be altered by a factor of threefold to fivefold; and (3) these vessels respond to *autoregulation* in addition to direct sympathetic stimulation. Autoregulation is the ability of the vessel to self-regulate based directly on the needs of the immediate tissues supplied by those vessels. Oxygen demand appears to be the single most important factor in this local self-regulation. As the tissue increases its use of available oxygen, the local vessels dilate to allow more blood, and thus more oxygen, to perfuse that area. The capillary bed also has a system by which blood can be shunted away from the primary capillary network. As it enters the capillary bed, the arteriole reduces in size and is referred to as a *metarteriole*. True capillaries arise from the metarteriole, but small muscular precapillary sphincters surround the initial portion of these true capillaries. These sphincters have the ability to open and close the flow of blood into the associated capillaries, and are controlled primarily by the local tissue needs, such as a lack of oxygen.

Alterations in blood pressure are largely controlled by the specific changes in the arteries, arterioles, venules, and veins as previously described. Generalized constriction of blood vessels leads to an increase in blood pressure, where generalized dilation results in a reduced blood pressure. Second- and third-line medication for those who are diagnosed as having hypertension or high blood pressure is predicated on these basic relationships. The first-line medication for hypertension is the use of diuretics, which theoretically reduce the sodium content in the walls of the arterioles. Second-line medication involves the use of adrenergic blocking agents, or agents that reduce sympathetic stimulation leading to a reduced degree of constriction. Finally, the third-line medication involves the use of direct vasodilators to achieve the reduction in blood pressure.

Blood

Any system of circulation must have a circulating medium. Blood and lymph serve this function, as they are responsible for transporting various materials between the different cells or tissues. The lymphatic system is extremely important relative to general health and coordinated physiological function, but it has little known relevance to the major focus of this book, so it will not be discussed.

Blood serves many useful purposes in the general regulation of normal body function. Of primary importance to the emphasis of this book are the following three functions: transportation, temperature regulation, and acid-base balance. With respect to its transportation function, blood carries nutrients and oxygen to the cell, and takes carbon dioxide, lactate, and other metabolic waste products from the cell to the lungs, liver, and kidneys. The blood also transports hormones from endocrine glands or their storage source to their respective target organs, i.e., that tissue or organ that reacts specifically to a particular hormone. Blood is critical in temperature regulation as it picks up heat from the core of the body or from areas of increased metabolic activity, and delivers it throughout the total body during normal environmental conditions, and to the periphery or skin when the total body is overheated. With regard to acid-base balance, the blood has the ability to buffer, or neutralize, the acids produced with anaerobic metabolism.

The composition of blood is highly variable from one individual to the next, and can even vary considerably within the same individual over time with alterations in plasma volume. Generally, however, the *plasma volume* constitutes approximately 55 percent of the total blood volume, with the red blood cells, white blood cells, and platelets constituting the remaining 45 percent. Of the blood plasma, approximately 90 percent of the content is water, 7 percent are the blood proteins (serum albumin, serum globulin, and fibrinogen), while the remaining 3 percent is comprised of cellular nutrients, salts, enzymes, hormones, antibodies, and

wastes. The ratio of the total blood cell mass to the total blood volume is referred to as the *hematocrit*, and typically varies between 40 to 50 percent. Total blood volume varies considerably on the basis of both the size and the state of training of the individual, with larger blood volumes being associated with increased size and high levels of physical conditioning. Values will range from 5 to 6 liters in men and 4 to 4.5 liters in women of average size and level of physical training. Since high levels of endurance training are typically reflected in increased plasma volumes, the resulting hematocrit will lead one to assume that the individual is anemic. What has happened instead has been an expansion of the plasma volume with only a slight increase in the cellular mass, or no change at all. Thus, the number of red blood cells is normal, or maybe even slightly above normal, but they are diluted in a much larger plasma volume. The table below illustrates this apparent paradox, using two individuals of exactly the same size. The hematocrit of the endurance-trained athlete would lead one to suspect that he has a low red cell count, and is possibly anemic, when, in fact, he has a high blood cell volume which has been diluted by a very high plasma volume.

The presence of a low hematocrit with a high plasma volume appears to have certain beneficial effects with respect to the transportation function of blood. Viscosity is that property of a fluid that resists internal flow. The more viscous a fluid, the more resistant that fluid is to flow. The viscosity of blood is normally about twice that of water. The higher the hematocrit, the greater the viscosity and the greater the resistance to flow. While an increase in red blood cells would appear to be highly desirable to increase the transportation of oxygen, this

Subjects	Age, yr	Ht, cm	Wt, kg	Total Blood Volume Liters	Plasma Volume Liters	Blood Cell Volume Liters	Hematocrit* %
Highly trained male athlete	25	180	80.1	7.4	4.8	2.6	35.1
Untrained male individual	24	178	80.8	5.6	3.2	2.4	42.9

*Hematocrit = (Blood cell volume ÷ total blood volume) × 100

increase in red blood cells, assuming no increase in plasma volume, would greatly increase the viscosity of the blood, and restrict the flow of blood. Thus, a low hematocrit in the presence of a normal or slightly elevated number of red blood cells would actually facilitate the transportation of oxygen.

With respect to oxygen transport, the red blood cell plays a vital role. The red blood cell contains approximately 34 grams of hemoglobin per 100 milliliters of cells, or 15 grams per 100 milliliters of whole blood. Each gram of hemoglobin is capable of combining with 1.33 milliliters of oxygen, or 20 milliliters of oxygen per 100 ml of blood (1.3 ml/gram $\times$ 15 grams/100 ml of whole blood). *Hemoglobin* is composed of a protein (globin) and a pigment (hematin). Hematin contains iron which binds with oxygen. Hematin also has a high affinity for carbon monoxide (approximately 250 times stronger than its affinity for oxygen), thus it is important not to breathe gas mixtures that contain moderate to high levels of carbon monoxide. Those who exercise out of doors in environments that have high carbon monoxide levels are warned to avoid exercising on days when the carbon monoxide levels are high.

Red blood cells continuously are undergoing production and destruction, with the normal life span of a red blood cell approximately four months. The rate of red blood cell production in the bone marrow is approximately equal to the rate of red blood cell destruction. In anemia, there is a marked deficiency of either total red blood cells and/or hemoglobin in the total blood volume. Obviously, oxygen transport capabilities would be greatly limited by anemia; general weakness and chronic fatigue would be typical side effects or symptoms of anemia. Anemia can result from excessive blood loss, red cell destruction, or a decrease in the rate of red cell production. When donating blood, the 500-milliliter withdrawal will represent approximately an 8- to 10-percent reduction in the total blood volume and in the circulating red cells. It will take up to a month or more to reconstitute the red blood cells, but plasma volume returns in twenty-four to forty-eight hours.

White blood cells are represented by only one out of every 500 blood cells. White blood cells function to protect the body against invasion by disease organisms. Since the body is continuously exposed to bacteria, many of which could cause serious disease if they invaded the deeper tissues, the white blood cells play an extremely important function in combating any infectious agent that tries to invade the body. The white blood cells act either by destroying invading agents through the process of *phagocytosis* or by forming antibodies against the invading agent where the antibodies destroy the agent. The adult human has approximately 7,000 white blood cells per cubic millimeter of blood, including polymorphonuclear neutrophils (62.0 percent), polymorphonuclear eosinophils (2.3 percent), polymorphonuclear basophils (0.4 percent), monocytes (5.3 percent), and lymphocytes (30.0 percent). In addition, blood platelets are fragments of a sixth type of white blood cell. Platelets are small, round or oval discs that are extremely important in the mechanisms of blood clot formation to prevent bleeding.

RESPIRATORY SYSTEM

Respiration is the process in which carbon dioxide is removed and oxygen is delivered to the tissues. Respiration can be differentiated into two separate processes: external and internal respiration. *External respiration* is the process of bringing air into the lungs, and the subsequent exchange of gases that takes place between the *alveoli* of the lung and the blood in the capillaries that supply the lung. *Internal respiration* refers to the process of gas exchange between the blood and the tissues to replenish oxygen and to remove carbon dioxide. Thus, external respiration identifies the process of gas exchange in the lung, and internal respiration identifies the process of gas exchange at the specific level of the tissue. External respiration is also referred to as *pulmonary ventilation*.

The anatomy of the respiratory system is illustrated in Figure 1–13. Air comes into the lungs through the nose, although the mouth must also be used when the demands for air exceed that which can be comfortably provided through the nose. There are certain advantages to bringing air in through the nose which are lost with mouth breathing. First, the air is warmed and humidified as it swirls through the turbinates inside the nose. Cold air or dry air can be very irritating to the lungs and the associated air passages, so this heating and humidifying process is very important. Of equal importance, the turbinates cause turbulence in the air flowing into the lungs, causing dust and other particulate matter to drop out against the nasal surfaces. This is a very efficient system that filters out almost all but the very smallest particles, reducing irritation and discomfort to a minimum. From either or both the nose and mouth, the air travels through the *pharynx, larynx, trachea, bronchi,* and *bronchioles,* until it finally reaches the smallest units, the *alveoli.* The pharynx is commonly referred to as the throat, and separates into the *trachea,* for the passage of air, and the *esophagus* for the passage of food. The ability of the body to differentiate between food and air is the result of nerve reflexes. Whenever food touches the surface of the pharynx, the vocal cords close and the epiglottis closes over the larynx, allowing the food to slide on into the esophagus. With certain accidents, injuries, or disease states, it becomes necessary to intubate or insert a tube into the trachea, usually at the larynx, to allow for breathing to continue or to provide for assisted breathing.

It is at the level of the alveoli where the gas exchange takes place. The capillaries in the lung form a network around the alveolar sacs. The distance between the air in the alveoli and the blood in the pulmonary capillaries is quite small (approximately 0.00016 inch), and the space is filled with

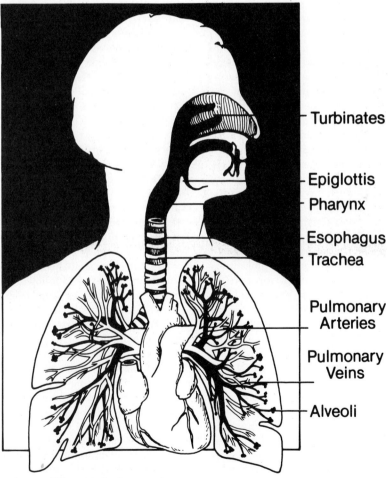

Figure 1–13   Anatomy of the respiratory system.

the epithelial cells of the alveoli and the endothelial cells of the capillaries. The red cells pass through the pulmonary capillaries in single file, thus each cell is exposed to the surrounding lung tissue. The close proximity of the alveoli to the capillary blood is responsible for the relatively stable concentrations of oxygen and carbon dioxide in the alveoli when compared to the relative large fluctuations at the level of the mouth between inspiration and expiration.

Inspiration is an active process involving the diaphragm, which is the primary muscle of respiration, and the muscles responsible for enlarging the thoracic or chest cavity, referred to as the *secondary muscles of respiration*. When the diaphragm contracts, it moves away from the lungs toward the abdominal cavity. This decreases the pressure within the thoracic cavity, creating a reduced pressure or vacuum within the lungs, which then allows outside air to flow into the lungs. *Expiration* is typically a passive process involving the relaxation of the diaphragm, which increases the pressure within the thoracic cavity forcing air out of the lungs. In forced or labored breathing, such as in exercise, the secondary muscles of respiration play a major role in inspiration, and the abdominal muscles play a major role in forced expiration. Contracting the abdominal muscles increases the intra-abdominal and intra-thoracic pressures and reduces the size of the thoracic cavity by pulling the rib cage down and inward.

These changes in intra-abdominal and intra-thoracic pressure assist not only in forced breathing, but they also assist the return of blood back to the heart. As the pressure increases, this pressure is transmitted to the great veins that are transporting blood back to the heart through the abdominal and thoracic areas, and provides an assist to the blood returning to the heart through a squeezing-like action. When the pressure decreases, the veins return to their original size and fill with blood. There is a related respiratory maneuver frequently performed in certain types of exercise that can be potentially dangerous. This is referred to as the *Valsalva* maneuver. The individual holds his or her breath, and increases the pressure in the intra-abdominal cavity by a forceful contraction of abdominal muscles, and in the intra-thoracic cavity by a forceful contraction of the diaphragm and the secondary muscles of respiration, with the glottis closed so the air

will be trapped in the lungs. This maneuver is typically performed in lifting heavy weights. The high intra-abdominal and intra-thoracic pressures restrict the venous return by collapsing the veins. This maneuver, if held for an extended period of time, can greatly reduce the volume of blood returning to the heart, a situation that can initiate a fatal chain of events. A similar maneuver is performed when one is attempting to defecate when constipated. While very helpful in certain circumstances, it is important to realize that this maneuver can be dangerous and should be avoided if one has hypertension or known heart disease.

The lungs can be divided into several anatomical and functional fractions, which are illustrated in Figure 1–14. The *tidal volume* is that volume of air that goes into or out of the lungs with each breath. It can vary from 0.5 liter at rest to 2.5 to 3.0 liters during heavy exercise. The respiratory rate refers to the number of breaths in a minute's period of time, and will vary from twelve breaths per minute at rest to forty to fifty breaths per minute during heavy exercise. Pulmonary ventilation, abbreviated $\dot{V}E$, is the product of the tidal volume and respiratory rate, and is also referred to as the *minute respiratory volume*. At rest, pulmonary ventilation values are in the range of 5 to 7 liters per minute. During exercise, pulmonary ventilation increases to levels in excess of 100 liters per minute, and can even exceed 200 liters per minute in very large, well-conditioned athletes. The control of ventilation is mediated through the respiratory centers in the medulla oblongata and pons of the brain stem.

The *vital capacity* is the largest volume of air that can be forcibly expired following a maximal inspiration. Normal values range from approximately 3 liters for small females to over 7 liters for the large, well-conditioned athlete. The *residual volume* represents that volume of air that remains in the lungs following a maximal expiration, i.e., at the end of the vital capacity maneuver. No matter how forcibly one expires, or how long one expires, the lungs will never completely empty or collapse. Normally, the residual volume is relatively small, varying between 0.8 liter to 1.6 liters, depending on the size of the individual. As a percentage of the total lung volume, which is simply the sum of the vital capacity and the residual volume, the residual volume should not exceed 30 percent. (Example: If the vital

Ventilation

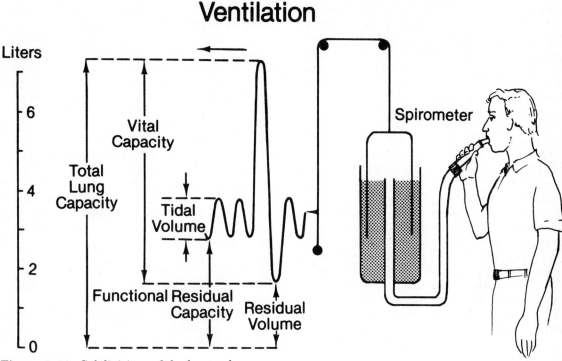

Figure 1–14 Subdivisions of the lung volume.

capacity = 4.0 liters, the residual volume = 2.0 liters, then total lung volume = 6.0 liters, and the ratio of residual volume to total lung volume = 2.0/6.0 = 0.33 = 33 percent.) This ratio, in addition to the vital capacity measure and several other tests to determine the speed with which the individual can empty one's lungs, are valuable screening tests for detecting chronic obstructive lung disease. It is important to recognize that almost all lung volumes are a function of body size as well as the disease state.

Gas exchange in the lung involves the removal of carbon dioxide from the venous blood returning from various parts of the body, and the replenishment of oxygen which has been removed at the tissue level. The process of gas exchange is a function of pressure gradients between the lung and the blood. Concentrations of various gases are typically described either relative to their percentage concentration, or their partial pressure. In the former, the air we breathe is composed of 79.03 percent nitrogen, 20.93 percent oxygen, and 0.04 percent

carbon dioxide. At sea level, the atmospheric pressure is approximately 760 millimeters of mercury (mmHg). This is considered the total pressure, or 100 percent. Each gas exerts pressure in direct proportion to its concentration. Thus, if the total pressure was 760 mmHg, then the partial pressure of nitrogen in air would be 600.6 mmHg (0.7903 × 760). Oxygen would be 159.1 mmHg (0.2093 × 760), and carbon dioxide would be 0.3 mmHg (0.0004 × 760). As we ascend from sea level to the higher elevations, the total atmospheric pressure decreases, the decrease being in direct proportion to the increase in elevation. As an example, at an elevation of 10,000 feet, the total atmospheric pressure is 523 mmHg, thus the partial pressure of oxygen in air would be reduced to 109.5 mmHg (0.2093 × 523). A gas will dissolve in a liquid in direct proportion to its partial pressure, assuming temperature remains constant. Thus, the gases and their movement from one part of the body to another are controlled by their partial pressures. The exchange of gases, e.g., between the alveoli and blood or between blood and the tissues, is influenced most by the pressure gradient between two areas or tissues. Refer to Table 1–1 for a general overview.

As an example of how gas exchange takes place, while the partial pressure in dry air is 159 mmHg, it drops to a level of 100 to 105 mmHg in the alveoli. The reason for this drop is the fact that considerable quantities of water vapor and carbon dioxide are found in the alveoli, with partial pressures of approximately 47 and 40 mmHg respectively. The alveolar gas concentrations remain relatively stable. The venous blood coming into the pulmonary capillaries from the right side of the heart has a partial pressure of oxygen which is typically 40 to 45 mmHg. The pressure gradient for oxygen between the alveoli and blood would then be typically between 55 and 65 mmHg. It is this pressure gradient that drives the oxygen from the alveoli into the blood. By the time the blood exits the lungs on its return to the heart, the partial pressure for oxygen will have nearly equilibrated with that in the alveoli. The greater the pressure or diffusion gradient, the more rapidly the gases will diffuse across the membrane. Carbon dioxide reacts in a similar manner; however, diffusion gradients aren't as important for carbon dioxide since it diffuses at a rate approximately twenty times faster than oxygen. At the tissue level, the same gas laws apply to the unloading of oxygen and the loading of carbon dioxide from the blood to the tissue and vice versa.

The influence of altitude on the transport of oxygen to the tissues can be better understood in light of the preceding discussion. At a 10,000-foot altitude or elevation, the partial pressure of oxygen in air is reduced to 109 mmHg, and in the alveoli to 69 mmHg. If the partial pressure of oxygen in the mixed venous blood remains at 40 mmHg, the diffusion gradient would drop from approximately 60 mmHg at sea level to 29 mmHg at altitude, which is more than a 50-percent reduction. This will have relatively little influence on the loading of oxygen at the level of the lungs, since the gradient is sufficient to nearly totally saturate the blood with oxygen. At the tissue level, however, the reduced pressure gradient will reduce the amount of oxygen that will be released from the blood to the tissues. Thus, altitude does present a significant challenge to the body, particularly during exercise. This will be discussed in much greater depth in Chapter 11.

METABOLIC SYSTEM

Metabolism is defined as the process by which energy is provided to the cells of the body. Food is ingested into the stomach, but the process of breaking down the food into its various components actually begins in the mouth, first through chewing, and second through the enzyme ptyalin which is found in saliva. Ptyalin acts to begin the breakdown or digestion of starches and other carbohydrates. Once in the stomach, ptyalin continues to breakdown the ingested carbohydrates. Enzymes of the stomach begin to act shortly after the food reaches

Table 1–1   *Composition of Atmospheric Air and the Consequent Partial Pressures of Respiratory Gases*

Gas	Percent in Dry Atmosphere	Partial Pressure in Dry Atmosphere	Partial Pressure in Alveolar Air	Partial Pressure in Mixed Venous Blood	Diffusion Gradient
Total	100	760	760	705	
H_2O	0	0	47	47	
O_2	20.93	159	100	40	60
CO_2	0.03	0.2	40	45	5
N_2	79.04	600.8	573	573	

From H. A. de Vries, Physiology of Exercise for Physical Education and Athletics, *2nd ed. (Dubuque, Iowa: William C. Brown Co., Publishers, 1974), p. 172. Reproduced by permission of the publisher.*

the stomach. Hydrochloric acid is the major sub-stance secreted by the stomach. It activates pep-sinogen to form pepsin, an enzyme that begins the digestion of proteins. Additional enzymes are re-leased from the stomach, and also from the pan-creas, liver, gallbladder, and small intestine. Diges-tion does not occur in the large intestine.

The energy resulting from metabolism must ul-timately come from the food ingested, which would include carbohydrates, fats, and proteins, in addi-tion to vitamins, minerals, and water. With respect to their concentration in the diet, carbohydrates are typically the major source of calories in the Ameri-can diet, constituting approximately 45 percent of the total calories consumed per day, while fats and proteins constitute 40 percent and 15 percent re-spectively. In other parts of the world where food supply is a major problem, up to 80 percent of the total calories come from carbohydrate sources. Car-bohydrates, fats, and proteins are converted into glucose, fatty acids, and amino acids respectively through the digestive processes. These basic nu-trients are used as fuel for immediate energy within the cell (glucose and free fatty acids almost exclu-sively); stored in the muscle and liver (glucose stored as glycogen), or in adipose tissue (free fatty acids stored as triglycerides), or in almost all cells (amino acids stored as small protein molecules); or used in the synthesis of protein molecules for specific cell structures (amino acids).

Energy is stored in the form of two high energy compounds: adenosine triphosphate (ATP) and creatine phosphate (CP). Whenever either ATP or CP are broken down within the cell, high levels of energy are released providing the energy necessary for normal cell function. The specific biochemical steps involved in the synthesis and breakdown of these high energy compounds are complex, and well beyond the scope of this book. A simplified schema-tic representation of the interaction of carbohy-drate, fat, and protein in the energy production cycle is presented in Figure 1–15.

As was discussed early in the chapter, muscle contraction results when ATP is reduced to adenosine diphosphate (ADP), and inorganic phos-phate, with the liberation of energy. CP is reduced to creatine and inorganic phosphate, providing the energy for the resynthesis of ATP. Oxidation, or *aerobic metabolism*, provides the energy to re-

synthesize CP. Those pathways up to the Krebs cycle can function in the total absence of oxygen, which is referred to as *anaerobic* metabolism. Anaerobic metabolism leads to the formation and accumulation of lactic acid, and this process is limited by the ability of the cell to either tolerate high lactate levels or low levels of pH, where pH is a direct measure of the degree of acidity or alkalinity. It is possible to survive for relatively short periods of time in the absence of breathing. However, this time is limited by the accumulation of lactic acid. Also, anaerobic metabolism is extremely inefficient in producing or generating ATP when compared to aerobic metabolism. One molecule of glucose when metabolized yields only two molecules of ATP when the reaction is confined to anaerobic metabolism. If the molecule of glucose goes through the complete cycle, there is a net yield of thirty-eight molecules of ATP.

In the presence of sufficient oxygen, metabolism can proceed through the aerobic stages to the point where oxygen is combined with hydrogen ions to form water and carbon dioxide. In the absence of sufficient oxygen, the hydrogen ions and hydrogen atoms accumulate and effectively block the aerobic cycle, causing the body to rely on anaerobic metabolism. During exercise at high work loads, the body is incapable of providing sufficient oxygen to regenerate the necessary ATP. Anaerobic metabolism begins to make its contribution and lactic acid starts to accumulate. It should be noted from Figure 1–15 that only glycogen is available as an energy source for anaerobic metabolism. Fat and protein enter the energy production chain at the Krebs cycle, which is a major phase of aerobic metabolism. Also, while proteins are available as an energy source, they are only used rarely, for they have far more important functions within the body, and the body attempts to spare protein whenever possible.

When discussing metabolism at the level of food intake and energy expenditure, it is traditional to refer to the caloric content of food and the caloric value of various levels of physical activity. The standard unit of measure of energy in nutrition is the *kilogram calorie*, or the Kcal. One Kcal is defined precisely as the amount of energy in the form of heat necessary to raise the temperature of one kilogram of water $1°$ centigrade from 15 to $16°$

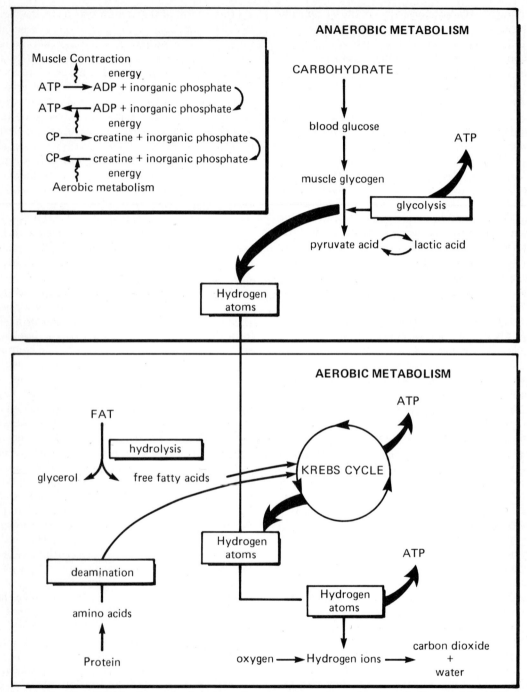

Figure 1–15 Simplified schematic drawing of anaerobic and aerobic metabolism, with ATP energy formation, in a single muscle cell.

centigrade. In nutrition research, a calorimeter is used to measure the absolute amount of heat produced when burning different food materials. When pure carbohydrate, fat, or protein is burned, each yields a net energy value of 4.10, 9.45, and 4.35 Kcal, respectively, of energy per gram of substance burned. Large human calorimeters have also been constructed which enable a very accurate analysis of the total calories expended in a twenty-four-hour period of time. The human chamber is extremely expensive to build, since one must have the ability to accurately assess small changes in temperature, as these changes indicate the metabolic rate of the individual.

The use of a human chamber has been largely replaced by indirect techniques for the assessment of energy expenditure—techniques which are almost as accurate, but much more versatile and much less expensive. The most accurate and widely used technique for indirectly assessing energy expenditure is to measure the volume of oxygen consumed. There is a direct linear relationship between the oxygen consumed, or what is referred to as *oxygen uptake*, and the level of energy expenditure. With carbohydrates, one liter of oxygen consumed is the equivalent of 5.0 Kcal. For fats, this value is 4.7 Kcal, and for proteins, 4.5 Kcal. On a normal mixed diet, a value of 4.8 Kcal is used. For the average man, a resting oxygen uptake is approximately 0.3 liter/min or 18 liters/hour (0.3 liter/min × 60 min/hr), which will total 432 liters of oxygen/day (24 hours × 18 liters/hour), for a total caloric expenditure of 2,074 Kcal/day (4.8 Kcal/liter × 432 liters/day), a value which is in close agreement with the average resting energy expenditure for a 154-pound or 70-kilogram man.

The basal metabolic rate (BMR) refers to the metabolic rate of the individual in a basal state, i.e., totally quiet and supine rest. The BMR will depend on the size of the individual, since the larger the person is, the more total calories expended in a day. While the average BMR will vary between 1,500 and 2,000 Kcal, the average metabolic rate of the individual who is engaged in normal daily activity will range from 1,800 to 2,700 Kcal. In highly active individuals this value can be much higher, approaching 10,000 Kcal/day in extremely large individuals performing many hours of exhaustive physical labor or exercise.

ENDOCRINE SYSTEM

The endrocrine system is composed of a series of glands referred to collectively as endocrine glands. Endocrine glands secrete *hormones*, which are potent chemical substances usually carried in the blood from the glands to other parts of the body where they assist in the control of specific body functions. Local hormones affect cells in the immediate vicinity of the organ that secretes the hormone, and include hormones such as acetylcholine, histamine, and the gastrointestinal hormones. General hormones are those that are emptied into the blood by the endocrine glands, and will be the primary focus of this discussion. General hormones vary in the general or specific effect they have on the body. Growth hormone, which is produced by the pituitary gland in the brain, has a generalized effect on all cells within the body, while another pituitary hormone, thyrotropin, has a very specific action solely on the cells in the thyroid gland. There is a great deal of similarity between the endocrine system and the nervous system relative to their regulation of body function. The nervous system, however, functions quickly and its effects are rather short-lived and localized, while the endocrine system functions much more slowly, and its effects are longer lasting and more general. Hormones are extremely potent, in that very small doses can have a marked physiological effect. In the following paragraphs, each of the major glands and their hormones will be briefly outlined and their functions defined. These are briefly summarized in Table 1–2. It should be recognized that this table and the following discussions are gross oversimplifications of a very complex and highly regulated system.

The *pituitary gland*, also referred to as the hypophysis, is a very small, marble-sized gland that lies in a bony cavity beneath the base of the brain. It was at one time considered to be the "master" gland of the human body. However, subsequent research has demonstrated that the *hypothalamus*, which lies immediately above the pituitary, is the major area of production of several of the pituitary hormones and controls the secretion of all of the pituitary hormones. Pituitary hormones are released into the blood in response to hypothalamic releasing and inhibiting factors. Specific releasing and inhibiting factors control the release or secretion of each of

Table 1-2 *The Endocrine Glands and Their Respective Hormones*

Endocrine Gland	Location	Hormone	Specific Action of the Hormone
Pituitary (hypophysis) Anterior segment	Brain	Growth hormone	promotes development and enlargement of all body tissues up through maturation; increases rate of protein synthesis; increases mobilization of fats and use of fats as an energy source; decreases rate of carbohydrate utilization
		Thyrotropin	controls the amount of thyroxin produced and released by the thyroid gland
		Corticotropin (ACTH)	controls the secretion of the hormones from the adrenal cortex
		Prolactin	stimulates breast growth and milk production during the last stages of pregnancy
		Follicle-stimulating hormone	initiates growth of follicles in the ovaries and promotes secretion of estrogen from the ovaries (female); promotes development of sperm (male)
		Luteinizing hormone	promotes secretion of estrogen and progesterone, and causes the follicle to rupture, releasing the ovum (female); causes testes to secrete testosterone (male)
Posterior segment		Antidiuretic hormone (vasopressin)	assists in controlling water excretion by the kidneys; elevates blood pressure
		Oxytocin	stimulates contraction of muscle in the uterus and breast
Thyroid	Base of the neck	Thyroxine	increases the rate of metabolism of all cells, resulting in a general increase in the total body metabolism; increases rate and force of contraction of the heart
		Triiodothyronine	similar to thyroxine
		Calcitonin	controls calcium ion concentration (decreases)
Parathyroid	Directly behind the thyroid gland	Parathormone	controls calcium ion concentration in extracellular fluid through its influence on bone, the intestine, and the kidneys (increases)
Adrenal Medulla	Directly above each kidney	Epinephrine (adrenalin)	mobilizes glycogen; increases skeletal muscle blood flow; increases heart rate and oxygen consumption
		Norepinephrine (noradrenalin)	elevates blood pressure; constricts arterioles and venules

Table 1-2 (Continued)

Endocrine Gland	Location	Hormone	Specific Action of the Hormone
Cortex		Mineralocorticoids	controls sodium retention and potassium loss through the kidneys
		Glucocorticoids	promotes synthesis of carbohydrate; protein breakdown; anti-inflammatory and anti-allergic action
		Androgens and Estrogens	causes the development of the male and female sex characteristics
Pancreas	Lies immediately beneath the stomach	Insulin	controls blood glucose levels through lowering of blood glucose; increases the utilization of glucose and the synthesis of fat
		Glucagon	increases blood glucose; stimulates the breakdown of protein and fat
Gonads			
Testes	Lie in the scrotum	Testosterone	promotes development of male sex characteristics, including growth of testes, scrotum and penis; facial hair and change in voice; promotes muscle growth
Ovaries	Lie above the uterus in the abdominal cavity	Estrogen	promotes development of female sex characteristics; provides increased storage of fat; assists in regulating the menstrual cycle
		Progesterone	assists in regulating the menstrual cycle

these hormones. The major pituitary hormones of significance for the focus of this book are: *growth hormone*, which promotes development and enlargement of the body tissues up to the point of full maturation, and influences the substrate or energy source in metabolism; *thyrotropin*, which controls the thyroid gland; *corticotropin*, which controls the adrenal cortex; and *antidiuretic hormone*, which controls water excretion by the kidneys and influences blood pressure.

The *thyroid gland*, located at the base of the neck, plays a critical role in regulating cellular and total body metabolism through the hormone *thyroxin*. As thyroxin is released, there is a proportional increase in metabolic rate. *Triiodothyronine* is a second thyroid hormone whose function is similar to thyroxin. The *parathyroids* control calcium ion concentration in the extracellular fluid through the hormone *parathormone*.

The adrenal glands are situated directly on top of each kidney and are composed of two parts: the *adrenal medulla* and the *adrenal cortex*. The adrenal medulla produces and releases two hormones, epinephrine and norepinephrine, which are collectively called *catecholamines*. They have a powerful effect on the cardiovascular and nervous systems, smooth and skeletal muscles, and metabolism. These two hormones prepare the individual for immediate action, "fight or flight," when that individual is suddenly aroused. The adrenal cortex produces and releases three general categories of hormones: *mineralocorticoids*, which regulate sodium and potassium; *glucocorticoids*, which influence carbohydrate metabolism; and *androgens* and *estrogens*, which regulate the development of male and female sexual characteristics. It is the release of androgens and estrogens from the adrenal cortex that allows males to acquire certain female characteristics, and females to acquire certain male characteristics, although the adrenal cortex typically releases only small amounts of the androgens and estrogens when compared to the levels released by the gonads. The *pancreas* regulates glucose levels in the blood through the interaction of its two hormones, *insulin* and *glucagon*. While glucagon increases blood sugar levels, insulin lowers these levels by assisting in the transfer of glucose from the blood into the cell. The high blood glucose levels in diabetics are due to the inability of the pancreas to produce sufficient insulin.

Hyperglycemia refers to elevated levels of blood sugar or glucose, while *hypoglycemia* refers to the opposite situation, where blood sugar levels are below normal.

The gonads are those glands that promote the development of the male and female sex characteristics. *Testosterone,* the major androgen or male sex hormone produced by the testes, promotes muscle growth, while estrogens, produced by the ovaries, promote the accumulation of body fat.

As was mentioned, this review of the endocrine system has been very brief and incomplete. Many other hormones have been identified, but either their functions have not been well defined, or their role during exercise is unknown.

GENERAL SUMMARY

In reviewing the brief description of each of the major body systems, one cannot help but be impressed, if not amazed, by the complexity of the human organism. Individually, even the most simple of the body systems is remarkably designed and engineered. Scientists are still attempting to unravel the many mysteries that prevent a better understanding of how each system functions independently. Attempting to understand how all of these systems operate in concert provides an even greater challenge. As this book progresses into other areas, using this chapter as a basic foundation in relating physiological function to sport and exercise, it is important to remember that the body functions as a total entity. Therefore, attempts must be made to study and understand any one area, e.g., nutrition for improved sport performance, within the context of the integration of function of the whole body. At times this requires three-dimensional thinking, but this approach is important in order to gain proper understanding and to avoid being misled.

STUDY QUESTIONS

1. How does growth in length and width occur in long bone?
2. Describe the contraction of muscle from the arrival of the neural impulse to the actual contraction of the individual sarcomere units.

3. What is a sarcomere, and what constitutes its basic structure?
4. What are the basic characteristics of fast-twitch and slow-twitch muscle fibers? Could a marathon runner be trained to develop more slow-twitch fibers?
5. What is the neuromuscular junction, and how do impulses cross this junction?
6. What is the role of cholinesterase and acetylcholine in the transmission of nerve impulses?
7. Describe the role of the muscle spindle in muscle contraction.
8. How does the heart contract, and how is heart rate controlled?
9. What is the difference between systole and diastole, and how does this relate to systolic and diastolic blood pressure?
10. How is blood flow to the various regions of the body controlled?
11. Describe the primary functions of blood.
12. With respect of respiration, how important is the partial pressure of a specific gas, e.g., oxygen?
13. How are carbohydrates, fats, and proteins used as energy sources?
14. What is the difference between aerobic and anaerobic metabolism?
15. Why is it important to understand the basic relationship of lactic acid and blood pH in metabolic function?
16. Briefly outline the major endocrine glands, their hormones, and the specific action of these hormones.

REFERENCES

Astrand, P. O., and Rodahl, K. *Textbook of Work Physiology*. 2nd ed. New York: McGraw-Hill Book Co., 1977.

Brobeck, J. R., ed. *Best and Taylor's Physiological Basis of Medical Practice*. 10th ed. Baltimore: Williams and Wilkins Co., 1979.

Burton, A. C. *Physiology and Biophysics of the Circulation*. Chicago: Year Book Medical Publishers, 1965.

Comroe, J. H. *Physiology of Respiration*. 2nd ed. Chicago: Year Book Medical Publishers, 1974.

Crouch, J. E. *Functional Human Anatomy*. 2nd ed. Philadelphia: Lea & Febiger, 1972.

deVries, H. A. *Physiology of Exercise for Physical Education and Athletics*. 2nd ed. Dubuque, Iowa: William C. Brown Co., 1974.

Ganong, W. F. *Review of Medical Physiology*. 2nd ed. Los Altos, Calif.: Lange Medical Publications, 1965.

Green, J. F. *Mechanical Concepts in Cardiovascular and Pulmonary Physiology*. Philadelphia: Lea & Febiger, 1977.

Guyton, A. C. *Physiology of the Human Body*. 5th ed. Philadelphia: W. B. Saunders, 1979.

Little, R. C. *Physiology of the Heart and Circulation*. Chicago: Year Book Medical Publishers, 1977.

Ross, G., ed. *Essentials of Human Physiology*. Chicago: Year Book Medical Publishers, 1977.

Shepherd, J. T., and Vanhoutte, P. M. *The Human Cardiovascular System: Facts and Concepts*. New York: Raven Press, 1979.

Turner, C. D., and Bagnara, J. T. *General Endocrinology*. 5th ed. Philadelphia: W. B. Saunders Co., 1971.

Tuttle, W. W., and Schottelius, B. A. *Textbook of Physiology*. 15th ed. St. Louis: C. V. Mosby Co., 1965.

West, J. B. *Respiratory Physiology: The Essentials*. Baltimore: Williams and Wilkins Co., 1974.

Winter, H. F., and Shourd, M. L. *Review of Human Physiology*. Philadelphia: W. B. Saunders, 1978.

2

Responses to Acute Exercise

INTRODUCTION

It was not until the early twentieth century that concerted efforts were made to gain insight into people's ability to functionally adapt to the stress of exercise. With the establishment of the Harvard Fatigue Laboratory in 1927 and the work of A. V. Hill in England in the 1920s, a group of dedicated scientists began a concerted effort to push back the frontiers in the area of exercise and sport physiology. While specific aspects of one's physical performance had been investigated by isolated research laboratories and in individual research experiments as early as the mid-to-late 1800s, the efforts in the 1920s marked the start of a new era in which scientists dedicated themselves to unlocking the mysteries of successful adaptation to the unique environment of exercise. Since this time considerable knowledge has accumulated about the ability to adapt to exercise. However, with the discovery of new knowledge, we realize that there is even more to be learned than was originally anticipated. The surface has been scratched, but this area of investigation is still in its infancy. With the availability of new techniques and bright young researchers, the period of rapid growth is quickly approaching.

ASSESSING THE RESPONSE TO EXERCISE

How are physiological responses to exercise determined? The highly skilled athlete or the recrea-tional jogger does not perform or exercise in environments that are conducive to monitoring the physiological responses to exercise. It is possible to monitor a few selected physiological parameters while one exercises in his or her natural environment. Telemetry and miniature tape recorders have been used to monitor heart rate and electrocardiogram, electromyography, respiration rate, and skin and deep body temperature. Most frequently, however, the individual is brought into the laboratory where he or she can be studied in much greater depth under highly controlled conditions. This dictates the use of specific laboratory exercise devices, typically referred to as *ergometers*.

One of the goals of studying exercise in the laboratory is to be able to produce a level of exercise that can be quantified and reproduced. In order to determine the functional relationship between exercise as a stimulus and the resulting adaptations of the body's different systems, one must be able to measure both the exercise and the response to exercise. There are a number of ways in which the individual can be exercised within the confines of the laboratory. The simplest form of exercise is bench stepping, in which the person steps up and down on a bench of standard height (usually between twelve and eighteen inches) at a fixed rate of stepping established by a metronome, e.g., twenty-four ascensions/min. This is the least expensive and most portable of the various testing devices, but it has several disadvantages. First, the total amount of work that is performed in a set period of time is totally dependent on the person's body weight, i.e., the heavier individual must lift more weight on each step. Second, the person's movements during a stepping test make it difficult to obtain certain physiological measurements.

A second device used for producing an exercise response in the laboratory is the bicycle *ergometer*. This can be used in either the normal, upright (Figure 2–1) or supine position (Figure 2–2). In addition, the bicycle ergometer can be used for arm cycling.

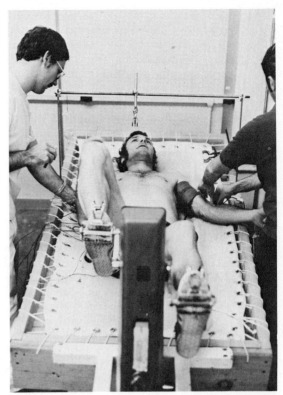

Figure 2–2 Supine bicycling on a bicycle ergometer.

Ergometers work on the basis of one of two principles: mechanical friction or electromagnetic resistance. With the mechanical friction devices, a belt surrounding the flywheel of the bicycle can be tightened or loosened to adjust the resistance against which the person pedals. The pedal rate must be kept constant to provide a constant level of work. With electromagnetic resistance, the flywheel moves through an electromagnetic field, and the strength of the field determines the resistance to pedaling. These electromagnetic devices are designed to provide a constant level of work independent of the pedaling rate, by using a feedback loop that increases the resistance when the rate slows, and decreases the resistance as the rate picks up. There are many advantages to using the bicycle ergometer. It is relatively inexpensive, portable, the work level or power output can be accurately defined, and the task is weight-independent, i.e., the work level can be set inde-

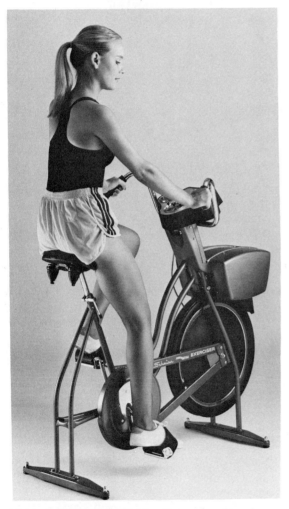

Figure 2–1 Upright bicycling on a bicycle ergometer. Photo courtesy of Mr. Keith Kingbay, Excelsior Fitness Equipment Company, 613 Academy Drive, Northbrook, IL 60062.

pendently of the individual's body weight. The bicycle ergometer does have the disadvantage, however, of causing the individual to become more fatigued from local, leg-muscle fatigue than from general, overall cardiovascular, respiratory, and metabolic fatigue. In addition, and closely related to the problem of local fatigue, the peak or maximum physiological parameters obtained on the bicycle ergometer are frequently lower than the peak parameters obtained during other forms of laboratory exercise.

Probably the most widely used laboratory exercise device is the motor-driven treadmill (Figure 2–3). The treadmill is a motorized device that drives a wide belt in one direction, while the individual walks, jogs, or runs in the opposite direction in an attempt to maintain the same relative position. The speed and elevation of the treadmill can be varied from a pace for very slow, level walking to the superhuman task of running up a 20-percent slope at a speed of 20–25 mi/hour. This device appears to provide the highest maximum physiological responses to exercise and maintains a constant work rate (the subject either keeps up with the rate of work or is thrown off the back of the treadmill). The treadmill is an expensive device, however, and lacks portability. In addition, it can be somewhat dangerous if the individual loses his or her balance.

Two unique laboratory work devices have been recently developed: the rowing ergometer and the swimming flume. The rowing ergometer (Figure 2–4) was devised to test competitive oarsmen in an activity that more closely approximated their competitive task. The swimming flume (Figure 2–5) was developed for the same purpose. Valuable research data had been obtained by instrumenting swimmers in a swimming pool. The problems of turns and of not having a stationary swimmer led to the use of tethered swimming. The athlete was placed in a harness that was connected to a rope and series of pulleys with attached weights. In this manner, the athlete would swim in a stationary position against different resistances. While the initial attempts provided useful data, they did not accurately duplicate the true environment of the swimmer. The swimming flume, while very expensive, has resolved this problem and has created many new opportunities to investigate almost all aspects of swimming.

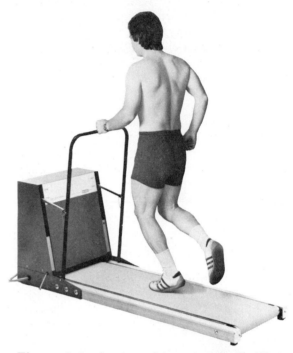

Figure 2–3 A motor-driven treadmill. Photo courtesy of Mr. Stan Peterman, Quinton Instrument Company, 2121 Terry Ave., Seattle, WA 98121.

Each of these laboratory modes of exercise makes it possible to exercise the individual from low to exhaustive levels, while maintaining one's body in a relatively stable position. This allows the person to be instrumented to measure a variety of physiological parameters. Expired air can be collected for the determination of the volume and rate of respiration as well as the amount of oxygen or energy used during exercise; electrodes placed on the chest allow the monitoring of the electrocardiogram to determine the normality and rate of the heart; blood pressure can be monitored either directly (arterial catheter) or indirectly (*sphygmomanometer*); arterial- and venous-blood samples can be drawn and analyzed for various components; body and skin temperature can be monitored; and many other specific parameters can either be recorded or observed. Advances in technology have made it possible to define an individual's responses to exercise quite explicitly, but even with these advances, there are still many

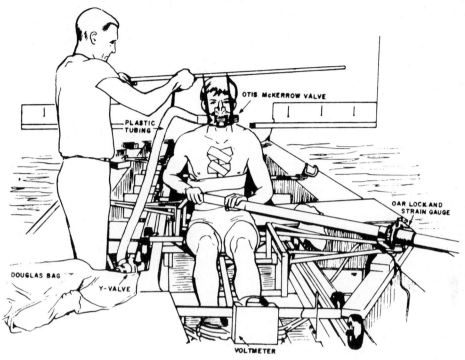

Figure 2–4 Rowing ergometer. (From F. C. Hagerman and W. D. Lee, "Measurement of Oxygen Consumption, Heart Rate, and Work Output During Rowing." *Medicine and Science in Sports,* 3 (1971). Reproduced by permission of the publisher.)

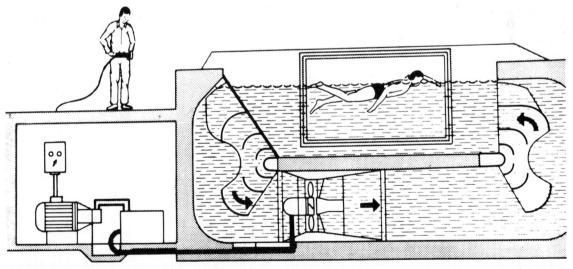

Figure 2–5 Swimming flume. (From P. O. Åstrand, "Do We Need Physical Conditioning?" *J. Phy. Ed.,* (March–April 1972). Reproduced by permission of the publisher.)

areas that cannot be accurately assessed or described. Only as technology pushes ahead will the total picture start to come more clearly into focus.

PHYSIOLOGICAL RESPONSES TO ACUTE EXERCISE

In the preceding chapter, a very brief review of anatomy and physiology was undertaken in an attempt to provide a basis for understanding how the human body reacts to various forms of exercise. This chapter and the next review people's basic responses and adaptations to the stress of exercise. Professor David R. Lamb, from Purdue University, in his book, "Physiology of Exercise: Responses and Adaptations," has defined the term *responses* as those sudden, temporary changes in function caused by an acute or single bout of exercise, which disappear shortly after the exercise period is completed. Examples of responses would include the increase in heart rate and blood pressure seen with exercise, with a return to resting values shortly following the cessation of exercise. Dr. Lamb defines *adaptations* as more or less persistent changes in structure or function following a period of physical training, which enable the body to better respond to subsequent exercise bouts. Examples would include increases in the size of muscle as a result of a six-month program of strength training, or the reduction in the heart rate response to a standard level of exercise with a twelve-week program of cardiovascular endurance training. The former adaptation allows the individual to exert greater levels of force, i.e., the person is stronger, while the latter adaptation allows the body to perform the same level of work, but at a lower cost to the heart.

The acute responses to exercise are influenced by a number of factors that must be considered when interpreting the results of these tests. First, the level of physical training, or the degree of conditioning of the individual, will greatly influence how one responds to a given level of exercise. The more highly conditioned the individual, the more efficiently he or she will be able to perform a given level of exercise. Factors such as too little sleep the night before the exercise bout, too much coffee, drugs, alcohol, tobacco, and general anxiety will all negatively influence how the individual will respond to a standardized exercise bout. Significant abnormalities in the electrocardiogram during exercise that are typically associated with advanced heart disease have been traced back in certain individuals to the fact that they had consumed four or five cups of coffee just prior to taking the exercise test.

Neuromuscular Responses

For purposes of review in this chapter, the muscular and nervous systems will be discussed concurrently, since they work in an integrative and supportive manner. Once movement is anticipated, the body prepares to spring into action. Either through reflex or conscious control, the appropriate motor units are stimulated and the muscles contract with the precise level of force producing an efficient and coordinated movement pattern. From available information, it appears that motor units are activated asynchronously, i.e. not all at the same time. Likewise, it appears that one can only recruit a certain fraction of the total number of motor units in a given muscle, even with a voluntary maximal contraction. Limited evidence exists to support this contention through the many examples of people who, under extreme emotional conditions, are able to perform superhuman feats of strength. The pattern of recruitment of motor units to participate in a voluntary contraction is an extremely important area in which there is very limited knowledge. Fortunately, research is being conducted at the present time in an attempt to better understand the process of motor unit recruitment.

Study of the muscle's activity through electromyography, the process whereby the electrical activity of the muscle can be monitored and recorded, has provided essential knowledge in the area of neuromuscular coordination, recruitment of motor units, and motor unit integration. New techniques allow the observation of isolated, single motor units. By using biofeedback techniques, individuals can be taught to selectively recruit specific motor units and to have these motor units contract in defined rhythms, e.g., drum rolls.

Closely related to the areas of motor-unit recruitment and strength is the area of muscular fatigue. Unfortunately, not too much more is known about muscular fatigue than is known about the expression of strength. *Muscular fatigue* is a term reserved strictly for that fatigue experienced in the local muscle or muscle group, as opposed to *overall fatigue*, which is probably cardiovascular in origin, or to *mental fatigue*, which is thought to be associated with boredom. These other types of fatigue will be discussed in later sections.

Studies by Merton in the 1950s found that when a person reached a state of extreme fatigue and was unable to move a certain muscle, electrical stimulation of that muscle did not elicit a response, and the action potentials (electrical impulses) received by the muscle were not diminished. He also found that if the blood supply to the active muscle was occluded, recovery from fatigue did not occur until the circulation to the muscle was restored. He felt that this indicated that muscular fatigue was not due to a failure of the central nervous system, but was due to peripheral circulatory factors, such as the build up of waste products that could not escape the muscle, or the lack of nutrients and oxygen. With maximal static or isometric contractions, the arterial blood flow through the contracting muscle will be either partly or totally restricted. Thus, the fatigue can be due to a lack of oxygen or nutrients from the arterial side, or to an accumulation of lactic acid, hydrogen ions, or heat, in the muscle.

Ikai et al. (1967), using repeated maximal contractions, one per second, of the same adductor pollicis muscle used in the studies of Merton previously cited, found strong, relatively increasing contractions as responses to short bursts of tetanizing stimuli applied every fifth second. These results indicated that central factors were an important aspect of muscle fatigue. Bigland-Ritchie et al. (1978), using the much larger quadriceps femoris muscle group, essentially confirmed the results of Ikai et al., pointing to central factors being important in muscle fatigue.

Asmussen (1979), in a general review of muscle fatigue, suggests the discrepancies between the aforementioned studies could be the result of different kinds of contraction, with isometric or static contraction being related to peripheral factors, and dynamic, repeated contractions being related to central factors. Asmussen concludes that there are actually two separate regions where fatigue can occur: a peripheral region distal to the stimulated motor nerves, and a central region proximal to the stimulated motor nerves. Peripheral muscle fatigue can occur in at least two different sites: the *transmission mechanism*, or the neuromuscular junction, muscle membrane, and endoplasmic reticulum; and the *contractile mechanism*, or the muscle filaments. Central fatigue can be an actual impairment of nerve cells in the central nervous system, or can be the result of an inhibition elicited by nervous impulses from receptors in the fatigued muscles, acting on the motor pathways anywhere from the voluntary centers in the brain to the spinal motor neurons.

Cardiovascular Responses

The major function of the cardiovascular system during exercise is to deliver blood to the active tissues, which includes the delivery of oxygen and nutrients and the removal of the metabolic waste products. If the exercise bout is prolonged, the cardiovascular system also assists in maintaining body temperature, so that the individual does not overheat. A series of complex interactions allow these cardiovascular adaptations to occur in an integrated manner.

Heart Rate. The heart rate (HR) is the simplest and one of the most informative of the cardiovascular parameters that can be measured. At rest, the heart beats at a rate of sixty to eighty beats/min. This is easily determined by locating the radial (thumb-side of the wrist) or the carotid (junction of the head and neck) artery pulses, counting for fifteen secs, and multiplying the result by four [HR = (beats/15 sec) × 4]. In very sedentary, deconditioned individuals, the resting heart rate can exceed one hundred beats/min, and in highly conditioned, endurance athletes, resting heart rates have been reported in the twenty-eight to forty beats/min range.

The lowest heart rate is found at rest in the supine position. It will be elevated slightly upon sitting and increase even further with standing. This is the result of the influence of gravity, which reduces the amount of blood returning to the heart when one shifts from a supine to an upright posture, thus reducing the stroke volume (SV). For cardiac output ($\dot{Q}$) to remain the same, the heart rate must increase, since $\dot{Q} = HR \times SV$. Resting heart rate is also influenced by age and the environment. It usually decreases with age and increases with extremes in temperature and altitude. Prior to starting the exercise bout, the pre-exercise heart rate may be increased well above normal resting values. This is referred to as an *anticipatory response* and is probably mediated through catecholamine secretion from the adrenal medulla. Reliable estimates of actual resting heart rate should be made under conditions that are conducive to the subject's total relaxation.

With an acute bout of exercise, the heart rate will increase in direct proportion to the intensity of the exercise, as is illustrated in Figure 2–6. In this figure, the intensity of exercise is represented by the oxygen consumption or uptake since for every increment in work there is an equal increment in oxygen uptake. When exercise is performed on a bicycle ergometer where the work can be accurately measured and can be identical for all individuals irrespective of their body weight, the oxygen uptake for any one level of work is very predictable from one individual to another. Thus, expressing the level of work or the intensity of exercise in terms of the oxygen uptake is not only accurate, but appropriate for comparing different individuals, or the same individual under different circumstances. From Figure 2–6, it is apparent that the heart rate increases in a direct or linear manner with increases in the intensity of exercise, until that point where the individual begins to reach exhaustion. As exhaustion is approached, there is a flattening out of the heart rate curve, indicating that the individual is approaching his or her maximum value. The maximum heart rate is a highly reliable value which remains constant from day to day and changes only slightly from year to year. Estimates of maximal heart rate have been made on the basis of one's age, since there is a slight but steady decrease in maximal heart rate with aging. Subtracting age in years from the figure 220 provides an approximation of the average maximum heart rate for that particular age group. However, individual

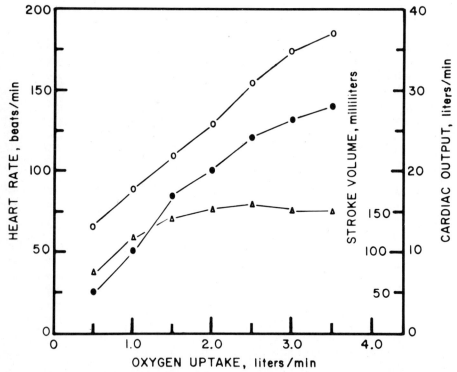

Figure 2–6 Heart rate (●), stroke volume (△), and cardiac output (○) response to increasing levels of work or intensity of exercise as reflected by the oxygen uptake.

values vary considerably around this average value with a standard deviation of approximately ±12 beats per minute.

At submaximal levels of work, when the level of exercise is held constant, the heart rate increases fairly rapidly until it levels off at what is called a *steady state level*. For each level of exercise, from very low to moderately high intensities of work, the heart rate will reach a steady state value within one to two minutes. However, the more intense the level of exercise, the longer it takes to achieve this steady state value. This concept of steady state values is important for several tests that have been developed to measure physical fitness. Individuals are placed on an exercise device such as a bicycle ergometer and are exercised at two or three standardized levels of work. Those who are in better physical condition on the basis of cardiorespiratory endurance capacity will have lower heart rates for the same level of work, thus indicating a more efficient heart. This will be discussed further under adaptations to chronic exercise.

Stroke volume, or the quantity of blood pumped per heart beat, is influenced by four factors: (1) return of venous blood to the heart, (2) ventricular distensibility, (3) ventricular contractility, and (4) aortic or pulmonary artery pressure. The first two factors influence the filling capacity of the ventricle, i.e., how much blood is available for filling the ventricle and the ease at which the ventricle is filled at the available pressure. The last two factors influence the ability of the ventricle to empty, i.e., the force with which the blood is ejected and the pressure against which it must flow in the arteries. These factors are important in understanding how the stroke volume responds to exercise.

Stroke volume will increase up to 40 percent when exercise is performed in the supine position, such as in swimming (Poliner et al., 1980). During upright exercise, however, stroke volume will increase nearly 100 percent with increasing levels of work up to approximately 40 to 60 percent of the individual's working capacity (Poliner et al., 1980), at which point it will level off and remain essentially unchanged up to the point of exhaustion (see Figure 2–6). When the body shifts from the reclining to the standing position, there is an immediate drop in the stroke volume and a compensatory increase in the heart rate in order to maintain a constant cardiac output. This decrease in stroke volume is due primarily to a pooling of the blood in the legs, which reduces the volume of blood returning to the heart. This pooling of blood in the lower extremities is the result of what has been termed the *hydrostatic pressure effect*. Gravity exerts a dramatic effect on any fluid column. The pressure of the fluid in the column is a direct result of where that pressure is measured, with the pressure being essentially zero at the top of the column, and reaching its highest value at the bottom of the column.

In the human body, gravity exerts a similar influence, which is most marked in the standing position. Thus, the pressure is highest at the level of the feet and lowest at the level of the head. This increased pressure in the lower extremities presents a barrier to the return of venous blood to the heart, and results in the pooling of blood in the legs and a reduced stroke volume. Interestingly, the highest stroke volume attainable in upright exercise is only slightly greater than the resting value in the reclining position (Poliner et al., 1980). Thus, the increases seen in stroke volume during low to moderate levels of work appear to be only compensating for or overcoming the hydrostatic pressure effect.

Stroke volume varies from 60 to 100 milliliters at rest and can increase to values approaching 200 milliliters or greater. The actual values, however, will depend almost entirely on both the size of the individual and his or her level of conditioning, with the bigger and better-fit individuals having the higher values. Also, it has been speculated that stroke volume may decrease at the very high heart rates (180 beats per minute or higher) since the time available to fill the ventricle is greatly reduced. However, there is little support for this theory.

The cardiac output, since it is the product of both the heart rate and stroke volume, follows a rather predictable course with increasing levels of work (see Figure 2–6). From a resting value of approximately five liters per minute, the cardiac output increases as a direct function of the level or intensity of the exercise to a maximal value of twenty to forty liters per minute or higher, with the absolute value again reflecting the individual's size and state of conditioning. During the initial stages of exercise, the increases in cardiac output are due to increases in both heart rate and stroke volume, but as the level of exercise exceeds 50 to 60 percent of the individual's capacity, any further increases are strictly the result of increases in heart rate, since stroke volume has plateaued.

Blood flow patterns change rather markedly as the individual goes from rest to exercise. Blood is redirected away from areas where it is not essential to those areas that are active during the exercise bout (Rowell, 1974). Of the resting cardiac output, only 15 to 20 percent goes to muscle, while in exhaustive exercise, the muscles receive 80 to 85 percent of the cardiac output. This shift in blood flow to the muscles is accomplished primarily by a decrease in blood flow to the kidneys, liver, stomach, and intestines. As the body starts to overheat, either as a direct result of the exercise or due to high environmental temperatures, an increasing amount of blood is redirected to the skin for the specific purpose of conducting heat away from the body core to its periphery where the heat can be lost to the environment. This will then reduce the amount of blood available to supply the muscles, and explains why most athletic performances in the heat are well below average. An additional problem that one faces with prolonged exercise, or exercise in the heat, is the reduction in blood volume due to sweating and the shifting of fluid out of the blood into the tissues (edema). The shift in blood flow, where flow is redirected to the active muscles, is accomplished through the dilation and constriction of the vessels in the active and inactive areas respectively, and is controlled through the autonomic nervous system as well as through the effects of increased metabolism at the site of the active tissue (Rowell, 1974). Increased metabolism causes an increase in the acidity at the local tissue level, which acts to open up additional arterioles and capillaries.

Systolic blood pressure increases in direct proportion to the increase in exercise intensity, with values ranging from approximately 120 mmHg at rest to 200 mmHg or greater at the point of exhaustion (Erikssen et al., 1980). Diastolic blood pressure changes little if any during exercise (Suzuki, 1980). In fact, an increase in diastolic pressure during exercise is considered to be abnormal, and is one of several criteria for stopping the test prematurely. Systolic pressure increases as a direct result of the increased cardiac output.

The oxygen content of the blood at rest varies from 20 milliliters (ml) of oxygen for every 100 ml of arterial blood to 14 ml per 100 ml of venous blood.

The difference between these two values, i.e., 20 ml − 14 ml = 6 ml, is referred to as the *arterial-venous oxygen difference*, and reflects the extent to which oxygen is extracted or removed from the blood as it passes through the body. With exercise, there is a progressive increase in the arterial-venous oxygen difference, which is a reflection of a decreasing venous oxygen content, with the arterial oxygen content remaining essentially unchanged. The venous oxygen content drops to values approaching zero in the active muscles, but the mixed venous blood in the right atrium of the heart rarely drops below 2 ml per 100 ml of blood, since the blood returning from the active tissues is being mixed with blood from inactive areas as it returns to the heart. (Åstrand and Rodahl, 1977). Therefore, the arterial-venous oxygen difference can increase approximately threefold from rest to maximal exercise.

The composition of blood changes as the individual goes from a resting to an exercising state. The red blood cell may actually undergo a decrease in size as the body is exposed to prolonged exercise that involves a substantial fluid loss (Costill et al., 1974). Proteins may also be lost from the plasma volume, although the results of studies at the present time are conflicting.

With substantial fluid loss in prolonged exercise due to sweating, there is a reduction in plasma volume, which results in a *hemoconcentration* of red blood cells and plasma proteins (i.e., since the fluid portion is reduced, the cellular and protein portion of the blood volume represents a larger fraction of the total blood volume). This hemoconcentration results in a substantial rise (20 to 25 percent) in the red blood cell count. At one time, it was thought that red blood cells were added to the circulation to facilitate oxygen transport. It is now recognized that the blood plasma is reduced with fluid loss and this causes an increase in the relative number of red blood cells, not in the absolute number (Costill and Fink, 1974). Plasma volume loss results from a shift of fluid from the plasma to the interstitial fluid (fluid between the cells).

At rest, the blood pH remains constant at a value slightly below 7.4. A pH of 7.0 is considered neutral; greater than 7.0, alkaline or basic; and less than 7.0, acidic. Thus, normal blood at rest is slightly alkaline. There is little change in blood pH up to about 50 percent intensity of exercise. As the intensity of exercise increases above 50 percent, the pH will start to drop, the blood becoming more acidic (Åstrand and Rodahl, 1977). This drop will be gradual at first, but it will become more rapid as the individual approaches exhaustion. Values of 7.0 or lower have been reported following maximal exercise. Tissue pH reaches levels even lower than 6.5 (Hermansen and Osnes, 1972). The lowering of the blood pH is primarily the result of an increased anaerobic metabolism and corresponds to the increase observed in blood lactate. Blood lactate levels range from an average of 10 mg/100 ml of blood (1.1 millimoles/liter of blood) at rest to 200 mg/100 ml (22 millimoles/liter of blood) within five minutes following exercise. Lactate values reach their maximum in the blood during the initial five minutes of recovery from exhaustive exercise. Large concentrations of lactate do not appear in the blood until the work load reaches or exceeds 50 percent of the individual's capacity, which is related to the concept of aerobic/anaerobic threshold, to be discussed later in this chapter.

Respiratory Responses

The pulmonary ventilation, or minute volume, increases from a resting value of approximately 6 liters/min to values above 100 liters/min during the end stages of exhaustive exercise in adult males, and can reach values in excess of 200 liters/min in large, well-conditioned male athletes. This is accomplished by an increase in both the tidal volume and the respiratory frequency. Tidal volume may increase from a resting average of 0.5 liter/min to 2.5–3.0 liters/min during maximal exercise. This would correspond to an increase in the fraction of the vital capacity from 10 percent at rest to 50 percent during exercise. The respiratory frequency can increase from 12–16 breaths/min at rest to 40–50 breaths/min during maximal exercise. There is a direct, linear relationship between the increase in pulmonary ventilation and the increase in work level up to about 60–80 percent of the individual's capacity. From this point through the end of maximal exercise, the ventilation increases at a much faster rate.

The movement of these large volumes of air during heavy exercise requires considerable work from the respiratory muscles. It also requires an additional expenditure of energy above that needed for the exercising muscles. At rest, the energy cost for

ventilation is approximately 1 ml of oxygen for each liter of air breathed (Åstrand and Rodahl, 1977). For 6 liters of air/min, this would amount to 6 ml of oxygen/min for ventilation, which is approximately 2 percent of the total oxygen consumed at rest. During the later stages of maximal exercise, the cost of breathing may increase to 10 percent of the total amount of oxygen consumed (Åstrand and Rodahl, 1977).

The fractional lung volumes also change with the transition from rest to maximal exercise. The increase in tidal volume comes primarily from the inspiratory reserve volume. Residual volume increases slightly, vital capacity decreases slightly, and total lung capacity remains the same. As the ventilation increases, there is also a better distribution of the ventilation in the lungs, i.e., the incoming air is more evenly distributed among the alveoli. Also, the increase in the pulmonary arterial pressure provides a better distribution of the blood (perfusion) throughout the lung. Again, due to gravity and the hydrostatic pressure effect, the perfusion of blood to the upper regions of the lung is poor while at rest; however, as exercise progresses and the pulmonary arterial pressure increases, the upper regions of the lungs receive proportionally more blood, which increases their efficiency.

Lung diffusion refers to the rate at which gases diffuse from the alveoli to the blood in the pulmonary capillaries. It is expressed in ml of the gas per minute per partial pressure difference between alveolar gas and the capillaries. Diffusion capacity for oxygen can increase threefold from a resting value of 25 ml/min/mmHg to a maximal value of 75 ml/min/mmHg.

Two practical respiratory phenomena exist in the athletic world that are poorly understood and almost impossible to duplicate in the research laboratory. These are the phenomena of "second wind" and "stitch-in-the-side," both brought on by running. The stitch-in-the-side is usually felt as a sharp, severe pain in the lower-thoracic or upper-abdominal area. Many theories exist to explain this phenomenon, but, to date, none have any conclusive scientific support. The two most logical explanations are: (1) ischemia, or lack of blood flow to the diaphragm; and (2) gastrointestinal gas, or ischemia of the large intestine. Whatever the cause, there is no simple remedy that works equally well for all people. Some can continue to run with their pain, while others find it necessary to slow down or stop. Specific dietary modifications have been suggested as a preventive measure, but sufficient evidence is not available to demonstrate their effectiveness.

Second wind is an equally confusing phenomenon. During a workout at a constant pace, the effort seems labored or the athlete is not "in the groove." Suddenly, the athlete feels a sense of freedom; the distress of labored breathing is gone; he or she has experienced second wind. The feeling of second wind does relate to a more comfortable pattern of breathing, but this is the result of a more basic physiological alteration, which has yet to be defined. It is possibly a result of more efficient circulation to the active tissues or of a more efficient metabolic process. The answer will have to await a much better understanding of how respiration is controlled during exercise.

Metabolic Responses

As the body shifts from rest to exercise, there is an increase in the total body metabolism. While this has been documented through direct calorimetry, much more data are available using indirect calorimetry, primarily through the assessment of oxygen consumption levels.

$\dot{V}O_2$ *max.* The increase in metabolism is in direct proportion to the increase in the level of work. As the index of metabolic activity, *oxygen consumption* ($\dot{V}O_2$) increases up to the last stage of exercise. At this point, the $\dot{V}O_2$ plateaus, even though the work level continues to increase (Figure 2–7). The value at which the $\dot{V}O_2$ plateaus is referred to as the *maximal oxygen consumption* ($\dot{V}O_2$ max). This value is a well-defined and reproducible physiological endpoint. $\dot{V}O_2$ max is regarded as the best cri-

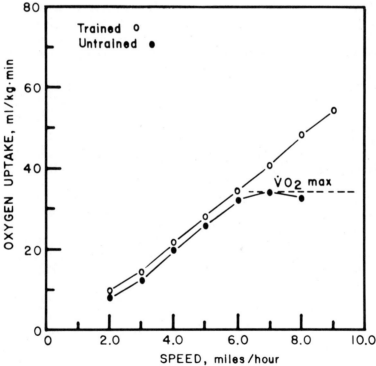

Figure 2–7 Oxygen uptake in relationship to different speeds of walking, jogging, and running illustrating the difference in response between a trained (o) and untrained (●) individual.

terion of cardiorespiratory endurance capacity or "physical fitness."

$\dot{V}O_2$ max values are influenced greatly by size, age, and level of fitness. To account for individual differences in size, $\dot{V}O_2$ max is frequently expressed relative to body weight (ml of oxygen/kg of body weight × min) or to lean body weight. This allows a more equitable comparison between individuals of different sizes. Mean $\dot{V}O_2$ max values decrease with age beyond fifteen to twenty years. This is probably due to a combination of true biological aging and a sedentary life style. In addition, females beyond ten to twenty years have mean $\dot{V}O_2$ max values considerably below those of males of similar ages. It is questionable whether these represent true differences between the sexes, or whether the female is a victim of her culture, which imposes a sedentary life style once she reaches menarche.

$\dot{V}O_2$ max varies from values as high as 80–84 ml/kg × min in long-distance runners and cross-country skiers to values in the mid-20's, or lower, for poorly conditioned, sedentary adults. The highest value recorded was 94 ml/kg × min for a champion Norwegian cross-country skier. The highest value recorded for a female was 74 ml/kg × min for a Russian cross-country skier. Values for athletes in various sports are presented in Chapter 9.

Oxygen Debt. Oxygen debt refers to the volume of oxygen consumed during the recovery period following exercise that is in excess of the volume normally consumed while at rest. A quick run down the block to catch the departing bus or a fast climb up several flights of stairs leaves one with a rapid pulse and an "out-of-breath" feeling. After several minutes of recovery, the breathing and pulse appear to return to normal. Most work or bouts of exercise are performed at levels well below one's endurance capacity ($\dot{V}O_2$ max). However, it is possible to perform work that requires considerably more energy/min than can be supplied by the body. This is accomplished through anaerobic metabolism, as discussed in Chapter 1 and illustrated in Figure 1–15. Pyruvic acid is unable to go through the Krebs cycle due to an accumulation of hydrogen ions and atoms and because of a lack of oxygen. Pyruvic acid is then converted to lactic acid, which allows glycolysis to continue until it results in the production of ATP. In addition, stored ATP and CP can be used to provide energy during this period of oxygen deficiency.

There is even an oxygen debt associated with low levels of exercise. This is due to the fact that oxygen consumption requires several minutes to reach the required or steady-state level (Figure 2–8), even

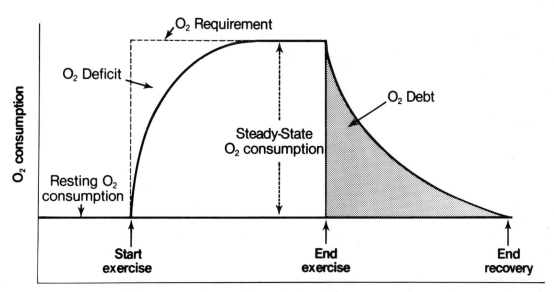

Figure 2–8 Oxygen debt resulting from a submaximal, steady-state exercise.

though the requirement to perform the exercise is constant from the very start of the exercise. This initial period, where the oxygen consumption is below the steady-state or required level, is referred to as the period of *oxygen deficit*. The deficit is calculated simply as the difference between the amount of oxygen that is required and that which is actually consumed.

Studies by Brooks et al. (1973) and Brooks and Gaesser (1980) raise serious questions as to the physiological explanation traditionally held for this excess postexercise oxygen consumption. For many years, the oxygen debt curve was mathematically described as having two distinct components: an initial fast component (alactacid portion), and a secondary slow component (lactacid portion). The classic theory postulated the fast component to be the result of the rephosphorylation of ATP and creatine phosphate. The slow component was theorized to be the result of lactate removal, with 80 percent of the lactate formed during exercise being converted to glycogen, and the remaining 20 percent being oxidized to CO_2 and H_2O, providing the energy necessary for glycogen repletion. The results from the two studies by Brooks et al. indicate that the slow component does not coincide with lactate removal. They concluded that the classical explanations of excess postexercise oxygen consumption are too simplistic, and that the physiological mechanisms responsible for the oxygen debt need to be much more clearly defined.

Energy Substrate. The *respiratory exchange ratio* (R) is the ratio between the amount of carbon dioxide produced and the amount of oxygen consumed, i.e., R = CO_2 produced/O_2 consumed. The R value will vary with the foodstuff or substrate that is being metabolized to provide the energy for work. When only fats are metabolized, the R = 0.71; for proteins, R = 0.82; and for carbohydrates, R = 1.00. By observing the R value at various stages of steady-state exercise, it is possible to estimate the type of substrate that is being metabolized to provide the necessary energy. As an example, if during 1 min of moderate exercise, the individual consumed 2.0 liters of oxygen and produced 1.8 liters of carbon dioxide, the R value would be 0.90 (R = 1.8/2.0 = 0.9). It has been demonstrated that the oxidation of 1 gm of glycogen uses 0.828 liter of oxygen and produces 0.828 liter of carbon dioxide.

Also, the oxidation of 1 gm of fat uses 1.989 liters of oxygen and produces 1.419 liters of carbon dioxide. Two equations can then be written, where x = gm of glycogen used, y = gm of fat used, and the assumption is made that no protein has been used.

$$2.0 \text{ liters of oxygen}$$
$$= 1.989y + 0.828x$$
$$(-)\ 1.8 \text{ liters of carbon dioxide}$$
$$= 1.419y + 0.828x$$

or

$$0.2 = 0.570y \ (x \text{ cancels out})$$
$$y = 0.2/.570$$
$$y = 0.35 \text{ gm of fat}$$

and substituting for y in either of these equations,

$$x = 1.57 \text{ gm of carbohydrate}$$

Thus, the energy for 1 min of moderate exercise was supplied by 0.35 gm of fat and 1.57 gm of carbohydrate.

The R value will usually vary from 0.75 to 0.81 at rest and will increase with exercise to reach values in excess of 1.0, as the individual reaches exhaustion. During recovery, R can be elevated to values of 1.5, or higher; this peak value tends to correspond to the peak appearance of lactate in the blood. When R values exceed 1.0, the body is relying, at least partially, on anaerobic metabolism, and the R value no longer provides an accurate estimate of the substrate being metabolized.

The major source of energy, or the fuel for muscular work, was previously thought to be carbohydrates, with fats serving only in a reserve, or secondary, role. It is now evident that fat is a major energy source during exercise. It appears that in aerobic work, where the intensity is below the individual's endurance capacity, from 50–70 percent of the energy used is provided by fats; the longer the duration, the higher the contribution of fat. With high levels of work, particularly in anaerobic work, the primary source of energy is from carbohydrates. The composition of the diet can have a rather remarkable influence on athletic performance, and this will be discussed in great detail in Chapter 10, Athletic Nutrition.

Anaerobic Threshold. While $\dot{V}O_2$ max is regarded as the best physiological criterion of endurance capacity, it does have certain limitations. With a group of endurance athletes, it is not possible to predict the order of finish in an endurance race by using only the $\dot{V}O_2$ max values. Likewise, correlations between endurance-running performance tests, e.g., Cooper's 12-min run, the Balke 1.5-mi run, the 2-mi run, and $\dot{V}O_2$ max are only moderately high ($r = 0.40$ to 0.89), indicating that there is more to a good performance than just $\dot{V}O_2$ max. It is also well documented that $\dot{V}O_2$ max will increase with physical training for only twelve to eighteen months, at which time it plateaus, even with continued, higher-intensity training. However, the individual can still improve running times for the various distances after the point at which the $\dot{V}O_2$ max stops increasing. Thus, performance can improve even though $\dot{V}O_2$ max has reached its peak.

Figure 2–9 illustrates one possible explanation for this apparent inconsistency. The athlete is able to improve performance even after reaching an upper limit or ceiling for one's $\dot{V}O_2$ max by developing the ability to work at a higher percentage of capacity for prolonged periods of time. Costill (1979) has found that most marathon runners complete the 26.2 mi with an average pace that corresponds to 75–80 percent of their $\dot{V}O_2$ max. Derek Clayton, former holder of the best time in the world for the marathon (2 hr, 8 min, 33 sec), had a measured $\dot{V}O_2$

max below that which would normally be expected on the basis of his world-record performance (69.7 ml/kg × min). Costill, however, found that Clayton was able to work at 86 percent of his $\dot{V}O_2$ max when running on the treadmill at his racing pace, a value considerably higher than the average world-class marathoner, and a value that probably accounts for his world-record running ability. It would appear that both $\dot{V}O_2$ max and the percentage of $\dot{V}O_2$ max that the athlete can maintain for a prolonged period of time are the determining factors in performance. This could explain the lower-than-expected correlations between $\dot{V}O_2$ max and endurance performance tests, and the ability of the athlete to improve performance despite the plateau in $\dot{V}O_2$ max.

Recently, investigators have introduced a new parameter that may be closely related to the percentage of the capacity that one can maintain for a prolonged period of time. Wasserman and McIlroy (1964) have termed this parameter the *anaerobic threshold*. It is defined as that point in an exercise of increasing intensity at which the body starts increasing anaerobic metabolism above resting levels and at which blood lactate concentration starts to increase. With the proper instrumentation, this threshold can be assessed very accurately by ob-

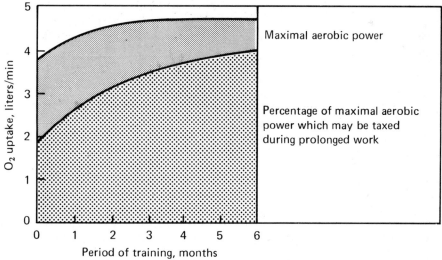

Figure 2–9 Influence of physical training on maximal oxygen uptake (maximal aerobic power), as well as on the fraction of maximal oxygen uptake that one can maintain during prolonged work. (From P. O. Åstrand and K. Rodahl, *Textbook of Work Physiology*. New York: McGraw-Hill Book Co., 1970. Reproduced by permission of the publisher.)

serving the ventilation, carbon dioxide production, and ventilatory equivalent for oxygen responses to exercise. All three processes increase linearly with increases in the level of work up to the point of the anaerobic threshold, at which time their rate of change increases. This increase in rate of change results in greater nonlinear increases in ventilation, carbon dioxide production, and ventilatory equivalent for oxygen, while the increases in the level of work remain linear (Figure 2–10). The anaerobic threshold can be expressed in terms of the percentage of $\dot{V}O_2$ max at which it occurs. An anaerobic threshold of 60 percent of $\dot{V}O_2$ max would indicate, theoretically, a greater performance potential for the same $\dot{V}O_2$ max than an anaerobic threshold of 45 percent of $\dot{V}O_2$ max. The higher percentage indicates that the individual can work at relatively higher levels of metabolism before having to rely on the inefficient, limiting process of anaerobic metabolism.

A recent study by Farrell et al. (1979) indicates that the anaerobic threshold, or the onset of plasma lactate accumulation as it is referred to in their paper, may well be the reason runners cannot run at a higher fraction of their $\dot{V}O_2$ max. They found that the best pace a marathon runner can maintain for the 26.2 mi race is very close to that pace corresponding to his or her anaerobic threshold. In other words, the experienced runner appears to be able to maintain a pace at just below that point where significant amounts of lactate start to accumulate in the blood.

Skinner and McLellan (1980), in their extensive review of the research literature on anaerobic threshold, have concluded that there are actually three phases during the progressive transition from exercise of low to maximal intensity, and that these phases are clearly defined by breakpoints in various physiological parameters that differentiate the first from the second phase, and the second from the third phase. The transition from Phase I to Phase II has been termed the *aerobic threshold*, and is characterized by a gradual increase in blood lactate, an increase in the fraction of expired oxygen (F_EO_2), and a break upward from linearity in ventilation and CO_2 production ($\dot{V}CO_2$). The transition from Phase II to Phase III has been termed the *anaerobic threshold*, and is characterized by a further increase in blood lactate, a sharp decrease in the fraction of expired CO_2 (F_ECO_2), and an additional break from

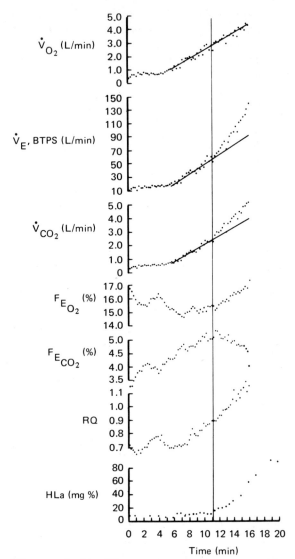

Figure 2–10 Illustration of the anaerobic threshold. (From James A. Davis, "Validity, Reproducibility and Effect of Endurance Training on the Anaerobic Threshold in College-Age Males," unpublished doctoral dissertation, University of California, Davis, 1975. Reproduced by permission of the author.)

linearity in ventilation. The aerobic threshold occurs at approximately 40 to 60 percent of $\dot{V}O_2$ max, at a blood lactate level of approximately 2 mmol·liter^{-1}. The anaerobic threshold occurs at approximately 65 to 90 percent of $\dot{V}O_2$ max, at a blood lactate level of approximately 4 mmol·liter^{-1}. The concept or the possibility of two thresholds rather than one is intriguing, and is certainly deserving of additional study.

Energy Cost of Various Activities. The amount of energy expended for different activities will vary considerably, depending on the intensity of the exercise, if factors such as duration and environmental conditions are kept constant. Many activities have been evaluated to determine the associated metabolic cost. This is usually accomplished by monitoring the oxygen consumption during exercise to determine an average oxygen cost per unit of time, which can then be converted to an energy expenditure in Kcalories/min. These values typically ignore the anaerobic aspects of exercise, since the oxygen debt is seldom used in these calculations. This is an important point, for an activity that costs a total of 300 Kcalories to perform may result in an additional 100 Kcalories expenditure above resting, during the recovery period; thus, the total cost of the activity would be 400, not 300, Kcalories. The body requires 0.2 to 0.35 liters of oxygen/min just to satisfy its resting energy requirements. This would amount to 1–1.8 Kcalories/min, 60–108 Kcalories/hour, or 1,440–2,600 Kcalories/day. Obviously, any increased activity above resting levels will add to the projected daily expenditure. Sedentary adult men and women of average weight will have an average caloric expenditure of 2,700 and 1,850 Kcalories/day, respectively. Football linemen, during preseason conditioning sessions, where two or three practice sessions are held per day, have been found to consume more than 10,000 Kcalories/day. The range of values for total daily caloric expenditure are, thus, quite varied and will depend on factors such as sex, age, weight, environment, and activity levels.

Sport activities differ with respect to their energy cost. Some require levels of energy expenditure that are only slightly greater than those at rest. Others have levels so high that they can be maintained for only short periods of time, e.g., sprinting. With regard to total energy expenditure, the total duration of the activity must be considered, in addition to the level of energy expenditure. While approximately 29 Kcalories/min are expended while sprinting at a speed of 15.5 *miles per hour* (mph), this level of

activity can be endured for only brief periods of time. Jogging at a 7-mph pace (approximately 8½ min/mi) will result in an expenditure of 14.5 calories/min, or only half of that expended in running at 15.5 mph, but jogging can be maintained for a considerably longer period of time, resulting in a greater total expenditure of energy. This is an important consideration for anyone contemplating the use of exercise to reduce weight. Table 2–1 provides an estimate of energy expenditure for various activities on the basis of the average mature male with an approximate body weight of 154 lb. Since most activities involve moving the body mass, these figures will vary considerably with the weight, age, and sex of the individual. The relative relationships of energy cost per activity, however, can be accurately evaluated.

Body Fluids and Temperature Regulation

As the length of the exercise period is increased, body fluid changes and temperature regulation become important to the efficient performance of the athlete. In activities that require several minutes or less, body-fluid changes and temperature regulation are of little or no practical importance. For the football player or the marathon runner, however, these processes are critically important, even to the point of being necessary for survival. Deaths have occurred during or as a result of various sport activities due to problems of dehydration (water deficiency) and hyperthermia (overheating).

Body Fluids. The body is divided into two major fluid compartments: the intracellular and extracellular compartments. The intracellular fluid compartment includes the fluid that exists within all of the cells in the body. The extracellular fluid compartment includes the plasma volume of the blood and the interstitial fluid, or that fluid that lies outside of and bathes the cells. The fluid volume is slightly larger than the water volume since fluid volume includes the water volume and those substances that are suspended or dissolved in the water.

With exercise, there is a loss of nonprotein fluid almost immediately from the plasma volume to the interstitial and intracellular fluid spaces, which is probably the result of increased hydrostatic pressure within the vascular system (Costill and Fink, 1974). The increase in blood pressure forces water

Table 2–1 *Typical Energy Expenditure for Various Physical Activities, Calculated on the Basis of a 154-Pound Man**

Activity	Kcalories/ min	Kcalories/ hour
Sleeping	1.2	70
Sitting	1.7	100
Standing	1.8	110
Walking		
2.0 mph	3.2	192
3.5 mph	5.0	300
4.0 mph	5.8	348
Jogging-Running		
7.0 mph	14.5	870
9.0 mph	16.8	1,008
12.0 mph	21.7	1,300
15.5 mph	28.8	1,728
Bicycling		
7 mph	5.0	300
10 mph	7.5	450
13 mph	11.1	666
Horseshoes	4.0	240
Baseball		
(except pitcher)	4.7	282
pitcher	6.5	390
Calisthenics	4.7	282
Dancing		
moderate	4.2	252
vigorous	7.0	420
Archery	5.0	300
Golf	5.0	300
Swimming		
Breast stroke, 1 mph	6.8	410
Crawl stroke, 1 mph	7.0	420
Back Stroke, 1 mph	8.3	500
Tennis	7.1	425
Weight Training	8.2	492
Basketball	8.6	516
Mountain Climbing	10.0	600
Football (American)	10.2	612
Squash	10.2	612
Fencing	10.5	630
Handball	11.0	660
Rowing, 3.5 mph	11.0	660
Gymnastics	11.5	690
Wrestling	13.1	790

*Adapted from L. E. Morehouse and A. T. Miller, Jr. *Physiology of Exercise.* 6th ed. St. Louis: C. V. Mosby Co., 1971.

from the vascular compartment to the nonvascular compartment. Up to a 10–20 percent or greater reduction in plasma volume can occur with prolonged work. If the exercise intensity or the environmental conditions are such that the individual starts to sweat, additional fluid loss can be expected from the plasma volume, although the major source of fluid for sweating is from the interstitial and intracellular spaces. This reduction in plasma volume with exercise results in an increased concentration of red blood cells, serum proteins, and hemoglobin. However, this is a relative, not an absolute, increase, as was mentioned earlier in this chapter.

The reduction in plasma volume is likely to be detrimental to performance. For long-duration activities, where heat loss is a problem, the total flow of blood to the active tissues must be such that an increasingly higher percentage of blood can be diverted to the skin to reduce body heat. If the plasma volume is already reduced by the hydrostatic pressure increase, this further reduction will have a negative influence on the performance of that activity. Also, the reduced plasma volume will result in more concentrated red blood cells, thus, increasing the viscosity of the blood. Recent evidence suggests that an increased blood viscosity can limit the oxygen-transporting ability of the blood (Horstman et al., 1980).

As sweating continues, there will be a loss of interstitial and intracellular fluid. This will create an increased osmotic pressure (higher concentration of solids) in the interstitial fluid, which will cause even more fluid from the plasma volume to diffuse into the interstitial fluid. While intracellular fluid volume is impossible to measure directly and accurately, research suggests that there is also a fluid loss from the intracellular fluid and even from the red blood cells, which may shrink.

Temperature Regulation. As the body starts to exercise, the rate of metabolism increases in direct proportion to the intensity of the exercise. The body, like a machine, is not 100 percent efficient, since it uses more energy than is actually needed for the exercise. The mechanical efficiency of the human body varies from 10 percent or less for activities such as swimming to over 30 percent for some other types of activities. The remaining energy that is not used in the process of muscular contraction is lost in the form of heat. This creates a considerable heat load within the body, which necessitates physiological adjustments to reduce body temperature. Exercise in a hot climate, particularly in one with elevated humidity, places additional heat stress on the body, and further temperature adjustments must be made.

The major physiological adjustment that promotes heat loss from the body is the shunting of blood to the periphery, as is evidenced by the red skin of an overheated athlete. When blood is brought to the body's surface, heat is lost more efficiently by convection and radiation. Convection is the process by which heat is lost or transferred from a body to a moving liquid or gas, e.g., cool air passing over the warm body. Radiation is the process through which heat is lost through electromagnetic waves. Two other forms of heat loss are important in the total attempt to regulate body temperature: conduction and evaporation. Conduction is the process in which heat is lost by direct contact with a cooler object or medium. Evaporation is a major form of heat loss at high body temperatures in a relatively dry environment. When water evaporates, 580 Kcalories of heat are lost for every liter of water that is evaporated. As one sweats, the sweat evaporates and cools the surrounding skin.

Body temperature is controlled in the brain by the hypothalamus and the adjacent preoptic area. At rest, even under considerably varying environmental conditions, body temperature is maintained at a relatively constant value of approximately 98.6° F. Temperature receptors in the skin assist the hypothalamus in maintaining this temperature constant. With exercise, body temperature increases in proportion to the intensity and duration of activity. Moderate exercise can raise the body temperature to over 100° F, and in severe exercise, temperatures can exceed 106° F (Costill, 1979).

Problems of temperature regulation become critical when the surrounding temperature equals or exceeds the skin temperature (approximately 92–93° F). Convection and radiation are ineffective avenues of heat loss and actually become avenues of heat gain when the surrounding temperature exceeds the skin temperature. The body must then rely on evaporative heat loss. This works well as long as the air immediately surrounding the body is dry, i.e., of low humidity. However, when air becomes saturated with water, the last major avenue of heat loss is closed and exercise must stop. Frequently, the micro-environment created by clothing, e.g., the football uniform or a rubberized sweat suit, can result in surrounding temperatures that are above the skin temperature and in air that is fully saturated with water vapor, creating a potentially dangerous situation. Problems of temperature regulation will be discussed in detail in Chapter 11, Environmental Factors and Athletic Performance.

Exercise in the cold presents certain problems, but these are not nearly as severe or frequent as those that occur in the heat. In the cold, one can always wear additional clothing, so heat that is normally lost in the body's metabolism is used to maintain body temperature. In addition, the blood vessels to and near the surface of the skin constrict, shunting blood away from the periphery and back to the center of the body to conserve the body's internal heat. Thus, body temperature during exercise in the cold is usually controlled effectively and efficiently.

Fluid Replacement. As a result of the need for adequate body fluid to maintain the sweating mechanisms necessary for temperature regulation in warm or hot climates, it is now recognized that fluid should be replaced during exercise. Costill (1979) has suggested that 100–200 ml of fluid be ingested at frequent intervals during prolonged bouts of exercise. This fluid should be relatively low in sugar and electrolyte content, since high levels decrease the absorption of fluid from the stomach and intestine. While glucose and electrolyte replacement are important, the replacement of the lost fluid appears to be of much greater importance for the purposes of fluid balance and temperature regulation. The quantity of fluid ingested should be approximately equal to the quantity of fluid lost. The body can lose up to 1–2 liters/hour under extreme conditions of exercise and environment, thus, replacement of the fluid during the activity is extremely important.

GENERAL SUMMARY

The field of exercise and sport physiology has advanced considerably since pioneering efforts began in the 1920s, although there is still considerably more knowledge to be gained than is presently available. The human body has demonstrated a remarkable physiological adaptability to the stress of exercise. Due to the limitations of field testing, these physiological adaptations are normally measured in the laboratory while the individual exercises on a stationary piece of equipment, such as a treadmill or bicycle ergometer.

The nervous system calls the body into action, either through conscious, central nervous system control or through sensory reflex action. Nerve impulses pass from the central nervous system to the motor neurons to activate the appropriate motor units. While strength is a function of the number of motor units activated simultaneously, endurance depends on adequate circulation to these active units. The cardiovascular system is, therefore, involved in supplying the working muscles with the necessary oxygen and nutrients and in removing metabolic waste products, in addition to serving as the body's cooling system in the regulation of body temperature. As the intensity of the exercise increases, the heart rate and stroke volume increase, although stroke volume tends to reach its peak and plateau at approximately 40–60 percent of the individual's capacity. The changes in the heart rate and stroke volume result in a large increase in cardiac output, allowing an increased blood flow to the active tissues. The increase in cardiac output is of much greater magnitude than the decrease in vascular resistance due to the dilation of the vessels in the active tissue. The net result is an increase in the systolic blood pressure with little or no change in the diastolic pressure. All of these changes are in direct proportion to the increase in exercise intensity.

The arterial-venous oxygen difference widens with increasing exercise intensity, indicating a greater extraction of oxygen at the tissue level. Plasma volume is reduced and the blood becomes hemoconcentrated. Blood pH decreases after exercise exceeds 50 percent of the individual's capacity, a change that is related to the appearance of lactate in the blood. Ventilation volume is increased to help meet the demands for increased oxygen consumption and carbon dioxide elimination. This is accomplished by an increase in both tidal volume and respiration rate, the increases again being directly related to the intensity of the exercise. Lung-diffusion capacity increases to facilitate oxygen loading, and the ventilation-perfusion ratio becomes optimized as the upper regions of the lung are better ventilated and better perfused with blood.

Metabolism also increases in direct proportion to the intensity of exercise, as reflected by the level of oxygen consumed. The peak or maximal level of oxygen consumed at or prior to reaching the point of exhaustion is referred to as the maximal oxygen consumption ($\dot{V}O_2$ max) and reflects the body's overall endurance capacity or cardiorespiratory fitness. Oxygen debt reflects anaerobic metabolism. The anaerobic threshold may play an important role in determining the individual's endurance performance potential when used in conjunction with his or her $\dot{V}O_2$ max value.

Last, fluid volume and temperature regulation are important aspects of prolonged exercise. Plasma volume may decrease by 20 percent or more as sweating reduces both plasma volume and interstitial fluid. The body relies on convection, radiation, conduction, and evaporation for heat loss to maintain body temperature. Evaporation appears to be the most critical avenue of heat loss in intense, prolonged exercise or in exercise in hot environments. Adequate fluid replacement during the activity is essential for both fluid balance and temperature regulation.

STUDY QUESTIONS

1. What are the major advantages and disadvantages of the bicycle ergometer and treadmill for producing a given level of exercise?
2. What is the difference between an acute response to exercise and a chronic adaptation to physical training?
3. What are the various theories that have been proposed to explain muscle fatigue?
4. How do HR, SV, and $\dot{Q}$ respond to increasing levels of exercise?
5. What are the major determinants of maximal heart rate and maximal stroke volume?
6. How does the body adapt to increasing levels of exercise to provide adequate blood flow to the active muscles?
7. What are the major cardiovascular adjustments made by the body when overheated?
8. What is the relationship between blood pH levels and levels of blood lactate as exercise progresses from low to high intensity?
9. What is the physiological significance of $\dot{V}O_2$ max and anaerobic threshold, and how are both determined?
10. Of what physiological significance is the respiratory exchange ratio?
11. What alterations occur in body fluids as one

progresses from low to high intensity exercise? From short to long duration exercise?

12. How is body temperature regulated during exercise?

13. Should an athlete be allowed to drink fluids during practice or competition? Why?

REFERENCES

Anderson, K. L.; Shepherd, R. J.; Denolin, H.; Varnauskas, E.; and Masironi, R. R. *Fundamentals of Exercise Testing*. Geneva: World Health Organization, 1971.

Asmussen, E. "Muscle Fatigue." *Med. Sci. Sports* 11 (1979): 313–321.

Åstrand, P.-O., and Rodahl, K. *Textbook of Work Physiology*. 2nd ed. New York: McGraw-Hill Book Co., 1977.

Bigland-Ritchie, B.; Jones, D. A.; Hosking, G. P.; and Edwards, R. H. T. "Central and Peripheral Fatigue in Sustained Maximum Voluntary Contractions of Human Quadriceps Muscle." *Clin. Sci. Molecular Med.* 541: (1978): 609–614.

Brooks, G. A.; Brauner, K. E.; and Cassens, R. G. "Glycogen Synthesis and Metabolism of Lactic Acid after Exercise." *Am. J. Physiol.* 224 (1973): 1162–1166.

Brooks, G. A., and Gaesser, G. A. "End Points of Lactate and Glucose Metabolism after Exhausting Exercise." *J. Appl. Physiol.: Respirat. Environ. Exercise Physiol.* 49 (1980): 1057–1069.

Carlsten, A., and Grimby, G. *The Circulatory Response to Muscular Exercise in Man*. Springfield, Ill.: Charles C. Thomas, 1966.

Clarke, D. H. *Exercise Physiology*. Englewood Cliffs, N.J.: Prentice-Hall, Inc., 1975.

Costill, D. L. *A Scientific Approach to Distance Running*. Los Altos, Calif.: Track and Field News, 1979.

Costill, D. L.; Branam, L.; Eddy, D.; and Fink, W. "Alterations in Red Cell Volume following Exercise and Dehydration." *J. Appl. Physiol.* 37 (1974): 912–916.

Costill, D. L., and Fink, W. "Plasma Volume Changes following Exercise and Thermal Dehydration." *J. Appl. Physiol.* 37 (1974): 521–525.

de Vries, H. A. *Physiology of Exercise for Physical Education and Athletics*. 2nd ed. Dubuque, Iowa: William C. Brown Co., 1974.

Edington, D. W., and Edgerton, V. R. *The Biology of Physical Activity*. Boston: Houghton Mifflin Co., 1976.

Erikssen, J.; Jervell, J.; and Forfang, K. "Blood Pressure Responses to Bicycle Exercise Testing in Apparently Healthy Middle-Aged Men." *Cardiology* 66 (1980): 56–63.

Falls, H. B., ed. *Exercise Physiology*. New York: Academic Press, 1968.

Farrell, P. A.; Wilmore, J. H.; Coyle, E. F.; Billing, J. E.; and Costill, D. L. "Plasma Lactate Accumulation and Distance Running Performance." *Med. Sci. Sports* 11 (1979): 338–344.

Fox, E. L. *Sports Physiology*. Philadelphia: W. B. Saunders Co., 1979.

Hermansen, L., and Osnes, J.-B. "Blood and Muscle pH after Maximal Exercise in Man." *J. Appl. Physiol.* 32 (1972): 304–308.

Horstman, D.; Weiskopf, R.; and Jackson, R. E. "Work Capacity during a 3-wk Sojourn at 4,300 m: Effects of Relative Polycythemia." *J. Appl. Physiol.* 49 (1980): 311–318.

Ikai, M.; Yabe, K.; and Ishii, K. "Muskelkraft und Muskuläre Ermündung bei Willkürlicher Anspannung und Elektrischer Reizung des Muskels." *Sportartz und Sportsmedizin* (1967): 197–211.

Johnson, W. R., and Buskirk, E. R., eds. *Science and Medicine of Exercise and Sport*. 2nd ed. New York: Harper and Row, 1974.

Karpovich, P. V., and Sinning, W. E. *Physiology of Muscular Activity*. 7th ed. Philadelphia: W. B. Saunders Co., 1971.

Knuttgen, H. G., ed. *Neuromuscular Mechanisms for Therapeutic and Conditioning Exercise*. Baltimore: University Park Press, 1976.

Lamb, D. R. *Physiology of Exercise: Responses and Adaptations*. New York: Macmillan Publishing Co., 1978.

Larson, L. A., ed. *Fitness, Health, and Work Capacity*. New York: Macmillan Publishing Co., 1974.

Mathews, D. K., and Fox, E. L. *The Physiological Basis of Physical Education and Athletics*. 2nd ed. Philadelphia: W. B. Saunders Co., 1976.

Merton, P. A., "Voluntary Strength and Fatigue." *J. Physiol.* 123 (1954): 553–564.

Morehouse, L. E., and Miller, A. T. *Physiology of Exercise*. 6th ed. St. Louis: C. V. Mosby Co., 1971.

Poliner, L. R.; Dehmer, G. J.; Lewis, S. E.; Parkey, R. W.; Blomqvist, C. G.; and Willerson, J. T. "Left Ventricular Performance in Normal Subjects: A Comparison of the Responses to Exercise in the Upright and Supine Positions." *Circulation* 62 (1980) 528–534.

Rowell, L. B. "Human Cardiovascular Adjustments to Exercise and Thermal Stress." *Physiol. Rev.* 54 (1974): 75–159.

Sharkey, B. J. *Physiology of Fitness*. Champaign, Ill.: Human Kinetics Publishers, 1979.

Shepherd, R. J. *Endurance Fitness*. Toronto: University of Toronto Press, 1969.

Shepherd, R. J. *Men at Work*. Springfield, Ill.: Charles C. Thomas, 1974.

Simonson, E., ed. *Physiology of Work Capacity and Fatigue*. Springfield, Ill.: Charles C. Thomas, 1971.

Skinner, J. S.; and McLellan, T. H. "The Transition from Aerobic to Anaerobic Metabolism." *Res. Quart. Exercise and Sport*. 51 (1980): 234–248.

Strauss, R. H., ed. *Sports Medicine and Physiology*. Philadelphia: W. B. Saunders Co., 1979.

Suzuki, Y. "Mean Arterial Pressure, O_2-Uptake, and Muscle Force Time during Dynamic and Rhythmic-Static Exercise in Man with High Percentage of Fast- and Slow-Twitch Fibers." *European J. Appl. Physiol.* 43 (1980): 143–155.

Wasserman, K.; and McIlroy, M. B. "Detecting the Threshold of Anaerobic Metabolism." *Am. J. Cardiol.* 14 (1964): 844–852.

Wilmore, J. H., and Norton, A. C. *The Heart and Lungs at Work*. Schiller Park, Ill.: Beckman Instruments, 1974.

3

Adaptations to Chronic Exercise

INTRODUCTION

The preceding chapter focused on the physiological adaptability of individuals to an acute bout of exercise. The present chapter looks at those changes that result from chronic exercise, i.e., physical training. These are changes that develop slowly after repeated bouts of exercise and that result in lasting physiological adaptations.

FACTORS INFLUENCING THE RESPONSE TO CHRONIC EXERCISE

Alterations resulting from chronic exercise will depend in magnitude on six basic factors (Pollock, 1973).

- Type of training activity
- Frequency of participation
- Duration of each training session
- Intensity of performance
- Duration of the total program
- Initial level of fitness of the subjects

Each of these factors is of considerable importance and will be discussed independently.

There are many ways in which physical exercise can be performed, e.g., just to name a few, bowling, golf, calisthenics, tennis, weight training, bicycling, and jogging. All activities, however, basically fall into one or a combination of several major categories: (1) flexibility or joint loosening, (2) strength and power, (3) speed and agility, (4) endurance, and (5) relaxation. The types of activities or exercises that are selected will depend to a large extent on the purpose of training. The forty-five-year-old who wants to "get back into shape" will emphasize endurance activities because of their ability to improve function of the cardiovascular and respiratory systems, both systems being susceptible to chronic, disabling and death-causing diseases. The young shot putter, however, would stress strength and power activities, with some attention to activities that would also develop speed and agility. Thus, the outcome of the conditioning program will be determined largely by the type of activity or activities that are selected.

The frequency of participation influences the magnitude of change or improvement. However, the change is highly dependent on the interaction between frequency, duration, and intensity. The forty-five-year-old "fitness seeker" can improve considerably with a training frequency of three days per week. Training programs of two days per week produce desirable changes, but they are substantially less than the changes that are produced by training programs of three or more days per week. Training more than four days per week will result in further gains, but, generally, they will not be worth the additional time invested, i.e., the degree of improvement decreases to a point where a great deal of time must be invested to achieve small, additional gains. Thus, for the "fitness seeker," three to four days per week appear to be optimal. For the competitive athlete, the small gain attained by working out an additional two or three days (a total of six or seven days per week) may be necessary, since it could mean the difference between first and second place.

The duration of each training session will depend largely on the purpose of the training program, i.e., for competition or for health and fitness, and on the type of activity. A minimum investment of twenty to thirty minutes per day is adequate to accomplish a good training response for general fitness. For the athlete, one to two hours on the track or field or five hours in the water might be necessary to prepare for the higher levels of competition. Similar to frequency, the magnitude of the change is dependent on the total time spent in training; the more time in training, the greater the degree of change.

The intensity at which the activity is performed is probably the most critical of the various factors that dictate the magnitude of change. Cardiovascular endurance changes begin to occur once the individuals start exercising at fifty percent of their endurance capacity or above. This appears to be a threshold below which changes will not occur. Again, the higher the intensity, the greater the change. With strength training, the muscle apparently must be taken to fatigue or near fatigue for significant strength changes to occur. Unlike cardiovascular endurance, training at 50–70 percent intensity will not result in any major gains in strength, although gains in muscular endurance might be found at these submaximal levels. The level of intensity needed to maximize gains in cardiovascular endurance has not been clearly established. Good improvement is possible both with interval training, where the intensity is close to maximum and rest or recovery periods are interspersed, and with long, slow distance (LSD) training, where an intensity of 60–80 percent of maximum is maintained for long periods of time. At the present time, neither of these two extremes appears to provide a distinct advantage over the other, although additional research in this area is certainly necessary (Saltin, 1975).

The duration of the total program will obviously make a difference as to how much change one might expect from a specific training regimen. From Figure 2–9 in Chapter 2, it can be clearly seen that the duration of training will substantially influence the improvement in $\dot{V}O_2$ max. Assuming that each individual has an innate, finite limit, or ceiling, that can be reached, but not exceeded (Ekblom, 1971), it seems reasonable to postulate that the closer the individual comes to attaining that limit, the more difficult it will be to elicit change, i.e., the rate of improvement will not be as great. As an example of this limitation, to train a 13.0 sec/100-yd-dash sprinter to lower one's time to 11.5 sec may take only three to six months, but to take a 9.4 sec/100-yd-dash sprinter and lower one's time to 9.2 sec may require a lifetime, or it may never occur. For every type of training program, the time needed to reach the peak or level of best performance will vary, according to which of the particular fitness components are being trained. $\dot{V}O_2$ max (endurance) may reach the individual's highest maximum, or peak, within six months to a year. With the anaerobic threshold (speed and endurance), it may take several years to reach the ultimate value. For strength and power, it may take many years to achieve the individual's best efforts. Unfortunately, little research has been conducted in this area. The present views are based largely on observations of how long it takes successful athletes to reach their peak performance.

Just as the time that is required to reach the level of peak performance varies, the subject's initial level of fitness also appears to have a marked influence on one's potential for change. It has been postulated that the closer one is to his or her ultimate performance, the more difficult it is to make substantial improvements (Pollock, 1973). Unfortunately, even though this postulate is sound, it is difficult to prove, since everyone has a unique, genetically determined, upper limit that can be reached (Ekblom, 1971). To assess this value would be extremely difficult. Using endurance capacity for illustrative purposes, it is clear that an individual with a $\dot{V}O_2$ max of 30 ml/kg × min should have both a greater absolute and a greater relative improvement in $\dot{V}O_2$ max than an individual of the same age who has an initial $\dot{V}O_2$ max of 50 ml/kg × min, providing that the two individuals are given the same duration, frequency, and relative intensity of training. Training at 75 percent capacity, three days/week, 30 min/day, for twenty weeks may improve the first individual from 30 to 40 ml/kg × min (10 ml/kg × min or 33.3 percent improvement), while the latter individual may improve from 50 to

55 ml/kg × min (5 ml/kg × min or 10 percent improvement). However, a third individual trained in the same manner could increase $\dot{V}O_2$ max from an initial level of 50 to a final level of 65 (15 ml/kg × min, or 30 percent improvement). The individual who improved from 50 to 55 may have had an ultimate ceiling or capacity of 58 ml/kg × min, while the individual who improved from 50 to 65 may have had an ultimate ceiling of 85 ml/kg × min. Thus, individual differences make it extremely difficult to predict an individual's ultimate potential or even his or her basic potential for improvement. While these illustrations are limited to endurance capacity, similar principles apply to each of the other areas, e.g., strength, power, and speed.

BONE, CONNECTIVE TISSUE, AND NEUROMUSCULAR CHANGES WITH TRAINING

It appears that chronic exercise is necessary to maintain normal bone strength and function (Booth and Gould, 1975). Studies in which subjects are placed in bed for prolonged periods of time show a substantial loss of calcium and phosphorus from the bone. Lack of exercise or activity is associated with a bone structure that is deficient in mineral content, a condition that results in weak and brittle bones. It is not at all clear whether physical training will make bones any stronger or larger than bones that undergo only normal levels of activity, e.g., walking and lifting. Some evidence suggests that high levels of activity, particularly those that involve carrying or lifting heavy objects, may increase the breadth or width of bones with little or no effect on their length. Even during periods of bone growth, chronic exercise has not been found to facilitate long-bone growth or to increase height.

Chronic exercise does have a facilitative effect on cartilages, tendons, and ligaments (Booth and Gould, 1975). Cartilages appear to increase in thickness with additional exercise. This provides a better cushion, or shock absorber, for jarring types of activities, e.g., running or jumping, and results in a better, more functional joint through better articulation of the bones that form the joint. Ligaments and tendons become stronger and larger with chronic exercise, thus, providing a greater degree of protection to the joints. While stronger ligaments and tendons will not give absolute protection against injury, the incidence and severity of injury should be greatly reduced.

With chronic exercise, there are a number of adaptations that occur in the neuromuscular system (Clarke, 1973). First, the extent of these adaptations will depend on the type of training program that was followed. If training was of a cardiorespiratory endurance nature, e.g., jogging or swimming, then modest gains in strength will occur, but only in those muscle groups that were used. Likewise, a program of stretching to increase flexibility combined with light calisthenics will produce only small to moderate gains in muscular strength. Strength training programs, where increased strength is the primary goal, will produce substantial gains in strength, ranging from 25 to 100 percent improvement, or greater, within a period of three to six months (Wilmore, 1974). When one stops strength training, however, the strength that was gained is rapidly lost, thus basic maintenance programs must be established once the individual has achieved the desired goals for strength development. Maintenance programs are designed to provide sufficient stress to the muscles to maintain the existing levels of strength, which allow the individual to reduce the intensity and/or the duration of the program as well as the frequency. Preliminary research indicates that one or two exercise sessions per week is sufficient to maintain strength, but is probably not adequate to stimulate further increases in strength (Clarke, 1973). Strength training procedures and programs will be discussed in more detail in Chapter 4.

How does one become stronger? What physiological adaptations take place that allow the individual to exert greater levels of strength? For many years it was assumed that strength gains were directly the result of increases in muscle size. This increase in the size of the muscle with training is referred to as *hypertrophy*. This was a logical assumption since those men who trained regularly with free weights, or other strength training modes, developed large, bulky muscles. In addition, when a broken limb is placed in a cast and immobilized for weeks or months, it is only a matter of a few days before the muscles start to lose strength and decrease in size, a process referred to as *atrophy*. With gains in the size of a muscle paralleling its gains in strength as a result of training, and with losses in the size of a muscle correlating with its losses in strength when immobilized, it was only natural to conclude a cause-effect relationship, i.e., gains in strength are the result of increases in the size of the muscle. However, observations and recent research suggest that there is more involved in understanding the basic mechanisms of strength gains than a simple relationship with the size of the muscle.

First, there have been numerous stories in newspapers and magazines where individuals have performed superhuman feats of strength at times of great psychological stress. Women have reportedly lifted automobiles off their husbands or children who were suddenly trapped beneath the car when the car slipped off the jack or blocks. Straight jackets were designed to control patients in mental hospitals who would suddenly go berserk and were literally impossible to restrain. Even in the world of sport, there have been isolated examples of superhuman athletic performances, such as Bob Beamon's long jump of 29 feet 2½ inches at the 1968 Olympic Games held in Mexico City, a jump which exceeds the previous world record by nearly 2 feet! World records are usually broken by inches, or more often by fractions of inches. His performance was incredible, and is still over a foot better than anyone has been able to do since that time. An additional fact that has recently surfaced also casts doubt on the simplistic view that strength gains are solely the result of increases in the size of the muscle. Studies of women involved in highly structured and controlled strength training programs have found that women experience similar gains in strength when compared to men on the same program, but they do not experience the same degree of hypertrophy (Wilmore, 1974). In fact, several subjects in these studies doubled their levels of strength in the absence of any change in the size of the muscle. Thus, strength gains can occur in the absence of hypertrophy!

How, then, does one explain gains in strength? The preceding examples should not be taken to imply that muscle size is not an important factor in the ultimate strength potential of the muscle. All other things being equal, size is extremely important, as is illustrated by the world and Olympic records for competitive weightlifting. From the lightest to the heaviest weight classification, there is a progressive increase in the record for total

weight lifted. However, these examples indicate that the mechanisms associated with strength gains are very complex, and as of this time not very well understood. There is accumulating evidence to indicate that motor unit recruitment is an important area that may well be involved in explaining those gains in strength that occur in the absence of hypertrophy as well as those episodic superhuman feats of strength (Moritani and deVries, 1979). As was mentioned, motor units appear to be recruited asynchronously, i.e., they are not all called on to contract synchronously or simultaneously. There is evidence that motor units are controlled by a number of different neurons, or interneurons, that have the ability to produce both excitatory as well as inhibitory impulses.

The final decision as to whether a motor unit will fire and contribute to the contraction, or remain in the relaxed state, depends on the summation of these many impulses. If the inhibitory impulses equal or exceed the excitatory impulses, no contraction will occur. If the excitatory impulses exceed the inhibitory impulse, the unit will be activated and contribute to the contraction of that muscle. Gains in strength may well be the result of the ability to recruit additional motor units to act synchronously to facilitate the contraction, increasing the ability to generate force or to demonstrate strength. The improvement in recruitment patterns could be the result of a blocking of or reduction in the number of inhibitory impulses, thereby allowing more motor units to be activated simultaneously. This is an attractive theory since it allows for an explanation of superhuman feats of strength and for those instances where strength gains are obtained in the absence of hypertrophy. It is only a theory at this point, and must undergo the rigors of scientific testing before we can accept it as fact.

When hypertrophy does occur with strength training, what basic adaptations are taking place that lead to an increase in the size of the muscle? Since males experience a significantly greater increase in muscle size for the same strength training program and for the same relative increase in strength when compared to females (Wilmore, 1974), it is hypothesized that the male androgen, testosterone, is responsible, at least in part. In the first chapter, in the discussion of the endocrine system, one of the functions ascribed to testosterone was its promotion of muscle growth. Some women will experience considerable hypertrophy with strength gains, while others experience essentially no change in muscle girth. It is speculated that the testosterone/estrogen ratio is higher in the former group, thus resulting in an increase in muscle mass. Some male athletes in certain events have been using anabolic steroids, which have the muscle-building qualities of testosterone, in an effort to increase muscle size and strength. While this practice does appear to produce the desired results, it is not without its risks. First, the use of anabolic steroids for this purpose is illegal. Second, the medical risks associated with this practice are rather significant, including cancer, and possible kidney and liver disease (American College of Sports Medicine, 1977). Still, certain athletes foolishly continue this practice with little concern for ethics or their health. This will be discussed in more detail in Chapter 12, Ergogenic Aids.

While testosterone appears to be essential to the process of hypertrophy, what actual changes occur within the muscle? The size of the whole muscle increases, but how is this accomplished? First, there are two types of hypertrophy: transient and chronic. *Transient hypertrophy* is that "pumping-up" of the muscle that takes place during a single exercise bout. This is largely the result of fluid accumulation or edema in the muscle, which is probably caused by fluid being forced from the blood to the interstitial spaces in the muscle. Transient hypertrophy, as its name implies, lasts only for a short period of time, as the fluid will eventually return to the blood within a matter of hours. *Chronic hypertrophy* refers to that hypertrophy that results from strength training, although it should be recognized that even chronic hypertrophy will be lost if the individual does not continue to train that muscle. Chronic hypertrophy is the result of structural changes in the muscle, and can be explained either as an increase in the number of muscle cells or fibers (hyperplasia), or an increase in the size of existing fibers. For many years, research tended to demonstrate that the number of muscle fibers is established at birth or shortly thereafter, and that this number remains fixed throughout life. If this is true, then chronic hypertrophy would be the result of muscle fiber hypertrophy, which could be explained by an increase in the number of myofibrils and/or filaments, sarco-

plasm, or in the connective tissue. An increase in myofibrils and filaments has been demonstrated in many research studies, and this would provide more cross bridges to produce force during a maximal contraction.

Recent research has pointed to the possibility that hyperplasia may be a factor in total muscle hypertrophy. Studies on cats have provided fairly clear evidence that with extremely heavy weight training, there is actually a splitting of fibers that takes place (Gonyea, 1980). Cats are trained to use their forepaw to move a heavy weight a fixed distance in order to get their food. These cats learn to generate considerable amounts of force. With this intense strength training, selected muscle fibers appear to actually split in half, with each half then increasing in size to that of the parent fiber. The possible role of fiber splitting in human muscle in response to strength training is at this time unknown. It would appear that individual fiber hypertrophy accounts for most, if not all, of the hypertrophy seen in the whole muscle.

The ability to change one muscle fiber type to another with physical conditioning is a topic of current interest. Based on the simple classification system of slow-twitch and fast-twitch fibers (see Chapter 1), it appears that neither heavy strength and power (anaerobic) training, nor endurance (aerobic) training, will alter the basic fiber types (Costill, 1979). As an example, an individual who possesses 75 percent slow-twitch fibers and 25 percent fast-twitch fibers will have these same proportions even after intensive anaerobic training, which, theoretically, would promote an increase in fast-twitch fibers, if fibers could change characteristics. The fibers will, however, begin to take on certain characteristics of the opposite fiber type if the training is of the opposite kind, though actual conversion from one fiber type to the other appears to be impossible. This has led researchers to postulate that if fiber types are established genetically, it might be possible to perform muscle biopsies on young children to determine their relative fiber types. In this way, children could be placed in activities in which the muscular demands were matched to their relative fiber types. While this idea is intriguing from the scientific viewpoint, it is not practical and would tend to destroy the fun and enjoyment of sport.

CARDIOVASCULAR CHANGES
WITH TRAINING

Training causes a number of changes that improve the transportation function of the cardiovascular system during exercise. These changes, which occur following endurance conditioning programs, will be discussed under several major categories.

Heart Rate

The heart rate at rest will decrease markedly as a result of endurance conditioning (Clausen, 1977). For a sedentary adult with an initial resting heart rate of 80 beats/min, the resting heart rate will decrease by approximately 1 beat/min for each week of training during the first few weeks. Following ten weeks of modest endurance training, the resting rate should drop to 70 beats/min. Highly conditioned endurance athletes typically have resting heart rates of 40 beats/min or lower, and occasionally have values lower than 30 beats/minute.

During exercise, the heart rate will be less for the same level of work as the individual becomes more highly conditioned. Figure 3–1 illustrates changes in heart rates for a constant level of work in five men who underwent twenty days of deconditioning (total bedrest) followed by sixty days of retraining. The submaximal heart rate for that constant level of work provides an excellent insight into the functional status of the cardiovascular system for each of these five subjects, who were studied longitudinally. Unfortunately, the heart rate from a single submaximal test on any one individual provides relatively little insight into the status of the cardiovascular system of that individual in comparison with others, since people of identical cardiovascular fitness will respond with substantially different heart rates to the same level of work. Comparing the individual with himself at varying points in time, however, provides valuable information about any changes that might be taking place within that individual as a result of changes in activity patterns. It is not unusual to observe a 20 to 40 beat/min decrease in submaximal heart rate at a standardized work load following a six-month training program of moderate intensity (Clausen, 1977). Since the work performed by the heart has a high correlation with the resting and exercise heart rates, the reduced submaximal heart rate indicates

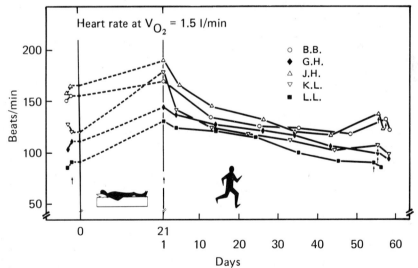

Figure 3–1   Response of submaximal heart rate to a constant level of work, following a period of bed rest and a subsequent period of retraining. (From B. Saltin et al., *Response to Exercise after Bed Rest and after Training,* American Heart Association Monograph, No. 23 (1968): 20. Reproduced by permission of the American Heart Association, Inc.)

that the heart is working more efficiently, i.e., doing less work.

At maximal levels of exercise, the maximal heart rate will remain approximately the same following endurance training (Pollock, 1973). Several studies have suggested that there is a slight reduction in HRmax in those individuals who have HRmax values in excess of 180 beats/min. There is also a tendency for highly conditioned endurance athletes to have HRmax values lower than untrained individuals of the same age.

The heart rate recovers from exercise at a much faster rate following endurance conditioning (Åstrand and Rodahl, 1977). This is true following exercise such as standardized, submaximal work bouts as well as maximal bouts of work. Under both submaximal and maximal conditions, there is a faster return of the heart rate to the pre-exercise level. The faster heart rate recovery following endurance training has led to the use of the pulse rate recovery as an index of cardiovascular fitness, i.e., the more fit individual will recover faster from a standardized level of work. As was mentioned in the case of the submaximal heart rate during standardized bouts of exercise, the heart rate recovery curve is an excellent way to quantify changes in cardiovascular conditioning of an individual at varying points in time, but it is not a very accurate means of comparing one individual with another. Too many factors other than cardiovascular fitness are involved when absolute heart rate recovery values are compared among different people.

Stroke Volume, Cardiac Output, and Heart Volume

Changes in stroke volume are closely related to the changes in heart rate that result from training. At rest, the stroke volume is substantially higher following an endurance training program. Similarly, stroke volume is higher at submaximal, standardized levels of work and also at maximal levels of work (Clausen, 1977). This increase is probably due to a more complete filling of the heart during the period of diastole, which results in a greater ventricular blood volume. In addition, the walls of the left ventricle tend to hypertrophy, which indicates a greater ventricular muscle mass, and the power of contraction (contractility) is increased, i.e., the ventricle contracts more forcefully, reducing the volume of the residual blood that remains following the contraction. Thus, a stronger heart and the availability of a greater blood volume appear to account for these increases in resting, submaximal, and maximal stroke volumes. In turn, it appears that the increased stroke volume allows the heart to beat at a slower rate, both at rest and during submaximal levels of exercise. It is also possible that the increased stroke volume is the result of the decreased heart rate, rather than the reduced heart rate being the result of an increased stroke volume. Resting stroke volumes can range from 70 ml for the untrained to 90 ml for the trained and up to 130 ml for the highly trained, endurance athlete. Likewise, maximal stroke volumes will vary from 125 ml to 150 ml and up to 220 ml for individuals in the same three classifications of training status.

Cardiac output is not greatly changed either at rest or for standardized levels of submaximal work following training (Clausen, 1977). For the same metabolic workload, e.g., 1.5 liters of oxygen/min, there may even be a slight decrease in the cardiac output, due to a more efficient extraction of oxygen, i.e., larger $a-\bar{v}O_2$ diff, or to better mechanical or metabolic efficiency. At maximal levels of work, however, the cardiac output is increased considerably. This is the result of an improved maximal stroke volume, since HRmax changes very little, if at all. Maximal cardiac output ranges from 14–16 liters/min in sendentary to 20–25 liters for trained and up to values in excess of 40 liters/min in highly conditioned, large, endurance athletes.

The weight of the heart and the heart volume are both increased as a result of training. Figure 3–2 illustrates the changes in heart volume with inactivity (bedrest) and with activity (retraining). Cardiac muscle, like skeletal muscle, appears to undergo hypertrophy as a result of chronic endurance training. Once there was great concern over the possible pathological consequences of cardiac hypertrophy induced by exercise, or "athlete's heart," as it was called. It is now recognized that this is a normal adaptation to chronic endurance training (Longhurst et al., 1980). The left ventricle, which does most of the work, is the chamber most affected.

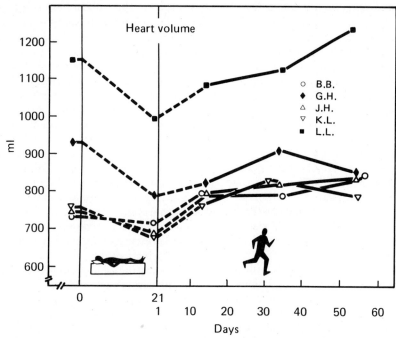

Figure 3-2 Changes in heart volume, following bed rest and a subsequent retraining program. (From B. Saltin et al., *Response to Exercise after Bed Rest and after Training,* American Heart Association Monograph, No. 23 (1968): 16. Reproduced by permission of the American Heart Association, Inc.)

Blood Flow, Blood Pressure, and Peripheral Vasculature

Blood flow through the muscles appears to be enhanced by endurance training (Clausen, 1977). This could be due to an increased number of capillaries in the muscle. Recent evidence suggests that there is an increase in the number of capillaries with training (Andersen and Henriksson, 1977). Also, the muscle fibers tend to increase in size during training, and the muscle fibers and capillaries are closer together, which results in a more favorable capillary-to-fiber ratio. It is also possible that the increased blood flow is the result of the existing capillaries in the muscle opening up wider to provide better perfusion of the muscle. Since endurance training also increases the blood volume, this latter adaptation can occur without severely compromising the venous return (Oscai et al., 1968).

Arterial blood pressure is altered very little dur-ing standardized, submaximal levels of work as a result of chronic exercise. Likewise, maximal systolic and diastolic blood pressure are not substantially altered with training. Resting blood pressure, however, is reduced with training in those individuals who are hypertensive or who have abnormally high resting blood pressures prior to training (Pollock, 1973). Resting blood pressure appears to remain stable in those who are considered normal prior to training. Unfortunately, few studies have actually measured blood pressure directly before and after training. Most studies have used indirect measurement techniques which are difficult to interpret during exercise.

Blood Volume and Composition

Blood volume increases with endurance training. This is accomplished through an increase in both plasma volume and in red blood cell volume (Åstrand and Rodahl, 1977; Oscai et al., 1968). However, the increase in plasma volume is so much greater than that of the red blood cell volume that the hematocrit (ratio of cell volume to total blood volume) actually decreases. It can decrease to the point where the trained athlete appears to be anemic on the basis of the relative concentration of red cells and hemoglobin. In fact, the total amount of hemoglobin and the total number of red blood cells (their absolute values) are typically above normal in the trained athlete, even though the relative values are below normal (Brotherhood et al., 1975). This condition leads to a reduction in the viscosity of the blood, which facilitates its movement through the blood vessels. Recent research has pointed to the importance of a low blood viscosity for enhancing the delivery of oxygen to the active muscles (Horstman et al., 1980).

The oxygen content of the arterial blood changes very little with training. Even though total hemoglobin is increased in absolute terms, the amount of hemoglobin per unit of blood is the same, or even slightly reduced (Åstrand and Rodahl, 1977). The $a-\bar{v}O_2$ diff is changed, however, with training. This may, or may not be evident at rest or during submaximal levels of exercise, but the $a-\bar{v}O_2$ diff is widened or increased at maximal exercise, although the change is not of a very great magnitude. Since the arterial blood oxygen concentration is unaltered, this increase in $a-\bar{v}O_2$ diff implies a greater extraction of the available oxygen, which results in a lower oxygen content of the mixed venous blood.

Blood lactate levels are lower for each level of submaximal exercise following training, but they increase to higher levels at the point of exhaustion (Åstrand and Rodahl, 1977). This suggests a greater tolerance to the pain associated with anaerobic metabolism. Recent studies indicate that anaerobic threshold can be increased consequent to endurance training, which is undoubtedly related to the reduced levels of blood lactate for standardized levels of submaximal exercise (Skinner and McLellen, 1980).

RESPIRATORY ADAPTATIONS TO TRAINING

The static lung volumes change very little with training (Åstrand and Rodahl, 1977). There is a tendency for vital capacity to increase slightly and for residual volume to decrease by approximately the same amount. Thus, the total lung capacity remains unchanged.

Pulmonary ventilation is unchanged at rest, but is slightly reduced at standardized submaximal levels of work, indicating a greater efficiency of the respiratory system (Åstrand and Rodahl, 1977). Maximum pulmonary ventilation is increased substantially with training, typically increasing from 100 to 125 liters/min. Large, endurance athletes can exceed 240 liters/min. Tidal volume is unchanged at rest and during submaximal exercise, but appears to increase at maximal levels of exercise. Respiratory rate is usually lowered at rest and during submaximal exercise, although the change is small. During maximal work, this rate is substantially increased.

Pulmonary blood flow appears to be increased following training, particularly the flow to the upper regions of the lung when the individual is sitting or standing (Carlsten and Grimby, 1966). This results in increased perfusion of the lung. Lung diffusion is unaltered at rest and during submaximal exercise, but is increased during maximal exercise. This increase is probably due to both the enhanced perfusion and ventilation of the lung, which provides a larger and more efficient area for gas exchange.

METABOLIC ADAPTATIONS TO TRAINING

Oxygen consumption at rest is either slightly decreased or unaltered following endurance training. At submaximal levels of exercise, $\dot{V}O_2$ is either unchanged or slightly reduced. A decrease in $\dot{V}O_2$, either at rest or during submaximal exercise or at both times, would suggest an increase in metabolic efficiency or in mechanical efficiency. While this might be a postulated change, conclusions from studies are divided as to whether this change does, in fact, occur. It is possible that researchers in those studies that demonstrated a reduced $\dot{V}O_2$ for the same level of submaximal work following training may have observed a practice effect on their testing devices. If not allowed prior practice on the bicycle ergometer, treadmill, or other appropriate testing device, the subject may perform at a lower energy cost ($\dot{V}O_2$) the second time he or she performs on the same device simply because of being more relaxed, accustomed to performing on the device, and knowing what is expected. Thus, the observed change may not be due to training.

$\dot{V}O_2$ max is increased substantially with endurance training. Increases from 4–93 percent have been reported in the literature (Pollock, 1973). An increase of 16–20 percent is more typical for the average individual who was sedentary prior to training and trained at 75 percent of one's capacity, 3 times/week, 30 min/day, for six months (Pollock, 1973). The $\dot{V}O_2$ max of a sedentary individual might increase from an initial value of 35 ml/kg × min to 42 ml/kg × min as a result of such a program. This is far below the values for world-class, endurance athletes, whose values generally range from 75–94 ml/kg × min.

The factors responsible for this change have been identified, but there presently is extensive controversy as to their relative importance. On the one hand, logical arguments have been raised and supported with documented research that suggest that a substantial portion of the increased $\dot{V}O_2$ max is the result of increases in the size and number of mitochondria, as well as an increase in the quantity of enzymes available in the mitochondria. On the other hand, it has been traditionally stated, with good supporting evidence, that the predominant factor in the $\dot{V}O_2$ max increase is the delivery of more oxygen to the active tissue through an increase in both maximal cardiac output and in local perfusion. The latter theory states that it is an inadequate oxygen supply or delivery that limits maximal performance; the former contends that, for the most part, the oxygen supply is adequate, but that the number, size, and content of the mitochondria are insufficient to utilize the available oxygen. Saltin and Rowell (1980) have stated in a recent review article that increases in $\dot{V}O_2$ max are attributable primarily to increased maximal muscle blood flow and increased muscle capillary density, while augmentations in the capacity for submaximal work are the result of increased oxidative potential in the muscle.

As was mentioned earlier in this chapter, and also in Chapter 2, Responses to Acute Exercise, the $\dot{V}O_2$ max will reach its peak value within six months to two years following the start of an endurance training program, even though the intensity of the training program and the individual workouts continue to increase. Yet, the individual will still note improvements in endurance performance after the $\dot{V}O_2$ max has leveled off and can no longer increase. Few people are able to run at a level of work that requires their $\dot{V}O_2$ max for more than a minute or two; thus, those who run for distances that require more time than this are competing at a level that is less than or below their $\dot{V}O_2$ max. Marathon runners typically run for periods of time in excess of two hours and are able to maintain their pace at approximately 75–80 percent of their $\dot{V}O_2$ max. It is theorized that once the peak $\dot{V}O_2$ max is attained, further performance improvements are made by being able to compete at a higher percentage of the $\dot{V}O_2$ max. Some athletes are able to work for prolonged periods of time at levels approaching 90 percent of $\dot{V}O_2$ max.

As an example, a young runner who starts training with an initial $\dot{V}O_2$ max of 52.0 ml/kg × min reaches one's genetically determined peak $\dot{V}O_2$ max of 71 ml/kg × min two years later and is unable to increase it to a higher level, even with more intensive workouts. At this point, the young runner is able to run at 75 percent of the $\dot{V}O_2$ max (0.75 × 71.0 = 53.3 ml/kg ×min) in a six-mile race. Following an additional two years of intensive training, the $\dot{V}O_2$ max is exactly the same, but the person is now able to compete at 88 percent of capacity (0.88 × 71.0 = 62.5 ml/kg × min). Obviously, by being able to sustain an oxygen consumption of 62.5 ml/kg × min, the runner will be able to run at a much faster pace than when he or she was able to sustain only 53.3 ml/kg × min. The mechanisms of this increased fractional utilization of the $\dot{V}O_2$ max cannot be explained at the present time, but they undoubtedly concern increased metabolic efficiency and are possibly related to shifts in the blood lactate and anaerobic threshold responses (Skinner and McLellen, 1980). It is also known that oxygen-debt capacity increases with training, a change that could also be associated with this phenomenon.

BODY COMPOSITION ADAPTATIONS WITH TRAINING

For purposes of simplicity and the convenience of discussion, the total body weight will be divided into two components: the lean body weight and the fat weight. When working with body composition data, the following relationships are important.

total body weight =
           lean body weight + fat weight
relative lean weight (percent) =
           (lean body weight/total body weight) × 100
relative fat weight (percent) =
           (fat weight/total body weight) × 100

Lean body weight refers to that part of the total body weight that remains after all of the body fat is removed. It is composed of muscle, skin, bone, organs, and all other nonfat tissue. It can be assessed in a number of ways, but the most common is through densitometry, using the underwater weighing technique (Behnke and Wilmore, 1974). The individual is weighed while totally submerged under water (Figure 3–3). The weight is measured when the individual has blown all the air out of the lungs and only the residual volume remains. The residual volume is also assessed and is used to correct the underwater weight. In this way, the increased buoyancy afforded by the trapped residual volume is also taken into account.

Several thousand years ago, Archimedes determined that a body immersed in a fluid experiences a loss in weight equal to the weight of the displaced fluid. In water, the weight of the displaced fluid can easily be converted to the volume of water that has been displaced; thus, the loss of weight in water is directly proportional to the volume of the water that is displaced or to the volume of the body that displaces that water (Behnke and Wilmore, 1974). Since density is equal to the ratio of mass to volume, or

$$D_{body} = \frac{mass\ or\ weight_{body}}{volume_{body}},$$

it is relatively simple to calculate the density of an individual's body. The density of fat is known, and the density of the lean tissue of the body has been calculated to be a relatively stable constant. By knowing the density of the body, the fat, and the lean tissue, it is a simple calculation to determine the relative fat weight and relative lean weight of the body.

As an example, two athletes are exactly the same age, height, and weight, and are competing for the position of middle linebacker on the university football team. Prior to the start of training camp,

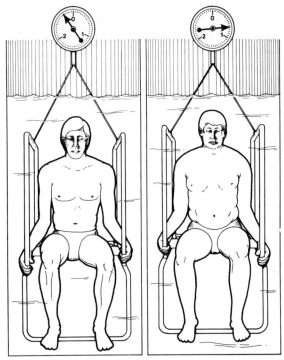

Figure 3–3   Underwater weighing technique for determining body density, allowing an estimate of lean and fat weight. Notice that the leaner individual on the left weighs more than the fatter individual on the right even though their scale weights are the same.

these two athletes undergo a series of tests, including the underwater weighing technique for determining body composition. The results of the body composition analysis are shown on the top of the next page. From this analysis, it is obvious that Ken is right at his desired weight while Dave is 19.1 pounds over his desired playing weight. The analysis would also indicate that Dave may be too light at his desired playing weight to play the middle linebacker position. He would have to emphasize an intensive weight training program to increase his lean weight.

With this in mind, the average college-age male and female will be approximately 15 and 25 percent fat, respectively (Behnke and Wilmore, 1974). With increased age and sedentary living, the relative percentages of fat increase. The endurance athlete

	Ken		Dave	
Height	74.0 in	188.0 cm	74.0 in	188.0 cm
Weight	205 lb	93.0 kg	205 lb	93.0 kg
Underwater weight		6.5 kg		5.0 kg
Volume (weight-underwater weight)		86.5 kg		88.0 kg
Density (mass or weight/volume)		1.075 gm/ml		1.057 gm/ml
Relative fat		10.5 %		18.4 %
Fat weight	21.4 lb	9.7 kg	37.7 lb	17.1 kg
Lean weight	183.6 lb	83.3 kg	167.3 lb	75.9 kg
Weight at 10% fat	204.2 lb	92.6 kg	185.9 lb	84.3 kg
Weight loss to achieve 10% fat	0.8 lb	0.4 kg	19.1 lb	8.7 kg

will have considerably lower values for relative body fat, while the large, football lineman or the shot putter usually will have values greater than the average for their ages.

With training, there are marked alterations in body composition. Strength training through weights or progressive resistance exercises decreases body fat and increases lean body weight, the latter due to increases in muscle mass (Wilmore, 1974). With endurance training, similar changes can occur (Pollock, 1973). If a 175-lb man were to jog 3½ miles in thirty minutes, he would expend approximately 500 Kcalories/session. If this routine were carried out an average of 3½ days/week, the weekly caloric expenditure would be 1,750 Kcalories, which is approximately equivalent to losing one-half pound of body fat/week. Studies have confirmed the fact that endurance programs reduce stores of body fat and increase the lean body weight, presumably due to hypertrophy of the active muscle mass. In a six-month training program of previously sedentary adult men, it is typical to observe a decrease of 6–8 pounds of fat and an increase of 2–3 pounds of lean weight when they jog an average of 3 miles in 24 minutes for 2½ days/week (Behnke and Wilmore, 1974; Pollock, 1973).

SPECIFICITY OF PHYSICAL TRAINING

Research into the value of various training programs and techniques has gradually led to the realization that training, to be most efficient, must be specific to the sport. The long-distance runner must run to maximize the conditioning process for this sport. Two hours of hard swim training each day will do little to improve running ability. Likewise, the golfer will gain little, if any, help for his or her golf game by shooting free throws on the basketball court. While these are obvious examples, there is a point at which both the coach and researcher are uncertain as to how valuable certain related activities are for various sports. For example, can the baseball player improve skills through strength training? Another question of considerable importance that relates to strength training is how valuable is strength training at slow speeds for activities that require a quick application of strength? Does bench pressing 350 pounds by a football lineman in a very slow and labored movement improve the explosive power needed in a game situation, where he has to apply his strength in a fast movement to catch his opponent off balance?

Unfortunately, research into the various aspects of specificity of training is limited, but what has been done underlines the need for further research. Clarke (1973), in his extensive review of the literature on adaptive changes in strength and muscular endurance with training, cites several examples where specificity of training was a major factor in interpreting the results of studies on various aspects of strength and endurance training. As one example, when comparing isometric and isotonic strength training, those subjects who train isometrically typically show the greatest improvement when they are tested isometrically, while the isotonic group shows the greatest improvement

Table 3–1 *Hypothetical Physiological and Body Composition Changes in a Sedentary, Normal Individual Resulting from an Endurance Training Program*, Compared to the Values of a World-Class Endurance Runner of the Same Age*

Variables	Sedentary Normal Pre-Training	Sedentary Normal Post-Training	World-Class Endurance Runner
Cardiovascular			
HR_{rest}, beats/min	71	59	36
HR_{max}, beats/min	185	183	174
SV_{rest}, ml**	65	80	125
SV_{max}, ml**	120	140	200
$\dot{Q}_{rest}$, liters/min	4.6	4.7	4.5
$\dot{Q}_{max}$, liters/min	22.2	25.6	34.8
Heart volume, ml	750	820	1,200
Blood volume, liters	4.7	5.1	6.0
Systolic BP_{rest}, mmHg	135	130	120
Systolic BP_{max}, mmHg	210	205	210
Diastolic BP_{rest}, mmHg	78	76	65
Diastolic BP_{max}, mmHg	82	80	65
Respiratory			
$\dot{V}_E$ rest, liters/min (BTPS)	7	6	6
$\dot{V}_E$ max, liters/min (BTPS)	110	135	195
f_{rest}, breaths/min	14	12	12
f_{max}, breaths/min	40	45	55
TV_{rest}, liters	0.5	0.5	0.5
TV_{max}, liters	2.75	3.0	3.5
VC, liters	5.8	6.0	6.2
RV, liters	1.4	1.2	1.2
Metabolic			
$a-\bar{v}O_2$ $diff_{rest}$, ml/100 ml	6.0	6.0	6.0
$a-\bar{v}O_2$ $diff_{max}$, ml/100 ml	14.5	15.0	16.0
$\dot{V}O_2$ rest, ml/kg × min	3.5	3.7	4.0
$\dot{V}O_2$ max, ml/kg × min	40.5	49.8	76.7
Blood $lactate_{rest}$, mg/100 ml	10	10	10
Blood $lactate_{max}$, mg/100 ml	110	125	185
Body Composition			
Weight, lbs	175	170	150
Fat weight, lbs	28	21.3	11.3
Lean weight, lbs	147	148.7	138.7
Relative fat, %	16.0	12.5	7.5

*Six-month training program, jogging three to four times/week, thirty min/day, at 75 percent of VO_2 max.

**Upright position.

(From J. H. Wilmore and A. C. Norton, The Heart and Lungs at Work. Schiller Park, Ill.: Beckman Instruments, 1974. Reproduced by permission of the publisher.)

when tested isotonically. Additionally, isometric training appears to be specific to the joint angle at which training occurs. If the subject trains at 90 degrees in the arm curl, the strength gained will be isolated to within a few degrees of that joint angle, and there will be little strength gain in the same movement at joint angles less than 60 degrees and greater than 120 degrees. Other studies have shown low or poor correlations between limb strength and the speed of movement or the muscular endurance of the limb.

Specificity of training has also been demonstrated in the area of cardiovascular endurance training. In one study, both an experimental and a control group were given maximal tests on a treadmill and also in a swimming pool, prior to participation by the experimental group in a swim-training program (Magel et al., 1975). On repeat testing at the conclusion of the twelve-week training program, the experimental group had a significantly higher swimming $\dot{V}O_2$ max compared with their pre-training values and with the post-training values for the control group. No improvement was found, however, in the treadmill $\dot{V}O_2$ max, which demonstrates the highly specific nature of the training program.

Another study (Holmér and Åstrand, 1972) illustrates the principle of specificity in an entirely different manner. A pair of identical twins were given a series of maximal tests under varying conditions: treadmill, swimming, arm work in the water, arm cycle work, etc. While both girls had been outstanding swimmers, one had stopped competitive swim training three years prior to this study. She had remained active in intramural-type sports while her sister continued with her competitive-level swim training. The peak $\dot{V}O_2$ max values attained in the maximal swim-type tests were considerably higher for the swim-trained sister, while the values on the treadmill were identical for the two girls. For the two cycling tasks (arm cycling and arm plus leg cycling), the differences between the sisters were only moderate, favoring the swim-trained sister.

Studies have demonstrated that specificity of training also exists at the histochemical and biochemical levels. Endurance training programs develop the slow-twitch muscle fibers and those enzymes associated with aerobic metabolism. Likewise, anaerobic training develops the fast-twitch muscle fibers and those enzymes associated with anaerobic metabolism (Costill, 1979).

From these studies, it is apparent that the body adapts to the specific type of stress under which it trains, and the adaptation is specific to the training activity. Thus, to maximize the training effect, one must train specifically for that sport or activity. Undoubtedly, there are certain general factors that contribute to success in a given sport or activity, but these appear to be secondary in importance to the theory of specificity.

GENERAL SUMMARY

Physical conditioning or training results in a number of changes within the body, all of which will depend to a great extent on the purpose of the training program. Weight training produces increases in muscular strength and endurance, but has relatively little influence on the respiratory and cardiovascular systems. Likewise, endurance exercise produces great changes in the cardiovascular and respiratory systems, but has relatively little effect on muscle strength. Training changes are specific to the activity being pursued and are also dependent on the frequency, duration, and intensity of participation.

Table 3–1 lists typical values before and after an endurance training program for a number of physiological and body composition parameters. In addition, the values for a world-class runner are listed for comparative purposes. This will illustrate the tremendous adaptability of humans, as well as demonstrate the great genetic differences between normally trained and highly trained and skilled athletes. It appears that athletes are born, and that training can take an individual only to the limit of one's genetic potential.

STUDY QUESTIONS

1. What factors influence the chronic physiological responses to exercise, and which of these is most important?
2. How is one's initial level of fitness, and one's genetic limit, likely to influence the magnitude of the response to training?
3. How are bone, ligaments, cartilage, and tendons altered with chronic endurance exercise?
4. What is the difference between hyperplasia and hypertrophy?

5. What is the relationship of gains in strength to hypertrophy?
6. Describe possible neural components to gains in strength.
7. What is the difference between transient and chronic hypertrophy?
8. What changes in fiber type result from chronic endurance training?
9. How do heart rate, stroke volume, and cardiac output change with endurance training? Describe these changes both at rest and during exercise.
10. What changes are observed in blood volume with chronic endurance training?
11. How does $\dot{V}O_2$ max respond to endurance training, and what factors are responsible for changes in $\dot{V}O_2$ max?
12. Define: lean weight, fat weight, and relative body fat.
13. How does one's body composition change with endurance conditioning?
14. What is meant by "specificity of training"? Is there such a thing as specificity of training? If so, cite examples.

REFERENCES

American College of Sports Medicine Position Statement. "The Use and Abuse of Anabolic-Androgenic Steroids in Sports." *Med. Sci. Sports.* 9 (1977): xi–xiii.

Andersen, P., and Henriksson, J. "Capillary Supply of the Quadriceps Femoris Muscle of Man: Adaptive Response to Exercise." *J. Physiol.* 270 (1977): 677–690.

Åstrand, P.-O., and Rodahl, K. *Textbook of Work Physiology.* 2nd ed. New York: McGraw-Hill Book Co., 1977.

Behnke, A. R., and Wilmore, J. H. *Evaluation and Regulation of Body Build and Composition.* Englewood Cliffs, N.J.: Prentice-Hall, Inc., 1974.

Booth, F. W., and Gould, E. W. "Effects of Training and Disuse on Connective Tissue." In *Exercise and Sport Sciences Reviews*, vol. 3, edited by J. H. Wilmore. New York: Academic Press, 1975.

Brotherhood, J.; Brozovic, B.; and Pugh, L. G. "Hematological Status of Middle- and Long-Distance Runners." *Clin. Sci. Mol. Med.* 48 (1975): 139–145.

Carlsten, A., and Grimby, G. *The Circulatory Response to Muscular Exercise in Man.* Springfield, Ill.: Charles C. Thomas, 1966.

Clarke, D. H. *Exercise Physiology.* Englewood Cliffs, N.J.: Prentice-Hall, Inc. 1975.

Clarke, D. L. "Adaptations in Strength and Muscular Endurance Resulting from Exercise." In *Exercise and Sport Sciences Reviews*, vol. 1, edited by J. H. Wilmore. New York: Academic Press, 1973.

Clausen, J. P. "Effect of Training on Cardiovascular Adjustments to Exercise in Man. *Physiol. Rev.* 57 (1977): 779–815.

Costill, D. L. *A Scientific Approach to Distance Running.* Los Altos, Calif.: Track and Field News, 1979.

de Vries, H. A. *Physiology of Exercise for Physical Education and Athletics.* 2nd ed. Dubuque, Iowa: William C. Brown Co., 1974.

Edington, D. W., and Edgerton, V. R. *The Biology of Physical Activity.* Boston: Houghton Mifflin Co., 1976.

Ekblom, B. "Physical Training in Normal Boys in Adolescence." *Acta Paediat. Scand.* Suppl. 217 (1971): 60–62.

Falls, H. B., ed. *Exercise Physiology.* New York: Academic Press, 1968.

Fox, E. L. *Sports Physiology.* Philadelphia: W. B. Saunders Co., 1979.

Gonyea, W. J. "Role of Exercise in Inducing Increases in Skeletal Muscle Fiber Number." *J. Appl. Physiol.: Respirat. Environ. Exercise Physiol.* 48 (1980): 421–426.

Holmér, I., and Åstrand, P.-O. "Swimming Training and Maximal Oxygen Uptake." *J. Appl. Physiol.* 33 (1972): 510–513.

Horstman, D.; Weiskopf, R.; and Jackson, R. E. "Work Capacity during 3-wk Sojourn at 4,300 m: Effects of Relative Polycythemia." *J. Appl. Physiol.: Respirat. Environ. Exercise Physiol.* 49 (1980): 311–318.

Johnson, W. R. and Buskirk, E. R., eds. *Science and Medicine of Exercise and Sport.* 2nd ed. New York: Harper and Row, 1974.

Karpovich, P. V., and Sinning, W. E. *Physiology of Muscular Activity.* 7th ed. Philadelphia: W. B. Saunders Co., 1971.

Knuttgen, H. G., ed. *Neuromuscular Mechanisms for Therapeutic and Conditioning Exercise.* Baltimore: University Park Press, 1976.

Lamb, D. R. *Physiology of Exercise: Responses and Adaptations.* New York: Macmillan Publishing Co., 1978.

Larson, L. A., ed. *Fitness, Health, and Work Capacity.* New York: Macmillan Publishing Co., 1974.

Longhurst, J. C.; Kelly, A. R.; Gonyea, W. J.; and Mitchell, J. H. "Echocardiographic Left Ventricular Masses in Distance Runners and Weight Lifters." *J. Appl. Physiol.: Respirat. Environ. Exercise Physiol.* 48 (1980): 154–162.

Magel, J. R.; Foglia, G. F.; McArdle, W. D.; Gutin, B.; Pechar, G. S.; and Katch, F. I. "Specificity of Swim Training on Maximum Oxygen Uptake." *J. Appl. Physiol.* 38 (1975): 151–155.

Mathews, D. K., and Fox, E. L. *The Physiological Basis of Physical Education and Athletics.* Philadelphia: W. B. Saunders Co., 1976.

Morehouse, L. E., and Miller, A. T. *Physiology of Exercise.* 6th ed. St. Louis: C. V. Mosby Co., 1971.

Moritani, T., and de Vries, H. A. "Neural Factors versus Hypertrophy in the Time Course of Muscular Strength Gains." *Am. J. Physical Med.* 58 (1979): 115–130.

Oscai, L. B.; Williams, B. T.; and Hertig, B. A. "Effect of Exercise on Blood Volume." *J. Appl. Physiol.* 24 (1968): 622–624.

Pollock, M. L. "Quantification of Endurance Training Programs." In *Exercise and Sport Sciences Reviews*, vol. 1, edited by J. H. Wilmore. New York: Academic Press, 1973.

Saltin, B. *Intermittent Exercise: Its Physiology and Practical Applications*. Muncie, Ind.: Ball State University, 1975.

Saltin, B., and Rowell, L. B. "Functional Adaptations to Physical Activity and Inactivity." *Fed. Proc.* 39 (1980): 1506–1513.

Sharkey, B. J. *Physiology of Fitness*. Champaign, Ill.: Human Kinetics Publishers, 1979.

Shepherd, R. J. *Endurance Fitness*. Toronto: University of Toronto Press, 1969.

Shepherd, R. J. *Men at Work*. Springfield, Ill.: Charles C. Thomas, 1974.

Simonson, E., ed. *Physiology of Work Capacity and Fatigue*. Springfield, Ill.: Charles C. Thomas, 1971.

Skinner, J. S., and McLellen, T. H. "The Transition from Aerobic to Anaerobic Metabolism." *Res. Quart. Exercise Sport.* 51 (1980): 234–248.

Strauss, R. H., ed. *Sports Medicine and Physiology*. Philadelphia: W. B. Saunders Co., 1979.

Wilmore, J. H. "Alterations in Strength, Body Composition and Anthropometric Measurements Consequent to a 10-Week Weight Training Program." *Med. Sci. Sports* 6 (1974): 133–138.

Wilmore, J. H., and Norton, A. C. *The Heart and Lung at Work*. Schiller Park, Ill.: Beckman Instruments, 1974.

SECTION B

Fundamentals of Physical Training

The skilled performance of an athlete is the final result of many long hours of physical training. This final result does not happen by chance, but requires an intense dedication on the part of the athlete and exceptional insight by both the coach and athlete as to what the best training program may be for the athlete in that particular sport or event. Just as each sport is different and requires its own unique training program, each athlete is also unique and requires an individualized training program to maximize his or her potential. To individualize training programs requires a basic knowledge of those components that constitute the foundation of physical training. This section is devoted to a discussion of each of these individual components. Each component will be defined, an explanation will be given as to how it is measured or assessed, and finally, there will be a discussion of the importance of that component for various sports. The last chapter in this section will focus on the problems of deconditioning and the importance of off-season conditioning programs.

This section is intended to apply to all sports and activities. Unfortunately, however, much of the research has been conducted on a limited number of sports. As a result, the individual chapters may appear to be biased toward one or two specific sports or activities. Hopefully, the basic principles will be presented in such a way that readers will be able to apply them to their own sports. In addition, while the term athlete is used throughout this section, the information is equally applicable to the nonathlete or noncompetitive individual who pursues exercise for health-related purposes.

4

Strength, Power, and Muscular Endurance

INTRODUCTION

As the shot putter crouches low at the back of the circle in preparation for the next put, it is obvious that great muscular strength and power will be necessary for a successful performance. Likewise, as the wrestler assumes the referee's position, it is apparent that strength and muscular endurance will be critical if he is to beat his opponent. What about the basketball player, golfer, or long-distance runner? Are strength, power, and muscular endurance of major importance to them? The answer, here, is not so obvious, but it is indeed, yes! Training for strength, power, and muscular endurance gains was, at one time, considered taboo for all athletes other than those in competitive weight lifting, weight events in track and field, and, on a limited basis, for football players, wrestlers, and boxers. It is now recognized that strength, power, and muscular endurance are important to successful performance by almost all athletes. Consequently, such training is an integral part of the training programs for almost all sports and activities. This change in attitude or philosophy has been largely the result of innovations in training procedures that have taken place over the last few years.

What is the exact meaning of the terms *strength*, *power*, and *muscular endurance*? Are these terms synonymous, and can they be used interchangeably? The answer to this last question is no. Although the terms are interrelated, each has its own meaning. *Strength* can be defined as the maximum

ability to apply or to resist force. The individual who can press 200 pounds of weight over his head has twice the strength of the individual who can only press 100 pounds. *Power* is simply the product of strength and speed. If two individuals can each bench press 250 pounds, but one is able to do it in one half of the time of the other, the faster individual would have twice the power of the slower individual, providing the distance the weight moved was the same. While absolute strength is an important component of performance, power is probably even more important for most activities. *Muscular endurance* refers to the ability of a group of muscles to sustain repeated contractions, such as in the performance of sit-ups or push-ups, or to sustain a fixed or static contraction for an extended period of time, such as in hanging from a bar, or holding a heavy weight horizontally to the side. While strength appears to be a pure component, independent of power and muscular endurance, both muscular endurance and power are dependent on the individual's level of strength.

ASSESSMENT OF STRENGTH, POWER, AND MUSCULAR ENDURANCE

A better understanding of the concepts of strength, power, and muscular endurance can be gained through a knowledge of how each is assessed or measured. This information is also valuable in helping the coach and athlete design tests or programs of evaluation that will provide accurate estimates of the athlete's progress in each of these areas.

Strength

Strength is exhibited in various ways, which must be taken into consideration in evaluative techniques. The area of strength can be subdivided as follows:

- Static strength
    isometric
        concentric
        eccentric
- Dynamic strength
    isotonic
        concentric
        eccentric
    isokinetic
        concentric
        eccentric

Static or *isometric* strength is that strength that is applied against a fixed, nonmoving resistance. An attempt to move or push over a building would be an example of an isometric contraction. The building represents a fixed or immovable resistance, and no matter how much strength one applies, the building will not move. Thus, the muscle or muscle group may contract to its maximal potential without the resistance, the muscles and joints, moving.

Dynamic strength involves actual movement, both of the involved muscles and joints and the resistance. Dynamic strength can be applied and assessed either *isotonically* or *isokinetically*. In isotonic movements, the resistance is constant throughout the full range of movement. As an example, when the athlete curls 130 pounds, the constant resistance is 130 pounds. To accomplish the lift, the elbow flexors must apply a constant force greater than 130 pounds. Due to the mechanics of the elbow joint, however, the force of 130 pounds represents different fractions of the maximal potential at each angle in the range of motion. Strength is the result of the contractile force and the angle of pull, as is illustrated in Figure 4–1. Thus, the 130 pounds in the biceps curl may represent maximal strength at the angles of 60 degrees and 180 degrees, but only 75 percent of maximal strength at 100

degrees, where the contractile force and angle of pull are optimal. In isotonic movements, therefore, the muscle is not contracting at its capacity or at a constant percentage of its capacity throughout the entire range of motion.

Isokinetic strength can be defined as the maximal contraction of the muscle group at a constant speed throughout the full range of movement. This is a new concept that has tremendous potential in the area of muscular strength, power, and endurance development. The resistance device is controlled at a fixed speed, and no matter how much strength is applied, the resistance will not move any faster. An isokinetic testing device is illustrated in Figure 4–2.

With either dynamic or static movement, there can be both *concentric* and *eccentric contractions*. Concentric contractions refer to muscle shortening, while eccentric contractions involve muscle lengthening. With the biceps curl, lifting the weight from the arms-fully-extended position to a position of complete flexion at the elbow would be an example of muscle shortening, or a concentric

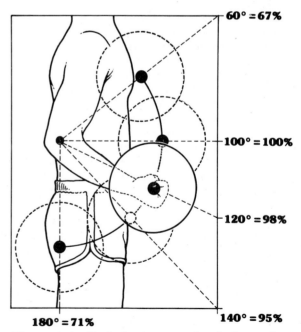

Figure 4–1   Variation in strength relative to the angle of contraction, with 100 percent representing the angle at which strength is optimal.

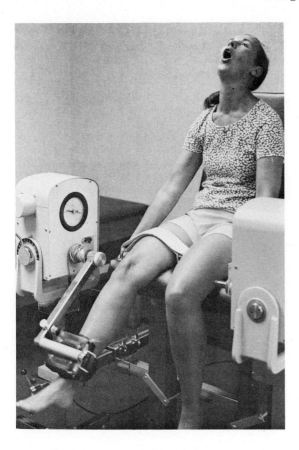

Figure 4–2 Isokinetic testing device. (Lumex, Inc., Bayshore, New York.)

contraction. Lowering the weight from the fully flexed to the fully extended position involves muscle lengthening, or an eccentric contraction. With static or isometric contractions, where there is no perceptible movement, a concentric contraction would be illustrated by a push or pull on an immoveable object or resistance, while eccentric contraction would be illustrated by an attempt to hold a heavy weight in a fixed position, i.e., the resistance is only immobile due to the force applied in the isometric contraction.

Strength can be assessed in a number of different ways. Static strength is usually measured by either a *dynamometer* or a cable tensiometer. The angle of the joint is fixed in a constant position and the individual exerts a maximal isometric contraction. The use of dynamometers has been primarily re-

stricted to measuring grip strength and strength of the back and legs (Figure 4–3). The cable tensiometer has been adapted to measure the strength of just about any muscle group or joint movement in the body (Figure 4–4). With both the dynamometer and the cable tensiometer, the magnitude of tension developed in the isometric contraction is sensed by the testing device and displayed on a meter. Strength can be measured very accurately with either of these devices, but only for the particular joint angle tested. On the basis of the data from Figure 4–1, it is obvious that the elbow strength measured at 90 degrees flexion will be quite different from that measured at 30 degrees or 150 degrees flexion. This is a basic limitation of static strength testing.

Dynamic strength can also be assessed in several different ways. The most popular way is to deter-

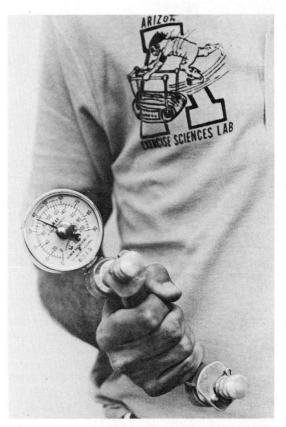

Figure 4–3 Grip strength measured with a hand-grip dynamometer.

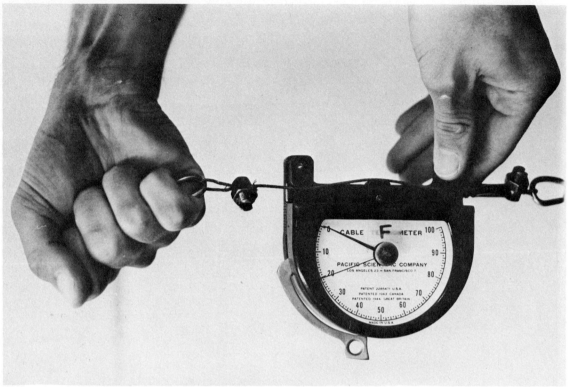

Figure 4–4   Cable-tensiometer for measuring isometric strength.

mine how much weight the individual can lift just one time. This is referred to as a *one-repetition maximum* (1-RM). As an example, to test elbow flexion strength, the individual would attempt to determine how much weight he could lift just one time. He might start at 75 pounds and find that it is too light, go to 90 pounds and find that it is too heavy, and back off to 85 pounds, which he would be able to lift just once. His 1-RM for the curl would then be 85 pounds. Like the static strength tests, this test is accurate, but it only gives an indication of the individual's strength at the weakest point in his range of motion, i.e., he will not be able to lift any more than the weight that he can just lift through the weakest point in his range of motion.

A relatively new testing device, which is available commercially, utilizes the concept of isokinetics and allows the muscle to apply full force at each point in the range of motion and records the resulting strength curve. This allows an accurate quantification of the strength at each point in the

range of motion and also allows the peak strength in the full range to be identified. A typical strength curve is shown in Figure 4–5 using a testing device similar to the one illustrated in Figure 4–2.

There appears to be a high degree of specificity for strength. A single strength test of an isolated muscle group does not appear to be representative of total muscle strength. Several studies have shown that testing three or four selected sites provides an adequate estimation of total body strength (Clarke, 1974a).

Power

Power is a much more difficult component to measure. Several field tests of power have been devised, including the vertical jump, standing long jump, and softball throw for distance tests. While these tests are repeatable and reliable, their validity is questionable, i.e., do they really measure power? Margaria et al. devised a power test in 1966. In this

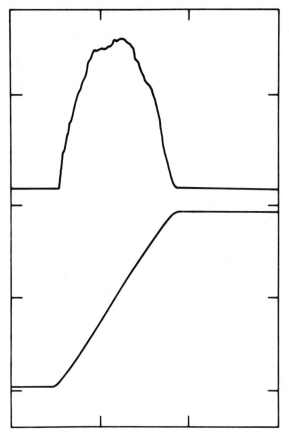

Figure 4–5 Strength curve (upper tracing) and joint angle curve (lower tracing) using the isokinetic testing device illustrated in Figure 4–2.

test, the individual runs up a flight of steps as rapidly as possible. After reaching full speed, the person is timed over a set distance that represents a certain vertical distance climbed. The vertical distance covered in a specific time, related to the weight of the individual, gives an absolute measure of power (see Appendix C, Field Tests for Assessing Physical Fitness). As an example, let us assume that the individual, who weighed 200 pounds, covered a vertical distance of 4 feet in 1 sec. He then performed 800 ft-lb (4 ft × 200 lb) of work in 1 sec, or 48,000 ft-lb of work/min. This would be the equivalent of 1.45 *horsepower* (hp) of work (1 hp = 33,000 ft-lb/min). This test, however, would reflect only the power of the legs, primarily the hip and knee extensors, and not of any other parts of the body.

The isokinetic testing device allows for an estimate of power from almost any muscle group or joint motion. By varying the speed at which the resistance moves, it is possible to estimate explosive power as well as general power. Explosive power can be defined as that initial burst of power that initiates limb movement (a ballistic movement) and can be estimated from the slope of the initial part of the strength curve, i.e., the steeper the slope, the greater the explosive power.

A new device, presently in the experimental stages, has been designed to provide an accurate assessment of power. This device attaches to a standard weight stack. The subject's name and the weight on the weight stack is entered into a small microprocessor, and the device measures the distance the weight travels and the time it takes to travel that distance. It then computes the power output.

Muscular Endurance

Muscular endurance can be measured by a number of field tests, including maximum number of pull-ups, push-ups and sit-ups. In the laboratory, muscular endurance can be measured by several different devices. The *ergograph*, a device developed in the early 1900s, provides a means for continuously lifting and lowering a constant weight through a fixed distance at a constant rate. The subject continues lifting the fixed weight at the established cadence until he or she is no longer able to lift the weight, i.e., until the point of exhaustion.

The same principle can be applied using fixed weights in standard weight training movements. As an example, a 100-pound weight could be used in the bench press and the total number of lifts or repetitions counted. This method has several drawbacks, however. Variations in arm length will influence the distance that the weight is lifted. Second, this technique does not allow for partial lifts.

The isokinetic testing device illustrated in Figure 4–2 gives a very accurate estimate of muscular endurance. The subject applies maximum force throughout the full range of motion and continues this as long as one can, until no further movement is possible. After the initial three or four contractions, there is a decrease in the peak strength attained. A summation of the peak strengths for each contraction, or a summation of the areas under each contraction curve, provides an accurate assessment of muscular endurance.

MUSCLE TRAINING PROCEDURES

Alterations in strength, power, and muscular endurance will result from muscle training programs. There are three basic types of muscle training: isometric, isotonic, and isokinetic. All three result in substantial increases in strength and power, but only isotonic and isokinetic procedures increase muscular endurance.

Isometric Procedures

Isometric training procedures follow the theory that strength can be efficiently gained by training the muscle or muscle group against a fixed, immovable resistance. The concept evolved in the early twentieth century, but gained great popularity and support in the mid-1950s as a result of the work of Hettinger and Müller (1953) in Germany. Their initial studies indicated that tremendous gains in strength would result from isometric training procedures, and, in fact, that these gains would exceed those resulting from the more traditional isotonic procedures. This caused a considerable change in the training patterns during this era; most athletes switched exclusively to isometric training or combined isometric training with isotonic training. Hettinger and Müller claimed increases of 5 percent of the original strength value per week as a result of one 6-sec contraction per day at only 67 percent of maximum contraction strength. Supposedly, little difference in improvement resulted when the tension was increased to 100 percent of maximum contraction strength or when repeated exercises totaling 45 sec were given.

Subsequent research has been unable to confirm the original work by Hettinger and Müller (Clarke, 1973). Most of the later studies demonstrated sizeable strength increases with isometric exercises, but not increases of the magnitude of 5 percent/week found in the original studies. However, it is difficult to use the percentage improvement as an objective evaluation of the value of any program. This is due to the widely accepted belief that the closer one is to theoretical maximum strength, the more difficult it is to show a high percentage improvement in strength. The farther one is from theoretical maximum, the easier it is to demonstrate substantial improvement. Thus, the same procedure or program may result in a 5-percent increase in a group of highly trained athletes and a 20-percent increase in a group of sedentary, deconditioned individuals.

Those early studies that followed the original work by Hettinger and Müller appeared to support their contention that it does not require a contraction of 100 percent of maximum contraction strength or more than one, 6-sec contraction to attain significant gains in strength (Clarke, 1973). One study compared two groups, one exercising at 67 percent of maximum contraction strength one 6-sec contraction per day, and the other at 80 percent of maximum contraction strength with five 6-sec contractions per day (Rarick and Larsen, 1958). Both groups made significant gains in strength, but there were no differences between the groups in their increases in strength. However, studies by Müller and Rohmert (1963) suggest that, while the 67-percent contraction held for 6 sec once per day will increase strength, the more demanding routine of 6-sec contractions at 100 percent of maximum contraction strength, repeated five to ten times, gives substantially greater strength gains. Obviously, additional work in this area will be necessary to gain an understanding as to which is the best routine for maximizing strength gains.

Thus, in the area of isometric training, it appears that the best results can be obtained by using maximum contractions, held for a period of 6 sec, repeated five to ten times per day (Clarke, 1973). In addition, the muscle group should be trained at more than one angle in the range of motion. Several studies have indicated that the strength gains are specific to the joint angle trained (Clarke, 1974a). As an example, performing isometric training at a 90-degree angle in the biceps curl will lead to substantial strength gains at that angle, but will result in only small increases at 45 degrees and 135 degrees, in that same range of motion. To optimize training, it seems justified to suggest that the athlete perform a series of five to ten 6-sec maximal contractions at each of three angles in the full range of motion. Otherwise, strength gains will be limited to a rather small portion of the total range of motion. Specific isometric exercises will not be reviewed in this book, since they can be easily designed to fit the specific needs of the athlete. Also, since there are no equipment needs, simple props, such as chairs and doorways, can be improvised to provide suitable resistance. An isometric power rack can be constructed inexpensively and used for a wide variety of exercises. All that is needed are two 4 × 4-inch posts with holes drilled every 2–3 inches, and several bars to insert into the holes to provide the static resistance to the exercise.

A new concept in the area of isometrics that was introduced in the early 1960s is referred to as *functional isometric training*. O'Shea (1969) has devoted an entire chapter to this concept in his book, *Scientific Principles and Methods of Strength Fitness*. The athlete applies maximum strength in one explosive movement and then sustains this effort in a fixed position for a short duration. A power rack is used. The barbell is placed on the bars of the power rack and additional bars, or pins, are placed 2–4 inches above the bars supporting the barbell. The athlete gets into the starting position, executes a fast isotonic movement through the 2–4 inches, and then holds the barbell isometrically against the upper bars or pins for 3–5 seconds. Thus, functional isometric training is a combination of both isometrics and a short explosive period of isotonics. In performing this system of training, it is important to isolate that muscle group that is to be trained. As an example, it is better to perform an overhead press in a sitting position to isolate the upper-body muscles and to eliminate unwanted assistance from the legs. To date, little, if any, research has been conducted on the advantages of functional isometric training over the more traditional procedures.

Isotonic Procedures

Traditionally, isotonic training has involved the use of weights in the form of barbells, dumbbells, and pulleys. Weight training procedures using the isotonic concept date back as far as recorded history and are even mentioned in Greek mythology. According to mythology, Milo of Crotona desired to become the strongest man in the world. When he was a young boy, he began lifting a young bull once a day and continued lifting it daily until the bull was fully grown. Milo eventually developed enough strength to lift the full-grown bull and to carry it around on his shoulders.

This story, although mythical, does illustrate two important, basic concepts in isotonic muscle training: the concept of overload and the concept of progressive resistance exercise. The concept of *overload* refers to the fact that to gain strength through muscle training procedures, it is necessary to load the muscles beyond that point to which they are normally loaded. Consider the example of a worker on an assembly line who must remove a seventy-five-pound object from a conveyor belt and place it into a packing carton. For his first few days on the job, this is a considerable stress and taxes his muscles nearly to capacity. As a result, his muscles increase in strength to the point where he can handle this task with ease, a process that may take several months. At this point, however, his muscle strength levels off and does not continue to increase. If the factory suddenly shifted to ninety-pound objects, this would constitute an overload, and he would then continue to gain in strength. Thus, the muscles must be taxed beyond so-called "normal" levels of work in order for significant increases in strength to occur.

The concept of *progressive resistance exercise* was illustrated earlier by Milo, i.e., as the muscles become stronger, they must work against a proportionately greater resistance to increase strength further. In essence, this is the systematic application of the overload principle. As an example, an individual who can perform only ten repetitions of a bench press using 150 pounds of weight, will, as he weight trains and gets stronger, be able to increase his repetitions for the same weight to fourteen or fifteen within a week or two. If he then adds 5 pounds of weight to the bar, giving him a total of 155 pounds, his repetitions will drop to eight to ten. As he continues to train, the repetitions continue to increase, and within another week or two, he is ready to add an additional 5 pounds of weight. Thus, there is a progressive increase in the amount of weight or resistance lifted.

DeLorme (1945), and later DeLorme and Watkins (1948), are credited with the initial efforts to systematize isotonic training procedures. Their initial interests were in the areas of physical medicine and rehabilitation. The DeLorme and Watkins system emphasized the use of heavy resistance and low repetitions to develop muscular endurance. Ini- of muscles, as opposed to light resistance and high repetitions to develop muscular indurance. Initially, it was suggested that the subject do seventy to one hundred repetitions divided into seven to ten sets of ten repetitions per set. Later, this was modified to the traditional DeLorme system in which three sets of ten repetitions are performed. The *ten-repetition maximum* (10-RM) is first determined. This represents the greatest resistance that can be lifted ten, but no more than ten, consecutive times. The first set is then performed at a resistance equal to 50 percent of the 10-RM, the second at 75 percent of the 10-RM, and the third at 100 percent of the 10-RM. The amount of weight used is adjusted, periodically, as strength increases. This is determined by the individual's success in the third set, when lifting one 10-RM. If one can lift this fourteen to fifteen times, it no longer represents one's 10-RM, and a new, heavier weight or resistance must be used.

Zinovieff (1951) proposed an alternate technique, since he felt the DeLorme technique had inherent weaknesses. He felt that it was difficult to maintain the quality of contraction in the last set at a full resistance of 10-RM, because of the impaired range of motion and painful joints with maximal contraction. He proposed the Oxford technique, which consisted of a total of one hundred contractions, divided into ten sets of ten repetitions each, the first being performed at 10-RM. Subsequent sets were performed at a lowered resistance to match the decrease in strength that accompanies fatigue. Theoretically, this allowed the individual to do all ten sets at 10-RM, since the decrease in resistance (theoretically) matched the decrease in strength.

Subsequent research has attempted to identify the best possible combination of sets, repetitions, and resistance to maximize strength gains. Clarke, in the January 1974 issue of the *Physical Fitness Research Digest*, summarized the many experiments of Berger in this area. The results include the following.

1. Training with loads as low as 67 percent of maximal strength, two times per week, combined with maximal loads one time a week, results in as much strength improvement as training maximally for three times per week. Training solely at 67 percent of maximal strength, three times per week did not increase strength.
2. The resistance was between 3-RM and 4-RM for training to provide optimum improvement in strength, when training three times per week.
3. Training with 2-RM for six sets, three times per week, was as effective in increasing strength as training with 6-RM for three sets, three times per week.
4. Training with 6-RM for three sets, three times per week, resulted in greater strength gains than training at either 2-RM or 10-RM for three sets, three times per week.
5. Training with 10-RM for three sets, two times per week, was as effective in gaining strength as training the same way three times per week.
6. Training with three sets per day improves strength more than the same training with only one or two sets per day.

Another study by Withers in 1970, compared three sets of 7-RM, four sets of 5-RM, and five sets of 3-RM. He found substantial strength gains in all three groups following a nine-week training program with exercises two days per week. He failed to find any differences between the groups.

From these findings, it would appear that weight training should be performed at 5- to 7-RM, with three sets being executed per training session, in order to maximize the strength gains. Training frequency should be three times per week, although this can be increased to five times per week if the muscles have been preconditioned to take this stress. Additional factors should be considered by the athlete when establishing a weight-training program. These would include the following:

1. Analyze the athlete's basic movements and identify those muscles or muscle groups that should be isolated for strength training.
2. Select exercises that train the identified muscles.
3. Perform at least three sets of each exercise, resting several minutes between sets.
4. Work out on alternate days.
5. Increase the resistance as rapidly as possible.

The length of the total work out will be determined by the number of exercises selected, and can vary from ten to ninety minutes. It has been determined from experience that with longer work outs, the specific exercises should be varied to alternate between upper-limb, trunk, and lower-limb exercises. To perform three consecutive upper-arm exercises only reduces the quality of the last two exercises. Selected isotonic exercises are illustrated in Appendix A, Strength Exercises.

Isokinetic Procedures

Isokinetic muscle training procedures are relatively new in concept and in practice. The concept, which was introduced by Perrine in 1968, was briefly explained in an earlier section of this chapter. First, in an isometric contraction, the contraction can always be performed at 100 percent of maximum contraction strength, but the strength gains are localized to that specific joint angle that is trained. In isotonic exercise, the resistance is constant, and since the maximum strength will vary according to the angle of pull and the length of the muscle throughout the entire range of motion, the contraction must be defined as submaximal through most of the range of motion, even if the resistance can be lifted only once. The lift would be maximal only at the weakest points in the range of motion. Isokinetic exercise attempts to utilize the advantages and eliminate the disadvantages of isometric and isotonic exercise.

In true isokinetic exercise, the resistance adjusts so that it is exactly matched to the force applied by the muscles. Thus, if the individual is able to motivate oneself to apply maximum force throughout the entire range of the lift, the resistance will vary directly with the force to allow a maximum performance throughout the same range. This is accomplished by having the individual exert force against a resistance that has a fixed speed of movement. No matter how much force is applied, the resistance will only move at a set speed and no faster. As an example of this behavior, if a car were placed on a hoist in a service station and raised to the chest level of a standing man, no matter how hard that man pushed on the hoist, the car would not move upward. If, however, the hoist was moved farther upward at a slow speed by its normal hydraulic operation, the man could then push upward with maximal force. The car and hoist would move upward, but no faster than the hoist was set to go. Isokinetic training equipment works on the same principle.

The ability to vary the speed of contraction is another interesting aspect of the isokinetic concept. Traditionally, strength training has been performed either at zero velocity (isometric contraction) or at very low velocities (traditional isotonic 6-RM to 10-RM sets). Athletic performances, however, are typically performed at very high velocities. The question must then be raised: Would muscle training at high velocities have a more favorable influence on the athlete's performance than the traditional, slow training procedures of isometric and isokinetic exercise? It would appear that high-velocity strength training would develop substantial muscle power. Unfortunately, since this concept is relatively new, only a few studies have been conducted on various aspects of isokinetic exercise.

Several studies have investigated the ability of isokinetic exercise to facilitate increases in muscle strength. Unfortunately, however, most of the limited work completed has been of a clinical nature.

During the past ten years, a number of new training devices have been designed which have attempted to provide either direct isokinetic training or variable resistance training. Figure 4–6 illustrates the Mini-Gym device, which utilizes a rope that, when pulled, is released at a pre-set speed. The speed of the rope is controlled internally and is essentially independent of the force exerted during the exercise movement. As illustrated, this device can be used in a number of different configurations to simulate basic sport activities. Nautilus strength training machines (Figure 4–7) have become very popular for the training of athletes. Special cams are designed which attempt to duplicate the variations in force-producing capabilities of the muscle group as it contracts through the range of motion. Universal Gym and Paramount have developed a variable resistance system which allows the use of their traditional weight stacks (Figure 4–8). Finally, the CAM II system utilizes pneumatic resistance which is achieved with compressed air and pneumatic cylinders. Rather than "pumping iron," the athlete is "pumping air"! This system is illustrated in Figure 4–9.

Comparison of Isometric, Isotonic, and Isokinetic Procedures

From the results described in the preceding sections, it is obvious that substantial strength gains

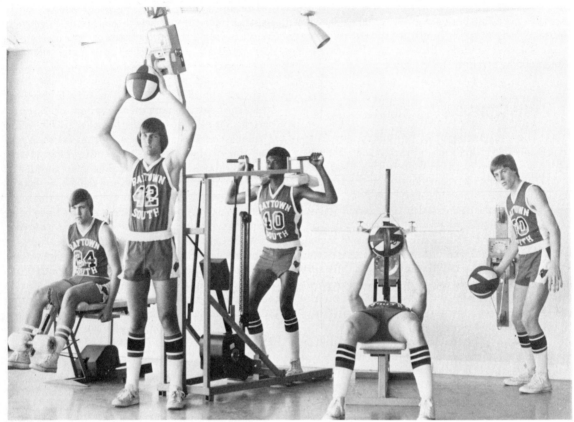

Figure 4–6   Mini-Gym specialized circuit for basketball. Photo courtesy of Mr. Glen Hensen, Mini-Gym, Inc., P.O. Box 266, Independence, MO 64051.

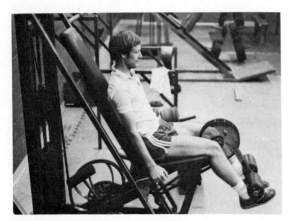

Figure 4–7   Nautilus variable resistance weight training machine.

can be obtained from each of the three different muscle training procedures. Does any one of the three offer a distinct advantage over the other two? Do all three provide equal gains in strength, power, and muscular endurance for an equal quantity of time and effort invested? These are questions that should be asked by the coach and the athlete, since they are both interested in obtaining the greatest benefit in the shortest time possible.

The majority of research that has been conducted to date in evaluating these three types of muscle training has dealt only with isometric and isotonic training. This is to be expected, however, since isokinetic training is a relatively new concept and has not been explored more than superficially from a research standpoint. As was discussed in an ear-

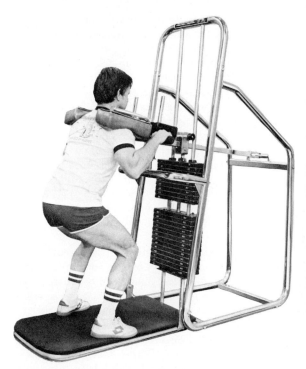

Figure 4–8 Universal Gym "Centurion," single station variable resistance training system. Photo courtesy of Mr. Norman Barnes, Universal Gym, Box 1270, Cedar Rapids, Iowa 52406.

lier section, the potential of the isokinetic concept is particularly impressive; thus, the concept probably will be extensively tested by researchers in the very near future.

A number of studies have compared isometric with isotonic training procedures. The problem in making this comparison, however, is in equalizing the intensity of training by equating isometric and isotonic work loads. Because of the principle of isometrics, i.e., static contraction, to accurately equate work loads is nearly impossible. Irrespective of this problem, many studies have attempted to equate the two, for purposes of accurate comparison, with reasonable success. These studies can be summarized as follows.*

1. Both isometric and isotonic procedures produce substantial gains in muscular strength. While most studies indicate little or no difference be-

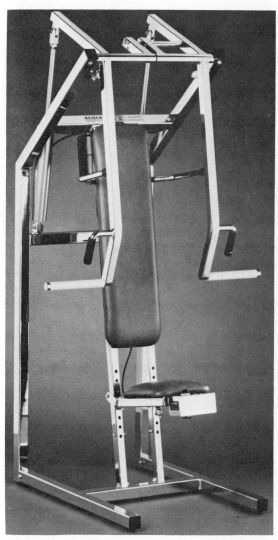

Figure 4–9 The CAM II pneumatic variable resistance machine. Photo courtesy of Mr. Randy Keiser, Keiser Sports Health Equipment, 1627 E. Street, Fresno, CA 93706.

*Adapted from H. H. Clarke, "Development of Muscular Strength and Endurance," *Physical Fitness Research Digest*. President's Council on Physical Fitness and Sports. Washington, D.C.: U.S. Government Printing Office, January 1971.

tween the two procedures, several studies have suggested that isotonic exercise provides greater gains.

2. Muscular endurance is more effectively developed through isotonic procedures, and recovery from muscular fatigue is faster in muscles that have been trained isotonically. These results would be expected on the basis of the static nature of isometric exercise, and the fact that it is not a rhythmical, repetitive type of exercise.

3. Isometric procedures appear to develop strength in only a limited portion of the total range of motion; therefore, isotonic procedures will produce a more uniform development of strength.

4. Isometric procedures can be used during a period of convalescence from injury. Normally, the athlete with a joint or bone injury is completely immobilized, and the lack of exercise will result in a reduction in both muscle size (atrophy) and strength. Isometric contractions involve no joint movement and can be safely and effectively used during the period of recovery from injury, to prevent substantial loss of muscle function.

5. Isotonic procedures appear to cause a greater degree of muscle hypertrophy. This may or may not be a desired outcome of the muscle training program.

In addition to such research findings, there are several practical considerations. Isometric exercises can be performed with little or no supportive equipment, eliminating the need for expensive equipment. They also can be performed anywhere, at anytime, and the time requirement for completing a workout is considerably less than that for isotonic exercises. This would allow the coach the freedom to assign strength-conditioning exercises for athletes to perform at home, both in-season and off-season. On the negative side, isometric exercises present motivational problems. Unless the exercise is performed with elaborate testing equipment, it is impossible to quantify the amount of strength that is applied during the contraction. Furthermore, with training, it is difficult to demonstrate improvement. This lack of positive feedback has led many athletes to abandon their isometric programs. Last, isometric exercises are potentially dangerous

for older individuals and individuals who have diagnosed cardiovascular disease, such as coronary artery disease (heart disease), hypertension, or stroke. When performing isometric exercises, the individual typically closes the glottis, creating a very high pressure within the thoracic, or chest, cavity. This is similar to taking in a full breath of air and then trying to exhale it as forcefully as possible with the mouth and nose closed. The resulting high pressure in the thoracic cavity makes it difficult, if not impossible, for the blood to return from the lower extremities, since the intrathoracic pressure will exceed the pressure in the inferior vena cava. This results in an increased blood pressure and a reduced availability of blood to the heart and brain.

As was mentioned earlier, little research has been conducted in the area of isokinetic procedures. Of the few studies that have been conducted, two have shown the isokinetic procedure to be as effective as both isometric and isotonic procedures.

One advantage of isokinetic exercises over either isometric or isotonic exercises is related to the problem of muscle soreness. While extreme soreness is present a day or two following muscle training with isometric and isotonic exercises, little or no soreness has been noted with isokinetic exercises. The possible reason for this is discussed in one of the following sections.

Circuit Training

Circuit training, a relatively new and innovative type of conditioning program, was developed by R. E. Morgan and G. T. Adamson in 1953 at the University of Leeds, England. This type of conditioning incorporates almost all the training factors that have been described into a single routine. Circuit training can be designed to develop strength, power, muscular endurance, speed, agility and neuromuscular coordination, flexibility, and cardiovascular endurance. The concept has a built-in versatility, which allows the program to be varied to meet the needs of the group. Logically, circuit training should be one of the most popular of the many training programs. Unfortunately, it has not been rapidly accepted in the United States, probably because those individuals who develop and operate conditioning programs lack information about it.

Circuit training is a formal type of training in which an athlete goes through a series of selected exercises or activities that are performed in sequence or in a circuit. Circuits can be set up inside gymnasiums, exercise rooms, hallways, or outside on courts and fields or on tops of roofs. There are usually six to ten stations in a circuit. The athlete performs a specific exercise at each station and then proceeds to the next station. The idea is to progress through the circuit as rapidly as possible, attempting to improve either by decreasing the total time it takes to complete the circuit or by increasing the amount of work accomplished at each station, or both. The stations are distributed throughout the area assigned to circuit training. The greater the distance between stations, the greater the degree of cardiovascular conditioning as the individual runs from one station to the next. An example of a circuit training program is illustrated in Table 4–1.

Various levels are established, depending on the skill level and ability of the group. A group of highly skilled and well-conditioned athletes would have higher levels of accomplishment than a group of sedentary college students who were attempting to get into condition. The individual would start at the lowest level, i.e., level Red–1 for the example in Table 4–1. He or she would go through the circuit a total of three times without stopping. The total time it took to complete three repetitions of level Red–1 is recorded. If he or she is able to finish under the target time of twenty-three minutes, the individual can move to the next level, Red–2.

Circuit training offers a number of unique advantages. It combines a number of different components of training, thus total fitness is emphasized. It provides an interesting training environment for the athlete, and there are established times and levels to motivate the athlete to continue improving. The circuit can be modified to fit the needs of any one group or individual, it can be adapted within the time constraints of the individual, and it can accommodate large groups of individuals at a relatively low expense. Progression in all activities is assured.

In designing a circuit, first establish the training needs of the athletes who will be using the circuit. Adapt the circuit to fit the specific needs of the individuals, if possible. Identify an area that can be used for the circuit, ideally where permanent stations can be established. Next, determine the number of stations that can be accommodated in the space allotted. Arrange the stations in such an order that exercises for similar body areas do not follow one another sequentially. Alternate with an upper-body strength exercise, flexibility exercise, muscular endurance, lower-body strength exercise, and cardiovascular endurance exercise, in sequence. Place the station number and the specific instructions at each station. This information should also include a list of the various levels and the required weights and repetitions.

As mentioned, the trainer or coach who has a basic knowledge of the principles behind circuit training will find that it is one of the easiest train-

Table 4–1   *Example of a Circuit Training Circuit**

Target Times			Red—23 minutes			Blue—25 minutes			
Station Number	Exercise	Weight, lbs	Red Circuit Repetitions 1	2	3	Weight, lbs	Blue Circuit Repetitions 1	2	3
1	Bench press	60	8	10	12	80	8	10	12
2	Squat thrust		10	13	16		19	22	25
3	Chins		1	3	5		7	9	10
4	Stair climb		4	6	8		10	12	14
5	Two-arm curl	45	8	10	12	55	8	10	12
6	Half-squat	75	9	12	15	100	12	14	16
7	Sit-ups		10	14	18		20	25	30
8	Running lap		1	1	2		2	3	3

*Adapted from R. P. Sorani, Circuit Training. Dubuque, Iowa: William C. Brown Co., 1966. Reproduced by permission of the publisher.

ing programs to implement. Once established, it requires little or no supervision, and can be an excellent adjunct to any regular training program, or it can function as a complete off-season training program in itself.

In 1976, Allen et al. investigated a new concept in training that has a great deal of application for off-season conditioning. They merged the circuit training concept with traditional weight training into a form of training now referred to as *circuit weight training*. Traditional weight training is usually performed in a slow, methodical manner, with very short work intervals and very long rest intervals. With circuit weight training, individuals work at 40–60 percent of their 1–RM for periods of approximately thirty seconds, with fifteen-second rest intervals interspersed between work periods. They start at the first station, completing as many repetitions as possible in thirty seconds, take a fifteen-second rest during which they move to the next station, and then start their second thirty-second work period. This continues until they complete the six to eight stations in the circuit, i.e., the first set, and then they start their second set. This form of training has been demonstrated to provide modest increases in $\dot{V}O_2$ max; major increases in strength, muscular endurance, and flexibility; and substantial alterations in body composition, i.e., increased lean weight and decreased fat weight. Gettman and Pollock (1981) have prepared an excellent review article on all research that has been conducted in the area of circuit weight training. The major advantages of circuit weight training include: (1) it is an activity that attends to the major components of athletic fitness; (2) it can be conducted in a very small area (small room with a multistation weight training machine); and (3) the complete workout (three sets) can be completed in less than thirty minutes.

MECHANISMS OF STRENGTH, POWER, AND MUSCULAR ENDURANCE GAINS

The mechanisms that are responsible for gains in strength, power, and muscular endurance that result from muscle training programs are not at all clear. It was mentioned in earlier chapters that the ability to improve strength may be more of a neurological phenomenon than an actual change in the properties or quality of the muscle. Steinhaus (1968) believes that inhibitory mechanisms in the neuromuscular system are necessary to keep an individual from literally tearing oneself apart, i.e., breaking bones and pulling muscle tendons out of their bony attachments. Autogenic inhibition is a reflex inhibition of the lower, motor-neuron discharge to a specific muscle when the tension on that muscle's tendons and internal, connective tissue structures exceeds the threshold of the imbedded, Golgi tendon organs. At higher levels in the nervous system, the reticular formation in the brain stem and the cerebral cortex both have the ability to initiate and propagate inhibitory impulses. It is quite possible that these inhibitory impulses are gradually overcome or counteracted, which then allows the expression of higher levels of strength that typically occur following a muscle training program. This theory certainly deserves considerable scientific investigation.

The early work of Hettinger and Müller (1953) pointed to the possibility that strength gains resulted from lack of oxygen in the exercising muscle. This was referred to as the *hypoxia* theory of strength gains. This theory has subsequently been tested on several occasions and found to have no validity. Other attempts to identify the mechanism for strength gains at the level of the muscle fiber have likewise not been fruitful. It appears that strength is probably mediated or controlled by the nervous system, but changes in the muscle tissue itself cannot be ruled out at this time.

Power is simply the product of strength and speed; thus, any increase in power must be the result of improvements in either strength or speed, or both. Since muscle training substantially increases muscle strength and can also increase speed of movement (to be covered later in this chapter), the increase in power with muscle training is also substantial. Unlike strength, the mechanisms responsible for these increases in power are obvious.

It is generally accepted that muscular endurance is best increased through muscle training that emphasizes high repetitions and relatively low resistance (Clarke, 1973). Yet, there is also a high correlation between strength and absolute muscular endurance. This would tend to suggest that even programs designed to produce optimal gains in strength, i.e., low repetitions and high resistance, will provide some improvement in muscular endurance. It appears, therefore, that strength is one of the major determinants of muscle endurance. What are some of the others? Local patterns of circulation appear to be important. Since muscular endurance is a repeated or prolonged contraction of a muscle or a muscle group, substrate for metabolism becomes a factor as does the removal of waste products. The more efficient the circulation and the greater the development of circulatory capacity within that local area, the greater the potential for muscular endurance. Research has indicated that muscle training at 20- to 30-RM is the most efficient way to increase muscular endurance. This routine will have little effect on muscle strength and bulk. Thus, factors other than strength are important in the development of endurance. The ability to tolerate higher levels of pain or an increase in anaerobic threshold are two additional factors that might explain increases in muscular endurance independent of changes in strength.

MUSCLE SORENESS

Muscle soreness may be present either during the latter stages of an exercise and immediate recovery, or between twelve and forty-eight hours after a strenuous bout of exercise, or at both times. Pain that is felt during and immediately after exercise is probably due to the accumulation of the end products of exercise and tissue edema caused by the high hydrostatic pressures that force fluid to shift from the blood plasma into the tissues. This is the "pumped-up" feeling that the athlete is conscious of following heavy endurance or strength training. This pain and soreness is usually of short duration, disappearing within an hour following the cessation of exercise.

The muscle soreness that is felt a day or two following a heavy bout of exercise is the result of factors yet to be defined. There are several theories that have been presented to explain this form of muscle soreness, but they do not have universal support or agreement. One theory states that soreness is the result of small tears in muscle or connective tissue. While actual structural damage is a possible outcome of certain types of explosive or violent exercise, it is suspected that this would account for only a limited percentage of cases of muscle soreness. deVries (1974) has suggested a theory for muscle soreness, which he labels the "spasm theory." According to this theory, exercise brings about localized muscle ischemia (deficiency of blood), the ischemia causes pain, the pain generates increased reflex motor activity, greater motor activity creates even greater local muscle tension, which results in even greater degrees of ischemia. His research supports this theory, and he has also found that static stretching procedures help to prevent soreness, as well as to relieve soreness when it is present.

This is an attractive theory and probably is closely related to the basic cause. The theory fails, however, to explain two phenomenon. First, muscle soreness will usually haunt the athlete only during the initial stages of training, i.e., the first week or two. Following this initial period, the athlete has relatively little trouble with soreness, even though he or she may be working at substantially higher absolute and relative work loads. The spasm theory does not seem to explain this phenomenon.

Second, isokinetic strength training has produced an interesting and an unexpected outcome. Little or no muscle soreness has been found following exhaustive bouts of isokinetic exercise. Talag (1973) investigated the relationship of muscle soreness to eccentric, concentric, and isometric contractions, and she found that a group trained solely with eccentric contractions experienced extreme muscle soreness, while the isometric- and concentric-contraction groups experienced little soreness with their training. The fact that isokinetic procedures use only concentric contractions with a passive recovery, combined with the results from the preceding study, suggests that muscle soreness is unique to those activities that have a component of eccentric contraction. Again, this does not seem to support the spasm theory.

Most recently, Abraham (1979) has provided data supporting Hough's torn tissue hypothesis, which was originally formulated in 1902. He found muscle soreness to correlate with the appearance of myoglobin in the urine, with myoglobin being a marker of muscle fiber trauma. Since myoglobinuria is associated with all strenuous work, independent of muscle soreness, he also looked at hydroxyproline excretion, indicative of connective tissue breakdown. He found a significant correlation between the day of maximum hydroxyproline excretion and the day when the subjects experienced their greatest soreness.

The actual cause of muscle soreness, however, must still be considered as unknown, at this time. The recent clue that soreness appears to be related solely to eccentric contraction should help researchers determine the basic cause of this perplexing and aggravating problem.

SEX DIFFERENCES

There are considerable differences in strength, power, and muscular endurance between males and females, once they reach puberty. Prior to this time, they are nearly identical to each other in these characteristics at each age. The higher values expressed by the boys, once they are past puberty, can be traced to several factors, both cultural and genetic. As a result of genetic factors, the young boy starts producing increasingly greater amounts of testosterone once he reaches puberty. This produces large increases in muscle bulk and an associated increase in strength. For cultural reasons, although changing, at the onset of puberty in the female, it becomes less acceptable for her to be involved in large-muscle activities. Without the stimulus of exercise, the muscles will not continue to gain in strength or in size, except for the increases that accompany the normal growth curve. This topic will be covered in much greater depth and detail in Chapter 13, The Female Athlete.

MUSCULAR TRAINING AND ATHLETIC PERFORMANCE

Gaining strength, power, or muscular endurance simply for the sake of being stronger, more powerful, or possessing greater muscular endurance is of relatively little importance to athletes, unless it will also result in improvements in their athletic performance. The application of muscular training to field event athletes in track and to competitive weight lifters, intuitively makes a great deal of sense. What about the gymnast, distance runner, baseball player, high jumper, or ballerina? Will muscular training assist them in the preparation for their events, activities, or sport? Since training is costly in terms of time, athletes cannot afford to waste time on activities that will not result in better athletic performances. What do research findings indicate? Clarke (1974b) has recently summarized all of the research in this area.

With regard to specific sports, muscular training appears to be a highly desirable supplement to the general training program for almost any athlete. In three studies of baseball, muscle training as a supplement to regular baseball practice resulted in significant improvements in throwing speed and in the speed to sprint ninety feet. In a single study of softball, underhand throwing ability for distance was improved with functional, isometric exercises, as well as the endurance to maintain maximum distance for eighty underhand throws. In all of these studies, the improvements noted were significantly greater than those in other groups that did not supplement their practice with muscular training.

Several studies have used isotonic or isometric weight training to supplement swim training programs. Those groups that supplemented their swim training with muscle training, with one exception, exhibited greater improvement at distances of twenty-five and fifty yards. Dr. James Counsilman, swimming coach at the University of Indiana and recognized developer of many Olympic and world-record-holding swimmers, is a strong advocate of supplementing swimming workouts with strength training. He has developed a series of isokinetic exercises that he believes will substantially influence swim training procedures in the near future.

In football, the influence of both isometric and isotonic strength training on the speed and force of the offensive football charge was investigated in a single study. The isometric group and the isotonic group improved significantly in both speed and the force of the offensive charge, while the control group did not improve on either test.

A number of studies have observed the influence of muscular training on the speed of movement. At one time, it was felt that muscle training would result in a muscle-bound, inflexible athlete and that speed would actually be decreased. Most studies, subsequently, have shown that speed can be improved with muscular training, although there are several studies with conflicting results. A recent study using isokinetic exercises found a substantial improvement in forty-yard dash

Table 4–2 *Strength Training Activities for Various Sports or Events* *

Sport, Activity, or Event — with sub-groupings: *Swimming* spans Backstroke–Freestyle; *Track and Field* spans Sprinting–Discus and Shot Put.

Movement	Baseball	Basketball	Golf	Gymnastics	Football	Soccer	Rowing	Tennis	Wrestling	Skiing	Hockey	Backstroke	Breaststroke	Butterfly	Freestyle	Sprinting	Hurdling	Javelin	Long jump	Distance running	Pole vault	High jump	Discus and Shot Put
Neck flexion and extension					X	X			X		X												
Shoulder shrug					X				X	X	X								X		X		
Military or overhead press					X	X			X	X					X		X						X
Behind the neck press												X		X									
Upright rowing	X	X	X	X		X	X		X	X	X	X			X					X	X		
Bent rowing						X			X							X	X						
Lat machine		X	X	X		X			X	X	X	X	X	X		X							
Triceps extension	X			X					X	X	X	X	X	X	X		X	X	X				X
Lateral arm raise	X			X					X			X									X		
Bent-arm pull-over	X	X			X	X						X	X	X			X	X			X	X	
Biceps curl			X			X																	X
Dumbbell curl	X	X	X	X	X	X	X	X	X							X			X	X		X	
Bench press	X			X		X			X			X	X	X	X					X	X	X	X
Incline press	X		X	X	X				X			X	X	X			X	X	X		X	X	X
Parallel bar dip				X	X			X	X			X	X	X		X							
Back hyperextension				X	X		X		X				X			X	X				X		
Trunk extension	X								X			X	X	X			X						X
Weighted sit-ups	X	X	X			X	X	X	X	X	X	X					X	X		X	X	X	X
Hip flexion												X	X	X	X				X				
Stiff leg dead lift				X		X	X		X							X					X		
Knee flexion												X	X			X	X	X					
Knee extension		X			X	X			X	X	X	X				X	X	X	X			X	X
Squat	X	X	X			X	X	X		X													X
Hack squat				X	X			X	X	X	X	X	X	X	X	X	X	X	X	X	X	X	X
Toe raise	X										X					X	X	X		X		X	

Adapted from J. P. O'Shea, Scientific Principles and Methods of Strength Fitness. 2nd ed. Reading. Mass.: Addison-Wesley Publishing Co., 1976. Reproduced by permission of the publisher.

speed, from 5.3 to 5.1 sec, following eight weeks of training.

Many studies have investigated the influence of muscular training on the performance of general motor tasks. Most studies have found that isotonic training substantially improves vertical jumping ability, while isometric training does not. The standing long jump has also been found to improve with isotonic training. Campbell (1962) observed the effects of systematic isotonic exercise on the motor fitness of college football, basketball, and track and field squads during their competitive seasons. Motor fitness was assessed from a composite score consisting of performances for right grip, vertical jump, squat thrusts, pull-ups, sit-ups, 300-yard shuttle run, and 50-yard dash. Each team was divided into two groups: one group trained the first half of the season with isotonic exercises to supplement their normal training, while the other group used only normal training procedures. At the midpoint of the season, the groups switched procedures. Isotonic training resulted in large gains in motor fitness, but the group that stopped weight training at midseason had actually decreased in motor fitness when tested at the end of the season.

From such findings, muscle training does appear to have a great deal to offer to athletes who wish to improve their performances. A word of caution must be inserted, however. Only a handful of activities or sports have been studied. It is possible, but not too likely on the basis of the information presently available, that muscle training will not be beneficial for every athlete, event, activity, or sport. At this time, the best advice appears to be to proceed with caution, and if the results prove beneficial, a more aggressive approach can be taken. Refer to Table 4–2 for suggested exercise movements for selected sports.

GENERAL SUMMARY

The athlete's performance can be separated into a number of individual components. The components of strength, power, and muscular endurance appear to be extremely important for most athletic performances. Strength is defined as the ability to apply or to resist force. Power is the functional application of both strength and speed. Muscular endurance refers to the ability of a group of muscles to sustain either repeated or static contractions for an extended period of time.

Strength can be expressed either statically (isometric contraction) or dynamically (isotonic or isokinetic contraction), and muscular contractions can either be concentric (shortening) or eccentric (lengthening). With muscle training programs, there are generally increases in strength, power, and muscular endurance. Isometric and isotonic training procedures result in similar gains in strength, but isotonic training appears to produce substantially greater gains in muscular endurance. Isokinetic training may have the greatest potential of the three types of muscle training for gaining strength, power, and muscular endurance, but this will have to await confirmation following additional research.

Maximum gains in isometric strength appear to come from five to ten 6-sec isometric contractions at 100 percent of maximal strength, repeated at three different points in the full range of motion. Isotonic training apparently is maximized by performing three sets per day of each exercise at 5 to 7 RM. Research is too limited at this point to make recommendations relative to an optimal training procedure for isokinetic exercise. High-speed contraction does appear to be important, but again, it is too early to tell at this time. Training three to five days per week appears to be optimal for all three training procedures.

Circuit training was developed in England in the 1950s and spread throughout the United States in the 1960s. This is a unique concept, since it incorporates strength, power, muscular endurance, speed, agility and neuromuscular coordination, flexibility, and cardiovascular endurance. A circuit usually consists of six to ten stations, each focusing on one exercise, e.g., pull-ups, so that all areas of the body are covered in a complete circuit. The athletes go through the entire circuit as rapidly as possible, repeating the circuit three times. They are assigned a specific amount of work to accomplish at each station. As they become better conditioned, they are able to reduce their time through the circuit. In addition, the circuit is designed for different levels of competence so that athletes can move up to the next highest level, as they improve. Each level requires a greater amount of work at each of the stations.

Strength gains probably result from changes occurring within the central nervous system. While it is impossible to rule out changes in the muscle itself at this time, it does appear that the central nervous system plays the major role. Power is increased by gains in either or both strength and speed. Muscular endurance is increased through gains in muscular strength and probably through changes in local circulatory patterns as well.

Muscle soreness is a phenomenon that is poorly understood. One theory attempts to explain soreness on the basis of small tears in the muscle or its connective tissue. A second theory attributes soreness to localized muscle spasms. Neither theory appears to hold under all conditions. The recent findings that soreness results predominantly from eccentric contraction types of exercises, or from activities that use eccentric contractions, should direct the efforts of future research in this area into more productive avenues.

Finally, muscle training has been shown to have a significant influence on the performance of several sports and on a number of motor activities. It seems obvious at this time that almost all athletes, no matter what their sports, can gain substantial benefits from muscle training. For most sports, however, the specific programs have yet to be established, so the athlete should proceed with caution.

STUDY QUESTIONS

1. Define and differentiate between strength, power, and muscular endurance. How do each of these components relate to athletic performance?
2. How does one assess muscle strength? Power? Muscular endurance?
3. What is the difference between eccentric contraction and concentric contraction?
4. What is the importance of power in specific sports or events?
5. What is the optimal routine for isometric strength training?
6. Define the overload principle and the principle of progressive resistance exercise.
7. Describe two distinct advantages of isokinetic or variable resistance training.
8. How does a muscle increase its strength?
9. What is the physiological explanation for muscle soreness?
10. Should all athletes strength train? If your answer is no, what criteria should be used to determine who should strength train?
11. What is circuit training, and how does this differ from circuit weight training?
12. What advantages might circuit training, or circuit weight training, have over other training procedures used for developing strength, power, and muscular endurance?

REFERENCES

Abraham, W. M. "Exercise-Induced Muscle Soreness." *Physician Sportsmed.* 7 (1979): 57–60.

Allen, T. E.; Byrd, R. J.; and Smith, D. P. "Hemodynamic Consequences of Circuit Weight Training." *Res. Quart.* 47 (1976): 299–306.

Berger, R. A. "Effects of Varied Weight Training Programs on Strength." *Res. Quart.* 33 (1962): 168–181.

Berger, R. A. "Comparison of Static and Dynamic Strength Increases." *Res. Quart.* 33 (1962): 329–333.

Campbell, R. L. "Effects of Supplemental Weight Training on the Physical Fitness of Athletic Squads." *Res. Quart.* 33 (1962): 343–348.

Clarke, D. H. "Adaptations in Strength and Muscular Endurance Resulting from Exercise." In *Exercise and Sport Sciences Reviews*, vol. 1, edited by J. H. Wilmore. New York: Academic Press, 1973.

Clarke, H. H. "Development of Muscular Strength and Endurance." *Physical Fitness Research Digest*, President's Council on Physical Fitness and Sports. Washington, D.C.: U.S. Government Printing Office, January 1974a.

Clarke, H. H. "Strength Development and Motor-Sports Improvement." *Physical Fitness Research Digest*, President's Council on Physical Fitness and Sports. Washington, D.C.: U.S. Government Printing Office, October 1974b.

Costill, D. L.; Coyle, E. F.; Fink, W. F.; Lesmes, G. R.; and Witzmann, F. A. "Adaptations in Skeletal Muscle following Strength Training." *J. Appl. Physiol.* 46 (1979): 96–99.

DeLorme, T. L. "Restoration of Muscle Power by Heavy Resistance Exercise." *J. Bone Joint Surg.* 27 (1945): 645–667.

DeLorme, T. L., and Watkins, A. L. "Technics of Progressive Resistance Exercise." *Arch. Phys. Med.* 29 (1948): 263–273.

deVries, H. A. *Physiology of Exercise for Physical Education and Athletics.* 2nd ed. Dubuque, Iowa: William C. Brown, 1974.

Edgerton, V. R. "Neuromuscular Adaptations to Power and Endurance Work." *Canad. J. Appl. Sports Sciences* 1 (1976): 49–58.

Fox, E. L. *Sports Physiology.* Philadelphia: W. B. Saunders Co., 1979.

Gettman, L. R., and Pollock, M. L. "Circuit Weight

Training: A Critical Review of its Physiological Benefits." *Physician Sportsmed.* 9 (1981): 44–60.

Gonyea, W. J. "Role of Exercise in Inducing Increases in Skeletal Muscle Fiber Number." *J. Appl. Physiol.* 48 (1980): 421–426.

Hettinger, T. *Physiology of Strength*. Springfield, Ill.: Charles C. Thomas, 1961.

Hettinger, T., and Müller, E. A. "Muskelleistung and Muskel Training." *Arbeitsphysiol.* 15 (1953): 111–126.

Jensen, C. R., and Fisher, A. G. *Scientific Basis of Athletic Conditioning*. 2nd ed. Philadelphia: Lea and Febiger, 1979.

Jesse, J. P. "Misuse of Strength Development Programs in Athletic Training." *Physician Sportsmed.* 7 (1979): 46–52.

Lamb, D. R. *Physiology of Exercise: Responses and Adaptations*. New York: Macmillan Publishing Co., 1978.

Lesmes, G. R.; Costill, D. L.; Coyle, E. F.; and Fink, W. J. "Muscle Strength and Power Changes during Maximal Isokinetic Training." *Med. Sci. Sports* 10 (1978): 266–269.

Margaria, R.; Aghemo, P.; and Rovelli, E. "Measurement of Muscular Power (anaerobic) in Man." *J. Appl. Physiol.* 21 (1966): 1662–1664.

Morgan, R. E., and Adamson, G. T. *Circuit Weight Training*. London: G. Bell and Sons, 1961.

Müller, E. A. and Rohmert, W. "Die Geschwindigkeit der Muskelkraft Zunahme bei Isometrischen Training." *Internationale Zeitschrift Angewandte Physiol.* 19 (1963): 403–419.

O'Shea, J. P. *Scientific Principles and Methods of Strength Fitness*. Reading, Mass.: Addison-Wesley Pub. Co., 1969.

Perrine, J. J. "Isokinetic Exercise and the Mechanical Energy Potentials of Muscle." *J. Health Phys. Ed. and Rec.* 39 No. 5 (1968): 40–44.

Rarick, G. L., and Larson, G. L. "Observations on Frequency and Intensity of Isometric Muscular Effort in Developing Strength in Post-Pubescent Males." *Res. Quart.* 29 (1958): 333–341.

Rasch, P. J., and Morehouse, L. E. "Effect of Static and Dynamic Exercise on Muscular Strength and Hypertrophy." *J. Appl. Physiol.* 11 (1957): 29–34.

Sorani, R. P. *Circuit Training*. Dubuque, Iowa: William C. Brown Co., 1966.

Steinhaus, A. H. "Inhibitory Mechanisms Operative in the Expression of Human Strength." Paper presented at the Annual Meeting, American College of Sports Medicine, Pennsylvania State University, May 1968.

Talag, T. S. "Residual Muscular Soreness as Influenced by Concentric, Eccentric and Static Contractions." *Res. Quart.* 44 (1973): 458–469.

Withers, R. T. "Effect of Varied Weight-Training Loads on the Strength of University Freshman." *Res. Quart.* 41 (1970): 110–114.

Zinovieff, A. N. "Heavy Resistance Exercises: The Oxford Technique." *Brit. J. Phys. Med.* 14 (1951): 129–132.

5

Speed, Agility, Neuromuscular Coordination, and Flexibility

INTRODUCTION

The average spectator who observes various athletic events would conclude that to be successful the sprinter running the one-hundred-yard dash must rely on speed, that the soccer player must depend on agility, neuromuscular coordination, and skill, and that the gymnast performing free exercise must have exceptional flexibility. Are these qualities or components important to athletes in other sports, activities, or events? The answer to this question must be yes! For example, the football player, regardless of playing position, must be concerned with each of these components. Since he is dependent on high levels of power for successful execution of his assignment, speed is essential to his performance because speed and strength, by definition, constitute power. Agility and neuromuscular coordination are particularly important to those players who handle the ball, i.e., backs and receivers, but they are also of concern to the big linemen who must maneuver, pursue, and elude. Last, flexibility is important, not only for proper execution, but also for injury prevention, an area that will be discussed in detail later in this chapter. While this example illustrates the requirements for only one sport, equally impressive cases can be developed for practically all sports. The information in this chapter will, therefore, be applicable to all athletes.

Speed is easily defined as the rate of motion or the velocity of the body, or any one of its parts. For the sprinter, his or her time for a set distance, e.g., 9.6

sec for 100 yd, represents an average velocity (100 yd/9.6 sec) of 10.4 yd/sec. The average velocity, however, is the result of two independent factors, acceleration and maximal velocity. Thus, the sprinter with good acceleration, but only average maximal velocity, will excel in the short sprints of forty to one hundred yards, but will appear to fade with distances over one hundred yards. This is an important point, for some sports rely on the accelerative component of speed, while others are concerned only with maximal velocity. The running back in football must have good acceleration, or quickness, to break through the line, but maximal velocity would also become important once he broke into the open, twenty to thirty yards from the line of scrimmage.

Agility and neuromuscular coordination are much more difficult to define. *Agility* refers to the maneuverability of the individual, i.e., the ability to shift the direction of movement rapidly, without loss of balance or sense of position. It is, therefore, a combination of speed, strength, quick reactions, balance, and coordination, and can refer to the total body or to a specific part, such as the hands or feet. *Neuromuscular coordination* reflects the ability of athletes to perform their sports, activities, or events with a smooth, balanced, and fluid motion. This component is exemplified by the diver who performs a complex series of twists, bends, and somersaults, and concludes with a poised entry into the water, or by the gymnast who performs a complex routine on the balance beam.

93

Flexibility refers to the range of motion, i.e., looseness or suppleness of the body or specific joints, and involves the interrelationships between muscles, tendons, ligaments, and the joint itself. Limited flexibility is usually the result of muscles and tendons that are too tight, restricting the range of motion. A good example of this occurs in the hip and knee joint. The hamstring muscles, which are the flexor muscles of the knee and the extensor muscles of the hip, cross both the hip and knee joints. A tightness of the hamstrings and the associated muscle tendons seriously limits flexibility at the knee and hip joints. This can be simply illustrated by having the athlete sit on the floor with his legs extended in front of him. He then leans forward, grabs his ankles, and bends slowly as he attempts to touch his head to his knee. Few athletes can do this. Most can bend no further than 45° forward from the vertical position. Tightness and pain can be felt in the backs of the knees and thighs and in the lower back. Extremely large muscles and excessive quantities of fat also tend to limit joint flexibility, but these are not as frequent a cause of limited flexibility as muscle and tendon tightness.

ASSESSMENT OF SPEED, AGILITY, NEUROMUSCULAR COORDINATION, AND FLEXIBILITY

Speed can be assessed in a number of ways, varying from simple timing procedures to procedures that require elaborate and expensive equipment. The assessment can be restricted to a body segment, such as measuring the velocity of the arm in a particular movement; it can focus on the total body, as in timing an individual's speed in the one hundred-yard dash; or it can be applied to external objects propelled by the body, as in measuring the speed of a thrown ball or the speed of the head of a golf club. In addition, the assessment of speed can also be separated into two components: acceleration and maximal velocity.

The speed of individual body segments can be assessed in several ways. Two of the more widely used techniques involve elaborate timing devices or *cinematography*. With a timing device, the body segment, e.g., foot, is placed on, or pressed against, a microswitch. The instant the foot moves to initiate the movement, the microswitch is triggered and starts a timer. The foot travels a fixed distance and either contacts a target or crosses the path of a light beam, either of which stops the timer. Since the distance that the foot moves is fixed, the result of dividing this distance by the time to complete the task provides an estimate of the movement time of the segment for that task.

Reaction time, another component of speed, can be assessed in a similar manner. *Reaction time* is defined as the length of time that it takes to respond to a stimulus, i.e., the time elapsed between the presentation of the stimulus and the actual start of the movement. In the previous example, using an additional timer, the subject can be instructed to react as quickly to a stimulus, e.g., switching on a light, as possible, and then to move the foot as quickly as possible from the microswitch to the target. Switching on the light would start the second timer, and the initial movement of the foot would stop it, thus measuring the length of time it took the subject to react to the stimulus. A variety of visual, verbal, or tactile stimuli can be used. The timers must be extremely accurate, as the times are frequently recorded to the hundredth or thousandth of a second.

With cinematography, movements can be more natural, since they are actually measured during competition. A special high-speed movie camera is used to record movements. The camera is set at a fixed distance from the subject, with objects of known size included in the field of vision, so that accurate distance estimates can be made. The camera is calibrated to use film at a fixed speed, so that segment speed can be estimated from a knowledge of the distance moved per frame and the number of frames taken per second. This is a very useful way to look at not only speed, but also at acceleration. Camera location, with regard to planes of movement, is extremely important. Frequently, several cameras will be used to provide a three-dimensional analysis of the movement.

Speed of the total body is usually assessed by timing the athlete as he or she runs as fast as possible for a given distance. Traditionally, football players are timed over a distance of forty yards, and baseball players over a distance of ninety feet, or a full trip around the bases. The objective is to select a distance that has some relationship to the sport in which the athlete is competing. As was mentioned earlier, speed is the result of both acceleration and maximal velocity. For certain sports or events, it is advantageous to be able to differentiate between the two. Since maximal velocity is usually obtained within the first thirty to fifty yards of a sprint, maximal velocity can be measured by having the athlete run an all-out, one hundred-yard dash and timing the individual between the fifty-yard and one hundred-yard markers. This provides a fifty-yard dash time, which, theoretically, is run at maximal running velocity. To assess acceleration, a crude estimate could be made by measuring the time to complete the forty-yard dash. A better method of evaluation, however, would be to have the athlete run all-out for fifty yards, starting from either a standing or crouched start, with timers stationed at ten, twenty, thirty, forty, and fifty yards. It would then be possible to determine true acceleration from one ten-yard segment to the next, since acceleration is defined as the rate of change in speed.

Acceleration =
$$\frac{\text{(final velocity} - \text{initial velocity)}}{\text{time required to change velocity}}$$

As an example, if a sprinter went from a crouched start (defined as zero velocity) to the first ten-yard marker in 2.1 sec, he or she would have an average velocity of 4.8 yd/sec. This is the arithmetical average between a starting velocity of 0 and an unknown velocity at the ten-yard marker. Since the average and initial velocities are known, the final velocity at ten yards can be calculated, i.e., average velocity = (final velocity + initial velocity)/2, or

$$4.8 \text{ yd/sec} = (x + 0)/2$$
$$x/2 = 4.8 \text{ yd/sec}$$
$$x = 9.6 \text{ yd/sec}$$

The acceleration for the initial ten-yard segment would then be

$$\text{acceleration} = (9.6 \text{ yd/sec} - 0 \text{ yd/sec})/2.1 \text{ sec}$$
$$= (9.6 \text{ yd/sec})/2.1 \text{ sec}$$
$$= 4.6 \text{ yd/sec}^2$$

To continue with this example, if the athlete crossed the twenty-yard marker in 3.05 sec, the thirty-yard marker in 3.90 sec, the forty-yard marker in 4.73 sec, and the fifty-yard marker in 5.56 sec, he or she would have attained the following accelerations:

10–20 Yards

Calculate average velocity ($\bar{v}$):

$$\bar{v} = 10 \text{ yd in } 0.95 \text{ sec } (3.05 - 2.1)$$
$$= 10.53 \text{ yd/sec}$$

Calculate final velocity (v_f):

$$10.53 \text{ yd/sec} = (v_f + 9.6 \text{ yd/sec})/2$$
$$21.06 \text{ yd/sec} = v_f + 9.6 \text{ yd/sec}$$
$$v_f = 11.45 \text{ yd/sec}$$

Calculate acceleration (a):

$$a = (11.45 \text{ yd/sec} - 9.6 \text{ yd/sec})/0.95 \text{ sec}$$
$$= (1.85 \text{ yd/sec})/0.95 \text{ sec}$$
$$= 1.95 \text{ yd/sec}^2$$

20–30 Yards

Calculate average velocity ($\bar{v}$):

$$\bar{v} = 10 \text{ yd in } 0.85 \text{ sec } (3.90 - 3.05)$$
$$= 11.76 \text{ yd/sec}$$

Calculate final velocity (v_f):

$$11.76 \text{ yd/sec} = (v_f + 11.45 \text{ yd/sec})/2$$
$$23.52 \text{ yd/sec} = v_f + 11.45 \text{ yd/sec}$$
$$v_f = 12.08 \text{ yd/sec}$$

Calculate acceleration (a):

$$a = (12.08 \text{ yd/sec} - 11.45 \text{ yd/sec})/0.85 \text{ sec}$$
$$= (0.63 \text{ yd/sec})/0.85 \text{ sec}$$
$$= 0.74 \text{ yd/sec}^2$$

30–40 Yards

Calculate average velocity ($\bar{v}$):

$$\bar{v} = 10 \text{ yd in } 0.83 \text{ sec } (4.73 - 3.90)$$
$$= 12.05 \text{ yd/sec}$$

Calculate final velocity (v_f):

$$12.05 \text{ yd/sec} = (v_f + 12.08 \text{ yd/sec})/2$$
$$24.10 \text{ yd/sec} = v_f + 12.08 \text{ yd/sec}$$
$$v_f = 12.02 \text{ yd/sec}$$

Calculate acceleration (a):

$$a = (12.02 \text{ yd/sec} - 12.08 \text{ yd/sec})/0.83 \text{ sec}$$
$$= (- 0.06 \text{ yd/sec})/0.83 \text{ sec}$$
$$= - 0.07 \text{ yd/sec}^2$$

40–50 Yards

Calculate average velocity ($\bar{v}$):

$$\bar{v} = 10 \text{ yd in } 0.83 \text{ sec } (5.56 - 4.73)$$
$$= 12.05 \text{ yd/sec}$$

Calculate final velocity (v_f):

$$12.05 \text{ yd/sec} = (v_f + 12.02 \text{ yd/sec})/2$$
$$24.10 \text{ yd/sec} = v_f + 12.02 \text{ yd/sec}$$
$$v_f = 12.08 \text{ yd/sec}$$

Calculate acceleration (a):

$$a = (12.08 \text{ yd/sec} - 12.02 \text{ yd/sec})/0.83 \text{ sec}$$
$$= (0.06 \text{ yd/sec})/0.83 \text{ sec}$$
$$= 0.07 \text{ yd/sec}^2$$

These calculations are summarized in Figure 5–1. From these results, it is obvious that this athlete had finished accelerating after thirty yards, reached his or her peak acceleration during the first ten yards, and maintained maximal running velocity from the thirty-yard marker to the 50-yard marker, i.e., approximately 12.05 yd/sec. Had the individual been able to maintain maximal running speed for the full one hundred yards, he or she would have completed the one hundred yards in 9.7 sec, i.e., 5.56 sec for the first 50 yards and 0.83 sec/10 yd for each of the final ten-yard segments. A detailed analysis such as this enables the coach and athlete to analyze the performance to determine in which segments the athlete's running speed can be improved.

The speed of movement of external objects that are propelled by the body can also be assessed. The techniques that are used are identical to those described for measuring the speed of limb movement with cinematography, or for measuring maximal velocity and acceleration with precision measuring devices. These techniques have been used to measure the speed at which a baseball or football can be thrown, the maximal speed and acceleration of a baseball bat or the head of a golf club, and the acceleration of the discus or javelin. These measurements can be of tremendous assistance to the coach or athlete who is attempting to improve performance. As a practical example of their utility, suppose a baseball coach is faced with the problem that three pitchers want to change from a full wind up preparatory to the pitch to a no wind up position. Will this change alter their pitching effectiveness? One of the factors that must be considered is whether the pitchers will sacrifice or gain maximal velocity by making this change. With the ability to measure pitching velocity, the coach will be able to determine the influence of this change in style. Consider another example in a similar situation. A coach or athlete may want to determine whether an isokinetic weight training program that is designed for baseball pitchers will effectively increase maximal pitching velocity. With the ability to determine pitching speed accurately, this information can be easily attained.

While not a measure of speed, as such, the anaerobic capacity or power of the athlete is closely related to speed and burst-type activity. The sprinter trains to develop anaerobic power, as well as acceleration and maximal velocity, the components of speed. It is not yet clear as to how anaerobic power specifically influences performances that are of a speed or burst-type nature. However, it is suspected that a highly developed anaerobic power, or capacity, is related to the ability to maintain the maximal running velocity or to perform repeated runs up and down the court or field, without substantially decreasing the quality or speed of the runs. Thus, some appropriate measure of anaerobic power would be an important assessment to have

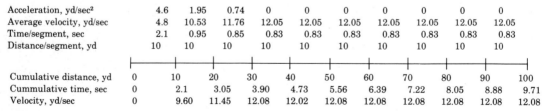

Acceleration, yd/sec^2		4.6	1.95	0.74	0	0	0	0	0	0	0	
Average velocity, yd/sec		4.8	10.53	11.76	12.05	12.05	12.05	12.05	12.05	12.05	12.05	
Time/segment, sec		2.1	0.95	0.85	0.83	0.83	0.83	0.83	0.83	0.83	0.83	
Distance/segment, yd		10	10	10	10	10	10	10	10	10	10	
Cumulative distance, yd	0	10	20	30	40	50	60	70	80	90	100
Cummulative time, sec	0	2.1	3.05	3.90	4.73	5.56	6.39	7.22	8.05	8.88	9.71
Velocity, yd/sec	0	9.60	11.45	12.08	12.02	12.08	12.08	12.08	12.08	12.08	12.08

Figure 5–1   Illustration of running speed, maximal velocity, and acceleration.

for any athlete who depends on speed. The Margaria Power Test was designed specifically to assess anaerobic power or capacity. This test was described in Chapter 4, Strength, Power, and Muscular Endurance, and is illustrated in Appendix C. This particular test is restricted to the legs and appears to be heavily dependent on body weight in order to attain a high score. As was mentioned in the first section of this book, the entire subject of anaerobic metabolism is just beginning to be explored in depth. With additional research, hopefully, additional tests of anaerobic power will be developed, which will provide more realistic estimates of the factors associated with anaerobic metabolism.

Agility and neuromuscular coordination are much more difficult to assess objectively. This is primarily due to the lack of adequate definitions for both agility and neuromuscular coordination. The definitions for these terms are likely to vary somewhat from one sport or activity to another. Neuromuscular coordination to the ballet dancer implies balance and sense of position, while the basketball player thinks of hand-eye coordination and the ability to control one's body in the air. As a result, test batteries have been devised to provide two or more specific tests, which, when combined into a single score, provide an estimate of either one or both of these two components. These tests have fallen into the general category of motor-fitness or motor-ability tests. Test batteries include the shuttle run, squat thrust, dodge run, obstacle race, balancing tasks, and specific sports-skill tasks. Two of the more comprehensive test batteries developed so far are the Iowa-Brace Test and the Fleishman Test. Opinion, at present, questions the usefulness of tests of "general" motor fitness or ability and favors the concept that skill or ability is specific to the individual task.

Flexibility is somewhat easier to measure than agility and neuromuscular coordination, but it is difficult to quantify objectively. In the past, simple tests such as the sit-and-reach test provided a fair estimate of general flexibility. In the sit-and-reach test, the individual sits on the floor with the feet extended forward in front of him or her (Figure 5–2), pressed flat against a box that supports the measuring device. With the back of the knees pressed flat against the floor, the individual leans forward and extends the finger tips as far as he or she can reach. The distance reached is recorded and serves as an approximation of one's flexibility at the hips. Several tests of this nature have been developed for assessing the flexibility of different parts of the body.

While tests such as these are adequate for mass screening, they do have inherent limitations. Most importantly, they do not allow for differences in limb length or proportional differences between the legs and arms. The individual with long arms and short legs will attain a good score on the sit-and-reach test, even if one has limited or poor flexibility. Likewise, the individual with short arms and long legs will be penalized and find it difficult to attain an acceptable score.

More accurate estimates of flexibility can be made with the Leighton flexometer or the ELGON, two devices that are available commercially. Both of the devices assess the degrees of rotation through the full range of motion.

The Leighton flexometer has a weighted 360-degree dial and a weighted pointer mounted in a case. The dial and pointer move independently and are both controlled by gravity. Both can be locked in position independently of each other. The segment is usually positioned at one extreme in the range of motion, the dial locked in position, and then the segment moved through the full range of motion. The pointer follows the movement of the segment, thus indicating the extent of joint movement in degrees. Since the length of limbs or seg-

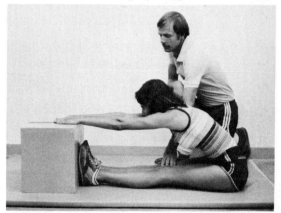

Figure 5–2 The sit-and-reach test to determine flexibility at the hip joint.

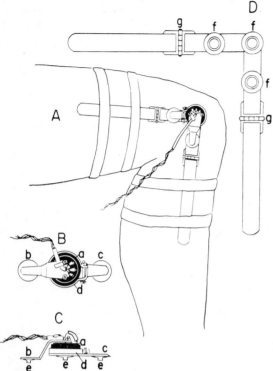

Figure 5–3 Electrogoniometer (ELGON). (From P. V. Karpovich and W. E. Sinning. *Physiology of Muscular Activity,* 7th ed. Philadelphia: W. B. Saunders Co., 1971. Reproduced by permission of the publisher.)

ment does not influence this assessment, the device provides a more accurate estimate of joint flexibility than cruder instruments or tests.

An electrogoniometer or ELGON is illustrated in Figure 5–3. A goniometer is a protractor-like device, which is used to measure the joint angle at both extremes in the total range of movement. With the ELGON, the protractor has been replaced by a potentiometer that can provide an electrical signal proportional to the angle of the joint. This device can give continuous recordings during a variety of activities. Assessments of movement have been made during jumping, running, basketball shooting, and general sports movements. The versatility of this unit allows a much more accurate and realistic assessment of functional flexibility, i.e., the degree of flexibility exhibited during an actual physical activity, as opposed to the more conventional measures of static flexibility, as previously described.

TRAINING PROCEDURES FOR DEVELOPING SPEED, AGILITY, NEUROMUSCULAR COORDINATION, AND FLEXIBILITY

Speed

The development of speed is not an easy task. While strength and endurance can be developed by 20 to 50 percent or more, it is unusual for speed to be increased more than 10 percent, even after years of specialized training. A fully mature boy who can run the one hundred-yard dash in 10.9 sec prior to extensive training or coaching, would be extremely fortunate to lower his or her time to 10.0 sec, a time that would represent an improvement in speed of slightly more than 8 percent. Speed appears to be primarily the result of a proper genetic combination, i.e., good sprinters are more than likely born rather than developed into good sprinters. An internationally famous college track-and-field coach once told a story of how a student from Africa, who attended his university as a freshman, wanted to run the sprints on the track team, although he had never competed or been coached previously. On his first time trial in the hundred-yard dash, he coasted to a 9.9-sec clocking, exhibiting the poorest possible form. Immediately, this coach knew that with proper coaching and training, he would be a world-record-setting sprinter. After four years of intensive training and diligent coaching, the athlete was able to sprint the hundred yards with outstanding form, great stamina, and a 10.1 sec clocking!

On the other hand, the Russian sprinter Borzov, who was outstandingly successful during the early 1970s, including winning gold medals in the 1972 Olympic Games, was developed by Russian sport scientists at one of the several Russian institutes for research in the sport sciences. The scientists, following an exhaustive analysis, established a comprehensive anthopometric, biomechanical, physiological, and performance profile of the characteristics that were necessary for an individual to become a world-class sprinter. A careful search and screening of athletes in Russia led to the discovery of Borzov, who was then a long jumper, and others. Following months of scientifically designed training within the confines of the Physical Education Institute at Kiev, Borzov was unveiled and immediately became one of the top sprinters in the world. Obviously, genetics were important in the initial selection process, but the important point to be made is that Borzov was developed through specialized training into a world-class athlete. The science of sport is just beginning to develop to the point where athletes can be preselected for their best sport or event on the basis of rigid scientific criteria and then placed on training programs that are individually designed to take advantage of their strengths and to develop those areas in which they are weak.

Training programs to develop speed must concentrate on the type of speed to be developed, i.e., total body, limb, acceleration, or maximal velocity. Speed is specific to the area being developed. The 9.3 sec/100-yd dash sprinter will not necessarily be able to fire a fastball into a catcher's mitt at 95 mph or throw a left jab into the face of his opponent with "lightning-like" speed.

The training program must be carefully selected to concentrate on those areas that are important to the athlete. deVries (1974) has stated that speed is the result of both positive and negative forces. Muscular contractions are positive forces, while air or water resistance, gravity, friction, and inertia are some examples of negative forces. Increases in speed can result from decreasing the influence of the negative forces or increasing the influence of the positive forces, or both. Thus, swimmers might shave their bodies free of hair to reduce friction and water resistance, and strength train their upper bodies to increase the force of the muscular contractions. Track sprinters might select a better pair of shoes, alter their forward lean to reduce friction and air resistance, and strength train their lower bodies to increase the force of muscular contractions. This illustrates the importance of individualizing training on the basis of the sport or event. Each sport, event, and position must be analyzed in the closest detail to determine how each positive and negative factor can be altered to maximize the performance potential of the individual.

While speed is highly specific to the movement, there are general factors that influence speed, which should be considered when designing a train-ing program. These include strength, reaction time, and flexibility. As was discussed in Chapter 4, Strength, Power, and Muscular Endurance, strength training does result in increases in speed, both specific speed of isolated limbs or body segments, as well as general body speed. One study cited an improvement from 5.3 to 5.1 seconds for the time to sprint forty yards, which could be considered a substantial improvement. Strength training has also been shown to decrease reflex time, which should facilitate overall speed. Reaction time can be improved by repeated practice of that specific movement. Last, flexibility can be greatly increased within a very short period of time, i.e., within several weeks. This could assist in the development of speed, although the value of increased flexibility is based more on logic than on objective, experimental evidence.

Biomechanical factors probably play the largest role in determining speed and the ability to increase speed. Stride length and stride frequency are two factors that are extremely critical. Research tends to point to stride length as the more critical of the two since stride frequency potential is much higher than is ever used in competition (Cavanagh et al., 1977). However, it must be realized that it is important to increase stride frequency and stride length when running, up to a certain speed. At a critical point, it will be necessary to increase either one or the other, since the resulting speed is too fast for both frequency and length of stride to be increased. In fact, increasing one of these factors may even lead to a decrease in the other, e.g., if the stride length becomes too long, it will take too much time to initiate the next stride, decreasing the stride frequency. Factors such as foot position relative to the center of gravity, knee lift, angle of the back leg at push off, and positioning of the various body segments are just some of many biomechanical factors that influence speed. Therefore, a detailed biomechanical analysis of each athlete would be necessary to determine individual strengths and weaknesses.

Increasing total body neuromuscular coordination is also an important goal of training for speed improvement. Running as rapidly as possible is an extremely complex task and requires intense concentration and coordination of all of the body movements. The movement patterns of the highly skilled sprinter appear to flow and are not at all forced. This is the result of perfectly integrated movement patterns. While this trait must be inherent, it is possible to improve the coordination of the movement patterns through repeated practice and intelligent coaching.

Recently, track and cross-country coaches have started using hill running to improve speed. This was one of the most important training concepts used by the Russians in training Borzov. A hill with a gradual 5–10-percent grade is used. The athlete runs up one side of the hill, a distance of 400 to 800 yards, and down the other side, as rapidly as possible. Running up the hill helps develop dynamic strength and power, while the downhill run helps develop rapid leg-movement patterns. While no formal research has been conducted on the advantages of this type of training compared to traditional sprint training, many coaches feel that it has been of tremendous value in training their runners for speed.

Several methods of speed training have been employed on the track, with varying degrees of success. Interval training is a form of training that alternates fast with slow periods of exercise. Using running as an example, for interval training, the variables that must be considered are the distance of the fast runs, the interval of recovery between the fast runs, the number of repetitions of fast runs, the duration of the fast runs, and the type of recovery activity (walking or jogging). An example of a typical, interval training program would be ten repetitions of 110 yards, each completed in 14 seconds, and 110 yards of jogging during the recovery, after each repetition. The athlete would sprint 110 yards in 14 seconds, jog 110 yards slowly, sprint a second 110 yards in 14 seconds, jog 110 yards slowly, etc., until the full ten repetitions are completed. Either slow or fast interval training can be effectively employed, the two differing only in the pace that is used in the sprint part of the interval program. Interval training will be discussed in greater detail in the next chapter.

Repetition running is similar to interval training, but involves repetitions of comparatively longer distances, with nearly complete periods of recovery. In comparision, the distances are shorter and the recovery is not complete in true interval training. In repetition running, the distances are normally 880 yards to two miles, with recovery being determined by a reduction in heart rate well below 120 beats/min.

Interval sprinting involves alternating sprints of fifty yards and jogs of sixty yards for distances up to three miles. The recovery period is quite short and the athlete fatigues quite rapidly. Acceleration sprinting is a gradual acceleration from jogging to striding and then to sprinting. As an example, the athlete would jog fifty yards, stride fifty yards, sprint fifty yards, walk fifty yards, and then repeat the entire sequence for a set number of repetitions.

The majority of the information in this section is geared toward improving running speed, primarily because this is the area in which most of the research has been conducted, to date. However, many of the principles covered can also be used to train the swimmer, bicyclist, or athlete in any other sport where speed, other than running speed, is important. To improve basic speed, the development of strength, reaction time, neuromuscular coordination, and flexibility would be equally important. It is somewhat ironic that, not too many years ago, weight training was not allowed in training programs for most athletes because it was felt that the gains in strength and muscle hypertrophy would limit flexibility and reduce speed. Fortunately, formal research and informal experimentation by the athletes have proven that strength training has just the opposite effect, i.e., increased strength and flexibility, in almost all sports. The importance of the different biomechanical factors vary with each sport and have to be carefully analyzed. Swimming, for example, is performed in water, a medium that involves a totally unique set of biomechanical factors and principles for successful performance. Several recent textbooks in biomechanics and review articles on specific activities or sports are listed in the reference section of this chapter for a detailed analysis of each sport, activity, or event.

Most of the specific training areas that have been discussed require individuals to use the activity that they are training for as the vehicle or mode of training. Track sprinters must run, sprint swimmers must swim, and sprint cyclists must ride their bicycles. They must all perform repetitious training in their specific activity. This has usually been accomplished through interval training. Interval training is used for both speed and endurance training and will be covered in greater detail in Chapter 6, Cardiovascular Endurance. Circuit training, another form of training that can influence the development of speed, was covered in depth in the previous chapter.

Agility and Neuromuscular Coordination

Agility and neuromuscular coordination in a particular sport can be improved by developing a training program that works on those specific components of agility and neuromuscular coordination that are unique to that sport or activity. The soccer player must work on eye-foot coordination and balance. The tennis player is more concerned about developing hand-eye coordination and a sense of position relative to one's opponent. Strength, power, reaction time, flexibility, mental alertness, and the ability to concentrate and focus on the task at hand, all contribute to agility and neuromuscular skill. Each of these components can be trained separately, or they can be integrated and practiced as a whole. As an example, basketball players can practice their fade-away jump shot as an integrated movement pattern, and also work on each of the specific components. They can weight train their hip and leg extensor muscles to develop strength and power, enabling them to jump higher and quicker. They can practice their reflexes to varying situations, attempting to improve reaction time. They can perform hamstring flexibility exercises to increase the flexibility of the hamstring muscle group. Mental alertness and concentrative powers can be greatly increased through optometherapy, an exciting new area that is presently being developed. Again, however, because of the specificity of training, the majority of the training must be specific to the sport or activity in which athletes are participating.

Optometherapy is an area with great promise for "fine-tuning" the athlete's neuromuscular coordination. Emphasis is placed on the visual system and its interaction with other body components and systems. Reilly, Harrison, and Lee (1973) summarized the results of their work in this area with professional athletes as follows:

- Increased concentration and span of attention
- Ability to cope with the negative influence of crowd noise, movements, visual stimuli, or other stresses during performance
- Ability to generate visual pictures and to use these in the acquisition and perfection of new skills, including preprogramming performance and anticipating plays and situations
- Relaxation before and during performance
- Development and maintenance of rhythm and timing
- More rapid and easier learning
- More efficient performance
- Improved balance and body control
- Ability to critically analyze performance
- More accurate perception of time, space, and direction

The development of conditioned reflexes appears to be an important part of this training. The skilled athlete is one who can immediately recruit a coordinated movement pattern without having to think it through. As the athlete develops in any skill, the recruitment of movement patterns changes from conscious control to conditioned reflexes. The more the activity is conditioned into a natural reflex action, the greater the athlete's degree of skill. This frees the mind to concentrate on more detailed aspects of the activity. Repetitious practice is the primary way in which motor patterns become conditioned reflexes. The athlete repeats the movement so often that the neural pathways become fixed and the movement becomes automatic. Once a skill is learned, it can be recalled with ease in a movement pattern that is coordinated and exact. A word of caution must be included at this point. Poor movement patterns or bad habits can be learned just as easily as good movement patterns. Therefore, the athlete must be observed closely at first, to make certain that he or she is performing the movement correctly. Constant repetition of an incorrectly learned pattern is extremely difficult to correct. This is the reason many tennis instructors dislike working with individuals who have attempted to learn tennis on their own. Frequently, they have already developed many bad habits that are difficult to correct. It is easier to start fresh with novices who have never held a tennis racquet in their hand prior to the first lesson.

As the basic skills are learned and become conditioned reflexes, the athlete can start to embellish his or her basic performance. Once the fast ball can be thrown accurately to the catcher, the pitcher can start working on the curve ball or slider. As the tennis player masters the backhand and forehand drives, he or she can start concentrating on how to vary the speed and the spin on the ball. The more movements the athlete can commit to conditioned reflexes, the more versatile will be one's performance and the greater one's potential for success.

Flexibility

A great deal can be done to increase the athlete's flexibility. Flexibility training is not difficult, requires little time and effort, and can be a pleasant experience. Most flexibility training can be accomplished during either the warm-up or cool-down phases of the daily work out.

deVries (1974) pioneered much of the work in the area of flexibility and athletics. He defines two types of flexibility: static and dynamic. Static flexibility refers to the range of motion of a particular joint. Dynamic flexibility refers to the flexibility of motion, i.e., the ease with which a joint moves through its range of motion during dynamic activity. If a muscle contracts quickly or in a jerky motion, it will stretch the antagonist muscles causing them to contract, thus limiting the range of dynamic motion. A firm, static stretch involves the inverse myotatic reflex, which results in an inhibition of the antagonist group of muscles, allowing them to relax, which enhances or increases the range of motion.

Methods of improving flexibility range from those involving rapid or ballistic types of movement, i.e., bobbing or jerking, to those that require slow positioning and static stretching. An example of each type can be illustrated using the hip flexion movement from the front sitting position. In the ballistic approach, the individual bends forward and attempts to touch one's toes with the fingers, and one's knees with the head, by using five or six rapid, jerking, or bouncing motions. In the static approach, the individual grabs his or her ankles with the hands and slowly stretches forward attempting to place the head on the knees. Although research has shown both methods to be equally effective, the static stretching method might be preferred, since there is less danger of injury and soreness and the antagonistic muscles are fully relaxed.

Since the early 1970s, coaches, trainers, and athletes have become more interested in flexibility training programs. Paul Uram, a high school physical education teacher and coach in Butler, Pennsylvania, has developed ideas about flexibility exercises since the early 1960s. His program, which has been adopted by a number of professional, college, and high-school teams, is fairly simple, requiring ten to fifteen minutes before each game or practice. The program is employed on a year-round basis, and all of the major muscle groups and joints are included in the workout. An example of a flexibility workout routine is illustrated in Appendix B, Warm-Up and Flexibility Exercises.

MECHANISMS OF GAINS

The way in which speed is increased is not clearly understood, primarily because those factors that determine an individual's speed have not been clearly defined or established. Speed increases are probably the result of changes in the central nervous system, which facilitate recruitment of motor units, allow a more rapid response to external stimuli, and provide a better, overall coordination of movement patterns. Improvements in strength and flexibility also play a major role. Athletes have stated that they feel that they can throw harder and faster with increased muscle and joint flexibility. This is attributed to the fact that they can get their arms back farther in the preparatory action, which results in a greater "whip-like" action on the ball.

Agility and neuromuscular coordination improvements also come from changes within the central nervous system, although the proprioceptors are important in any functional adaptations that result from training. Repetition of basic movement patterns appears to be the major consideration in improving these characteristics. Establishing learned patterns of movement that can be recalled quickly and integrated into the ongoing activity is the desired goal. The specific changes that occur within the nervous system are not clear at the present time.

Flexibility is gained through either passive, static-types of stretching, or through ballistic-types of movement. The muscles, tendons, and ligaments appear to be the site of any changes in flexibility, whether increased or decreased. The mechanism of change appears to be a simple stretching of the involved tissue.

RELATIONSHIP OF SPEED, AGILITY AND NEUROMUSCULAR COORDINATION, AND FLEXIBILITY TO ATHLETIC PERFORMANCE

Throughout this chapter, many examples have been given as to the importance of the factors of speed, agility and neuromuscular coordination, and flexibility to athletic performance. It is obvious that the track sprinter and the football running back rely on speed for success in their various sports. What about the other less obvious sports? Speed is a component found in just about every sport, with the possible exception of bowling. While baseball is a relatively slow sport, the sprint to first base to beat out a drag bunt or the attempt to break home on a hit-and-run play require bursts of speed. Fencing is an art of finesse and agility, but the weapon is moved with great speed in both offensive and defensive maneuvers, as well as in making quick advances and retreats. Speed, therefore, is an essential component that must be emphasized in every conditioning program.

Agility and neuromuscular coordination are critical to the success of any athlete. This area, more than any other, must receive priority attention when training programs are designed. It is important to use the activity itself in most phases of the training program, since this will help reinforce the movement patterns. Even with strength training, it is helpful and probably more beneficial if the type of training activity can be performed in a way that imitates the actual sport activity. Swimmers should duplicate their swimming motion, pitchers their throwing motion, and place-kickers their kicking motion. This will reinforce the movement patterns and should develop a more functional strength.

Flexibility is of major importance to the athlete. It is presently believed that the flexible athlete not only is more proficient, but less prone to serious injury. Flexibility in the antagonistic muscles is important in preventing muscle injuries, particularly with rapid limb movement. Muscle pulls and joint injuries occur when the muscles and joints have poor or limited flexibility. On the other hand, muscles and joints that are too loose or flexible also present a greater potential for injury. Thus, athletes must adjust their training programs to provide themselves with a degree of flexibility that prevents injuries, but is not so extreme that there is too much flexibility, leaving the muscles and joints in a vulnerable position.

GENERAL SUMMARY

Speed, agility, neuromuscular coordination, and flexibility are components of physical training that are extremely important for athletes in all sports and events. Speed is defined as the rate of motion or the velocity of the body or any one of its parts. While average velocity is the most frequently used measure of speed, speed can also be measured in terms of acceleration and maximal or peak velocity. Agility and neuromuscular coordination refer to the maneuverability of the individual and the ability to perform in a smooth, balanced, and fluid motion. Flexibility refers to the looseness or suppleness of the body or specific joints through their range of motion.

Speed can be assessed relative to a specific body segment, e.g., speed of the arm movement, to the total body, and to external objects propelled by the body. Assessment can be simple, such as timing the individual through a set distance, or it can be complex, using cinematography, elaborate timing devices, or fundamental equations to calculate acceleration, sequentially, at fixed segments in the total movement.

Agility and neuromuscular coordination can be assessed by a number of different tests of general motor fitness or motor ability. These tests generally contain test items, such as the shuttle run, squat thrust, dodge run, obstacle race, balancing tasks, and specific sports skill tasks. Flexibility can be assessed by a number of simple, stretching-type tests, such as the sit-and-reach test, but it is more accurately measured with either a flexometer or an electrogoniometer. While a flexometer measures static flexibility through the full range of motion, the electrogoniometer can measure continuous changes in the range of motion during a variety of activities, thus providing an assessment of dynamic flexibility.

Although speed is an inherent characteristic, determined largely through genetics, it is possible to train the sprinter to develop greater speed. The degree of improvement, however, is considerably less than would be found with either strength or endurance training. Since speed is specific to the activity, the training must be specific. In addition, since general factors such as strength, reaction time, and flexibility influence speed, training programs should include specialized development in these areas. Biomechanical factors are also extremely important in the development of speed and should be carefully analyzed to determine where the athlete should concentrate his training.

Agility and neuromuscular coordination must be developed specifically for the sport or activity, since each has its own unique demands. Considerable, repetitious practice is required to develop conditioned reflexes that respond in a smooth and integrated manner. In addition, attention should be given to developing strength, power, reaction time, flexibility, mental alertness, and the ability to concentrate on the task at hand.

Flexibility can be incorporated into the training program either through ballistic-types or static stretching-types of flexibility exercises. Both types appear to be equally effective; however, the static stretching exercises are less likely to result in injury and soreness.

This chapter considers the possible mechanisms of gains in strength, agility and neuromuscular coordination, and flexibility, in addition to how they are related to the athlete's actual performance. It is concluded that each of these factors is important for successful performance, no matter what the sport.

STUDY QUESTIONS

1. What are the two major components of speed?
2. How is acceleration measured in sprint-type activities?
3. What are the major factors that limit joint flexibility?
4. How can the speed of body segments or sports implements be measured?
5. Describe a training program for the development of sprinting speed.
6. Describe a training program for the development of arm speed.
7. Of what advantage is hill training for sprint speed?
8. How can one improve neuromuscular coordination?
9. Describe a circuit training program as it might be developed for a basketball team.
10. What are the basic advantages of circuit training over other forms of training for developing speed, flexibility, and agility?
11. What physiological adaptations occur to allow one to become faster?

REFERENCES

Atwater, A. E. "Cinematographic Analysis of Human Movement." In *Exercise and Sport Sciences Reviews,* vol. 1, edited by J. H. Wilmore. New York: Academic Press, 1973.

Barney, V. S.; Hirst, C. C.; and Jensen, C. R. *Conditioning Exercise.* St. Louis: C. V. Mosby Co., 1965.

Cavanagh, P. R.; Pollock, M. L.; and Landa, J. "A Biomechanical Comparison of Elite and Good Distance Runners." *Annals N.Y. Acad. Sci.* 301 (1977): 328–345.

Cooper, J. M., and Glassow, R. B. *Kinesiology.* 4th ed. St. Louis: C. V. Mosby Co., 1976.

Cretzmeyer, F. X.; Alley, L. E.; and Tipton, C. M. *Track and Field Athletics.* 8th ed. St. Louis: C. V. Mosby Co., 1974.

deVries, H. A. *Physiology of Exercise for Physical Education and Athletics.* 2nd ed. Dubuque, Iowa: William C. Brown Co., 1974.

Dillman, C. J. "Temporal and Kinematic Analyses of Running." In *Exercise and Sport Sciences Reviews,* vol. 3, edited by J. H. Wilmore and J. F. Keogh. New York: Academic Press, 1975.

Dyson, G. H. G. *The Mechanics of Athletics.* 7th ed. London: University of London Press, 1977.

Garrison, L.; Leslie, P.; and Blackmore, D. *Fitness and Figure Control: The Creation of You.* Palo Alto, Calif.: Mayfield Publishing Co., 1974.

Hay, J. G. *Biomechanics of Sports Techniques.* 2nd ed. Englewood Cliffs, N.J.: Prentice-Hall, 1978.

Hay, J. G. "Biomechanical Aspects of Jumping." In *Exercise and Sport Sciences Reviews,* vol. 3, edited by J. H. Wilmore and J. F. Keogh. New York: Academic Press, 1975.

James, S. L., and Brubaker, C. E. "Biomechanical and Neuromuscular Aspects of Running." In *Exercise and Sport Sciences Reviews,* vol. 1, edited by J. H. Wilmore. New York: Academic Press, 1973.

Jensen, C. R., and Fisher, A. G. *Scientific Basis of Athletic Conditioning.* 2nd ed. Philadelphia: Lea and Febiger, 1979.

Morgan, R. E., and Adamson, G. T. *Circuit Training.* London: G. Bell and Sons, 1961.

Reilly, R. E.; Harrison, W. D.; and Lee, W. C. *Introduction to Optometherapy.* Davis, Calif.: Vision Center for Sports, 1973.

Sorani, R. P. *Circuit Training.* Dubuque: William C. Brown Co., 1966.

6

Cardiovascular Endurance

INTRODUCTION

Of the various components that comprise the total physical training program, endurance is probably the most underrated. It is given relatively little attention in the training programs of most nonendurance athletes. The football player fails to understand why an endurance component is important in his total training program. Football is perceived as an anaerobic activity, consisting of repeated bouts of high-intensity work of short duration. Seldom does a run exceed forty to sixty yards, and even this is followed by a substantial rest interval. From all outward appearances, football is an anaerobic or burst-type of activity, and the need for endurance is not readily obvious. Sport scientists, however, are beginning to recognize the importance of endurance training to all activities, whether sprint-type, slow and skilled, or of an endurance nature. What the football player fails to realize is that this burst-type of activity must be repeated a number of times throughout the game. With a high level of endurance, the quality of the burst activity is maintained, and the athlete is still fresh at the start of the fourth quarter. It is now believed that those teams that fall apart in the final quarter are the teams that have ignored the endurance component in their training programs. A similar case can be made for athletes in most sports and will be presented in detail later in this chapter.

Endurance can be defined as the ability to perform prolonged bouts of work without experiencing fatigue or exhaustion. As was mentioned in Chapter 4, Strength, Power, and Muscular Endurance, endurance is comprised of two separate components, which are related but different in importance to athletic performance and in their manner of development through physical training. Muscular, or local, endurance refers to the ability of a single muscle or muscle group to sustain prolonged exercise. The exercise can be either of a rhythmical and repetitive nature, e.g., pull-ups, or of a static nature, e.g., sustained, isometric contraction. The resulting fatigue is confined to the local group of muscles that was exercised. General, or cardiovascular, endurance refers to the ability of the total body to sustain prolonged, rhythmical exercise. This type of endurance is typified by the long-distance runner who is able to run long distances at a fairly fast pace. Absolute muscular endurance is highly related to the muscular strength of the individual, while cardiovascular endurance is highly related to the development of the cardiovascular and respiratory systems. Muscular endurance was discussed in Chapter 4. Cardiovascular endurance is the topic of the present chapter.

Although cardiovascular endurance is one of the most neglected components in the athlete's training program, exercise physiologists recognize it as probably the most important component in the athlete's physiological profile. Cardiovascular endurance has become synonymous with the term *physical fitness*. A minimal level of cardiovascular endurance is essential for any sport or activity, and current opinion is that even higher levels can facilitate the athlete's performance and reduce chances for serious injury.

ASSESSMENT OF CARDIOVASCULAR ENDURANCE

Cardiovascular endurance can be assessed in the field or in the laboratory. The maximal oxygen consumption ($\dot{V}O_2$ max) is regarded by most sport scientists as the best objective laboratory measure of endurance capacity. As described in Chapter 2, Responses to Acute Exercise, $\dot{V}O_2$ max is defined as the highest attainable oxygen consumption value in maximal or exhaustive exercise. Just as the athlete reaches exhaustion, the volume of oxygen consumed ceases to increase and either plateaus or decreases slightly. It is felt that the attainment of this plateau signals the end of the exercise, since the athlete has taxed one's ability to deliver oxygen to the working muscles to its finite limit. This finite limit will dictate the level of work or the pace that the athlete can tolerate. One can continue for a brief period beyond the time at which $\dot{V}O_2$ max is attained by calling on one's anaerobic reserves, but these also have a finite capacity. With endurance training, this finite limit is increased, with improvements in $\dot{V}O_2$ max of 20 percent or more following a six-month training program (Pollock, 1973). This results in the athlete being able to work at higher levels of work or at a faster pace, thus improving one's athletic performance potential.

In the laboratory, the endurance capacity, or $\dot{V}O_2$ max, is determined while the athlete walks, jogs, or runs on a treadmill (see Figure 2–3), rides a stationary bicycle ergometer (see Figure 2–1), rows on a rowing ergometer (see Figure 2–4), or swims in a swimming flume (see Figure 2–5). While the $\dot{V}O_2$ max may differ by 10 percent or slightly more between these different modes of laboratory exercise, the principles of testing are similar. Using the treadmill as an example, the athlete is first instrumented for the test. This involves attaching a set of electrodes to one's chest and placing a mouthpiece in the mouth with a noseclip positioned to divert all inspired and expired air through the mouthpiece. The electrodes conduct electrical signals from the heart for transmission to an electrocardiograph which provides a recording of the heart's electrical activity i.e., electrocardiogram (ECG). An ECG is used to determine the normality of heart function and also to provide an objective assessment of the athlete's heart rate during exercise.

The mouthpiece is attached to a two-way breathing valve, which allows inspired air, i.e., normal room air, to come in from one side and expired air to be diverted through the other side. All expired air goes through a gas meter, which measures its total volume. Periodically, samples of the expired air are analyzed for oxygen and carbon dioxide content. This information and other factors, such as barometric pressure and temperature of the expired air, are used to calculate the volume of oxygen consumed, the amount of carbon dioxide produced, the respiratory exchange ratio, and the volume of air expired.

The athlete is placed on the treadmill and allowed to relax in the sitting position. Once resting measurements have been obtained, the athlete stands to the side of the treadmill, off the belt, while the treadmill is started. The athlete then steps on the treadmill and begins walking at a moderate speed. After several minutes of adjustment to the unique situation of walking on a treadmill, the speed of the treadmill is increased to a fast walk. There are many different tests that can be performed on the treadmill, but the principles are basically the same. The ultimate purpose is to gradually bring the athlete to a state of total fatigue or exhaustion within a period of eight to fifteen minutes. This can be accomplished by either increasing the speed of the treadmill, or the slope of the treadmill, or both. Changes in speed or slope usually occur every minute or two.

Testing on the bicycle ergometer, rowing ergometer, or swim flume all use the same basic approach to reach the end point of the test—exhaustion. Throughout these tests, continuous measurements are made of the athlete's physiological responses to the exercise. In many cases, it is only the final few minutes of exercise that are important in defining the physiological determinants of endurance capacity. However, the information collected during the early stages of the exercise bout can be of significance in indicating the athlete's efficiency in performing at submaximal levels of work. In fact, several laboratories have their athletes run at a fixed speed, e.g., 200 meters/min or approximately

7.5 mph at a 0-percent slope, and determine the average oxygen consumption once the athlete reaches a steady state. The lower the average oxygen consumption/kg of body weight, the more efficient the athlete (Costill, 1979). The actual significance of these differences in efficiency is not clearly understood at the present time, but they are of obvious importance to the endurance athlete's performance.

Additional tests of cardiovascular endurance capacity include those tests that are referred to as field tests, or performance tests. Over the years, researchers have found that certain field tests have a relatively high correlation or relationship with laboratory tests of endurance capacity, i.e., $\dot{V}O_2$ max. $\dot{V}O_2$ max is regarded as synonymous with the term *aerobic power*, indicating that endurance capacity is almost, or completely, dependent on the aerobic process. From Figure 6–1, it is possible to determine the relative contribution of aerobic and anaerobic metabolism on the basis of how long an individual exercises at full capacity for a particular length of time. For up to two minutes of maximal effort, the exercise is primarily of an anaerobic nature. Maximal effort that lasts between two and two and one-half minutes is divided nearly equally between aerobic and anaerobic work. Maximal effort that lasts more than two and one-half minutes is considered to be more of an aerobic work task. To predict maximal aerobic power, or $\dot{V}O_2$ max, it is necessary to have a field test that lasts substantially longer than two to three minutes. Theoretically, the higher the aerobic component of the total exercise metabolism, the better predictor that exercise test will be of $\dot{V}O_2$ max.

With this in mind, Dr. Bruno Balke developed one of the first field tests of endurance capacity ($\dot{V}O_2$ max), the 1.5-mile endurance run. In this test, the athlete attempts to run the 1.5-mile test distance as fast as possible. When the individuals taking this test have some experience with pacing, the results correlate reasonably well with $\dot{V}O_2$ max. Dr. Kenneth Cooper, in his book, *Aerobics*, proposed a slight modification of the Balke test. He proposed that the distance an individual could run in twelve minutes was a good predictor of $\dot{V}O_2$ max. He reported a correlation of 0.90 between the distance covered in twelve minutes and $\dot{V}O_2$ max in a large group of Air Force personnel. Subsequent studies have reported substantially lower correlations, but this could be

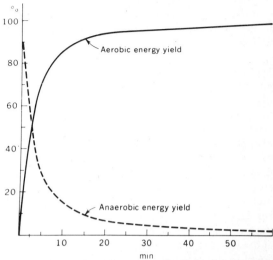

Figure 6–1   Relative contribution of anaerobic and aerobic metabolism to total energy expenditure in maximal work of up to sixty minutes' duration. (From P.-O. Åstrand and K. Rodahl, *Textbook of Work Physiology*. New York: McGraw-Hill Book Co., 1970. Reproduced by permission of the publisher.)

partially the result of using subjects that are unaccustomed to running and do not have any feel for the pace they should or could maintain over the twelve-minute interval. Instructions and scoring tables for both these tests are presented in the last section of this book.

Other tests have been proposed to predict cardiovascular endurance capacity. The American Alliance of Health, Physical Education, Recreation, and Dance has proposed the 600-yard walk-run as a test of endurance capacity. The California State Physical Fitness Test uses a six-minute walk-jog to test for endurance capacity. Both the 600-yard walk-run and the six-minute walk-jog test have been found to have low relationships to actually measured $\dot{V}O_2$ max, which would indicate that neither test is a good predictor of endurance capacity (Vodak and Wilmore, 1975). By referring to Figure 6–1, it is not difficult to determine why neither of these tests are successful predictors of endurance capacity. The six-minute walk-jog test relies on less than 80 percent aerobic effort, and the 600-yard walk-run test takes not more than three to four minutes to complete, which would require less than

60–65 percent aerobic effort. The running-type of field test should require a minimum of twelve to fifteen minutes, which would result in greater than a 90-percent aerobic effort.

Other field tests have been proposed over the years to provide an accurate estimate of cardiovascular fitness, aerobic capacity, or $\dot{V}O_2$ max. Probably the most popular and simple tests to administer are the step tests. Several different types of step tests have been proposed, but they are all similar in principle. The athlete steps up and down on a bench of a set height (usually twelve to twenty inches), at a fixed rate (usually eighteen to thirty-six steps/min), for a fixed time (usually between two and five minutes). An example of this type of test is the Harvard step test, developed at the Harvard Fatigue Laboratory in the early 1940s. The purpose of the test was to measure the ability of the body to adapt to and recover from hard physical work. The athlete would step up and down on a twenty-inch bench at a cadence of thirty steps/min for a period of five minutes, or shorter if he or she could not last the full five minutes. The athlete, following the exercise, would sit down and his or her pulse would be counted for three thirty-second intervals during the recovery period, i.e., from 1–1.5 minutes, from 2–2.5 minutes, and from 3–3.5 minutes. The index of fitness was calculated as follows

Fitness Index =

$$\frac{\text{Duration of exercise (sec)} \times 100}{2 \times (\text{sum of three 30-sec pulse counts})}$$

As an example, if the athlete stepped up and down for four minutes and twenty-five seconds, and his or her pulse count for the first thirty-second counting period was eighty beats, sixty beats for the second counting period, and fifty beats for the third, the individual's index would be

$$\text{Fitness Index} = \frac{265 \text{ sec} \times 100}{2 \times (80 + 60 + 50)}$$

$$= \frac{26,500}{2 \times (190)}$$

$$= \frac{26,500}{380}$$

$$= 69.7$$

This would place the athlete in the average category on the basis of standard scoring tables that have been derived for this test.

Unfortunately, the results from the Harvard step test, or any of the other modifications of the Harvard test, have not correlated very highly with laboratory measures of endurance capacity. The principle behind the tests is good, i.e., the better-conditioned individual will have a lower pulse rate during the period of recovery. However, there is simply too much variability between and within individuals to make this a valid test of endurance capacity.

A similar criticism can be made of another form of endurance capacity test: the physical working capacity (PWC) tests. The PWC tests are usually administered on a bicycle ergometer, and the athlete is exercised at increasing work loads, usually changed every two to three minutes, until he or she reaches some predetermined heart rate. As an example, in the PWC_{170} test, the athlete is exercised to a heart rate of 170 beats/min. The level of work that is required to get the heart rate to this level is referred to as the PWC_{170}. The athlete who is able to perform 1,500 kilopond-meters of work per minute at a heart rate of 170 has a greater endurance, or working capacity, than the athlete who can only reach 1,350 kilopond-meters of work per minute. Again, the principle is sound, i.e., the better-conditioned athlete will have a lower pulse rate for the same level of work or will be able to do more work at the same pulse rate, but the correlations with $\dot{V}O_2$ max are relatively low.

It is unfortunate that these tests are not better predictors of $\dot{V}O_2$ max, for they are very simple to administer and do not require a maximal or exhaustive effort by the subject. The heart rate both during submaximal exercise and recovery should be lower for the same rate or volume of work in the individual with the higher endurance capacity. The tremendous variability between subjects, however, precludes an accurate assessment of endurance capacity utilizing these relationships. But it should be mentioned that these tests can be used with fairly high validity to compare an individual with oneself at different points in time. If an athlete undergoes a strenuous conditioning program, or becomes relatively sedentary or inactive, these pulse rate response tests are sensitive to the resulting changes in one's cardiovascular condition. In fact, one of the last tests given to an astronaut prior to space flight and one of the first tests given immediately upon return from space is a variation of the PWC test. This has been found to be an accurate indicator of the degree of cardiovascular deconditioning that results from extended periods of weightlessness.

TRAINING PROCEDURES FOR DEVELOPING CARDIOVASCULAR ENDURANCE

There are a number of specific endurance training programs, ranging from interval training to long, slow distance (LSD) training, all of which provide similar results and take similar factors into consideration in their designs. The factors to be considered in the development of any cardiovascular endurance program would be progressive overload, duration of each training session, frequency of the training sessions, intensity of the training sessions, the ratio of intense work to rest intervals, and the purpose of the training program. Progressive overload was discussed in Chapter 4 as it applied to the development of strength, power, and muscular endurance. Progressive overload is also important to endurance conditioning and simply implies that the work load for each training session should be greater than the load that can be comfortably performed (overload), and that this work load should be gradually increased as the athlete becomes better conditioned (progressive overload).

The duration of the training session will depend on several factors, including the sport or activity that is being pursued and the intensity of the individual training sessions. The competitive swimmer may have to spend five hours per day in the water, while the football player, using jogging as a general conditioning activity, may work out for only twenty to thirty minutes. The frequency of the training sessions will depend on the endurance training program. For general endurance fitness, three to four days per week are sufficient, but for endurance competition, five to seven days per week are essential. The intensity of the training session will also depend on the purpose of the endurance training program, i.e., fitness or competition, as well as on the philosophy of training for each session, i.e., short-duration, high-intensity or long-duration, low-intensity training. The ratio of the work to the rest intervals also depends on the philosophy of the training program. High-intensity training will necessitate frequent rest intervals, while no rest intervals are needed with low-intensity, continuous training.

With these factors in mind, the basic foundations of several endurance training systems will be explored in the following sections.

Interval Training

Interval training, which was briefly discussed in Chapter 5 in relation to its use for the development of speed, will be discussed in much more detail in this section. The concept of interval training has existed for a number of years in one form or another. deVries (1974) credits the collaboration of a coach, Gerschler, and a physiologist, Reindell, both from Germany, with formalizing a structured system of interval training in the 1930s.

With interval training, short periods of work are alternated with short periods of rest or reduced activity. The concept has a firm foundation in physiological principles. Researchers have demonstrated that athletes can perform a considerably greater volume of work by breaking the total work into short, intense bouts with rest intervals interspersed between consecutive work bouts. The intervals of work and rest are usually equal and can vary from several seconds to five minutes or more. In addition to the work interval and the rest, or relief, interval, the vocabulary of interval training also includes the terms *set, repetition, training time, training distance,* and *frequency.* These terms are comparable to the same terms used in previous sections of this book and will, therefore, not require definition. Interval training is frequently prescribed on the basis of the above terms, as illustrated in this example,

> Set 1: 6 × 440 at 75 sec (90 sec jog)
> Set 2: 6 × 880 at 180 sec (200 sec jog-walk)

In the above example, for the first set the athlete would run six repetitions of 440 yards each, completing the work interval in 75 seconds and resting 90 seconds between work intervals with slow jogging. The second set consists of running six repetitions of 880 yards each, completing the work interval in 180 seconds and resting 200 seconds between work intervals with slow jogging and walking.

The interval training approach can be used in almost any sport or activity, but has received its greatest use in track, cross-country, and swimming. Interval procedures can be adapted to the sport or activity by selecting the form or mode of training and then manipulating the primary variables to fit the sport and athlete. Fox and Mathews (1974) have identified the following five variables that must be individually adjusted for each athlete.

- Rate and distance of the work interval
- Number of repetitions and sets during each training session
- Duration of the rest or relief interval
- Type of activity during the rest interval
- Frequency of training per week

Several methods can be used to determine a sufficient work rate. One that can be used for any form of physical activity is to monitor the pulse rate. The athlete can be assigned a training pulse rate on the basis of his or her maximal heart rate. Since few people have access to a treadmill and electrocardiograph, this can be determined fairly accurately by having the athlete run an all-out, 440-yard run, and then monitoring the pulse rate during the first fifteen seconds of recovery. It can be assumed that the athlete attained maximal heart rate during the 440-yard run, and it is known that the first ten to fifteen seconds of recovery provide an accurate reflection of the heart rate during the last few seconds of exercise.

This procedure can be accomplished quite easily by locating the carotid pulse at the juncture of the head and neck, the radial pulse on the thumb-side of the wrist, or by simply placing the hand directly over the heart. With the second hand of a watch, start by counting the first pulse beat as zero and then count the number of beats in the following fifteen-second interval. This value multiplied by four will provide a reasonably accurate estimate of the maximal heart rate (HRmax) in beats per minute. A set percentage of HRmax can then be used to guide the runner's rate or intensity of work during the work interval. A high-intensity work interval would be run at 95 percent of HRmax, and a moderate-intensity work interval would be run at a rate between 85 and 95 percent of HRmax. Frequently, the duration of the rest intervals is dictated by the return of the HR to a pre-set level, e.g., 120 beats/min. When the heart rate reaches this level, the athlete starts the next work interval.

Another method for establishing the rate or intensity of the work interval is to assign a specific duration for a set distance, e.g., thirty seconds for 220 yards. Wilt (1968) has derived a simple way of establishing these durations. The times for distances between 55 and 220 yards are established by adding between 1.5 and 5.0 seconds, respectively, to the fastest time the athlete can run those distances from a running start. For the distance of 440 yards, one to four seconds should be subtracted from one-quarter of the athletes fastest mile time, e.g., for a five-minute mile, 300 sec/4 = 75 sec − 4 = 71 sec. For distances over 440 yards, each 440 yards of the distance should be run at a speed equal to the average 880-yard time in the athlete's best three-mile run, minus four seconds, e.g., for an 880-yard interval and a fifteen-minute, three-mile best time, 300 sec/4 = 75 sec/440 yd − 4 sec = 71 sec/440 yd or 142 sec (2:22) for the 880 yd.

The distance covered during the work interval can be varied from 20 to 30 yards to distances in excess of several miles. The length of the interval will depend on the athlete. Athletes who run short distances, such as sprinters, basketball players, and football players, will utilize short intervals of 30 to 220 yards, although the 220-yard sprinter will frequently run over-distances of 330 or 440 yards. The miler may run intervals as short as 220 yards, but most of one's training would be at distances of 440 yards, 880 yards, one mile, and some over-distance work. In running over-distance intervals, the athlete extends the length of the interval beyond that distance normally run in competition. Theoretically, this type of training will allow the athlete to complete his or her racing distance at top speed, without experiencing fatigue or exhaustion toward the end of the run. While this is a widespread practice among coaches and the theory appears sound, no research is available to substantiate the value of its use.

The number of repetitions and sets will also be largely determined by the sport, activity, or event of the athlete. Generally, the shorter and more intense the interval, the greater the number of repetitions and sets. As the training interval is lengthened in both distance and duration, the number of repetitions and sets is correspondingly reduced. Fox and Mathews (1974) have established a series of guidelines that can be followed in the selection of the number of repetitions and sets.

The duration of the rest interval will depend on how rapidly the athlete recovers from the work interval. This period of rest can be determined individually, using the athlete's pulse rate to dictate at what time he or she is physiologically ready to start the next work interval. For athletes thirty years of age and younger, it is a common practice to allow the pulse rate to drop to 130–150 beats/min before starting the next repetition and to below 120 beats/min before starting the next set. For those over thirty years of age, since the maximum pulse rate declines with age, reduce the above pulse rate guidelines by 1 beat/min for every year over age 30. As an example, the forty-five-year-old, Masters-competition athlete would use 115–135 beats/min for a recovery pulse rate between intervals, and 105 beats/min for a recovery pulse rate between sets. Since absolute accuracy is not essential in determining these recovery rates, the pulse can be counted for a six-second period and multiplied by ten. This can result in a counting error as large as 10 beats/min, but this is acceptable for these purposes.

The type of activity performed during the rest interval can vary from slow walking to rapid walking and jogging, or the equivalent of these activities in other sports. Generally, the more intense the work interval, the lighter or less intense the work performed in the rest interval. As the athlete becomes better conditioned, he or she will be able to increase the intensity or decrease the duration of the rest interval, or do both.

The frequency of training will depend largely on the purpose of the interval training. The world-class sprinter or middle-distance runner will need to work out five to seven days per week. The athlete who plays team sports, where interval training is used only as a supplement to a general conditioning program, can obtain benefits from two to four days per week. For general conditioning or for off-season conditioning programs, two to four days per week appear to be adequate, although the improvement gained from two days per week programs will be minimal.

The coach or athlete who is interested in the specific details of how to organize and administer an interval training program should refer to the excellent text by Fox and Mathews (1974) cited in the reference section of this chapter. These authors have provided many excellent examples of how interval training can be utilized for various types of conditioning programs. The text by Costes (1972) also provides an excellent practical approach to interval training.

Continuous Training

Continuous training, as the name implies, involves continuous activity, without rest intervals. This has varied from high-intensity continuous activity of moderate duration to low-intensity activity of an extended duration, i.e., long, slow distance, or "LSD," training. High-intensity continuous activity is performed at work intensities that represent 85–95 percent of the individual's HRmax. As an example, the middle-distance runner may run a total distance of five miles, averaging approximately a 5 min/mi pace, with an average pulse rate of 180 beats/min (HRmax = 200 beats/min). The longer-distance runner maintains a pace that is just below his or her racing pace, although this will depend on the competition distance and the distance of the training runs. This has been a very effective way of training endurance athletes without requiring high levels of work that are stressful and uncomfortable for the athlete. One advantage of this type of training for the competitive runner is the constant pace at near-competition levels. Running at an even pace during a race appears to be the most efficient way, physiologically, to attain the runner's best time. Therefore, this type of training would greatly aid the runner in preparing for actual competition. A word of caution should be introduced at this point, however, since the demands of this type of training program are extraordinary, particularly when extended over weeks and months. It is suggested that slower-paced variations, such as LSD or Fartlek, be introduced periodically, e.g., twice per week, to give the athlete some relief from the exhaustive, high-intensity, continuous training.

LSD training became extremely popular during the latter part of the 1960s. Dr. Ernst VanAaken, a German physician and coach, is credited with introducing and popularizing this system of training. Dr. VanAaken's work in this area started in the 1920s, but received widespread support only recently. With LSD training, the athlete performs at a relatively low intensity, e.g., 60–80 percent of HRmax. Pulse rates seldom get above 160 beats/min for the young athlete and 140 beats/min for the older athlete. Distance, rather than speed, is the main objective. Endurance runners may train 15–30 mi/day using LSD techniques, with weekly distances of 100–200 miles. The pace of the run is considerably slower than the maximum pace the individual can sustain. The individual capable of running a 5 min/mi pace will train at a 7–8 min/mi pace. While the cardiovascular and respiratory stress is considerably less and much more tolerable compared to high-intensity continuous training, the extreme distances required can result in significant muscle and joint discomfort and actual injury.

LSD training is probably the most widely used form of endurance conditioning for the jogger who wants to stay in condition for health-related purposes, the athlete who participates in team sports and endurance-trains for general conditioning, and the athlete who wants to maintain endurance conditioning during the off-season. For these purposes, the pace is kept at 60–80 percent of HRmax, but the distance is reduced to three to five miles. This appears to be an excellent approach to general endurance conditioning, since it has been shown to be effective and can be performed at a comfortable level of work. For the middle-aged, or older, individual who is attempting to attain or maintain an acceptable level of physical fitness, this is also the most judicious way to train from a medical viewpoint. Vigorous exercise in the older individual is potentially dangerous and burst-types of activity should not be encouraged.

Fartlek training, or speed play, is another form of continuous exercise that has a flavor of interval training. This form of training was developed in Sweden and is used primarily by distance runners. The athlete varies the pace from high speed to jogging speed as his or her will dictates. This is a free form of training where fun is the main goal and distance and time are not considered. Fartlek training is normally performed in the countryside where there are a variety of hills. Each athlete is free to run whatever course and speed he or she prefers, although the speed should, periodically, reach high intensity levels. Many coaches have used Fartlek training to supplement either high-intensity continuous training or interval training, since it provides variety to the normal training routine. Fartlek runs are normally performed for durations of forty-five minutes or longer.

Interval-Circuit Training

A relatively new concept in training has been introduced in several of the Scandinavian countries. This concept combines interval and circuit training. The circuit may be one to five miles in length, with stations every 400 yards to one mile. The athlete jogs or sprints the distance between stations, stops at each station to perform a strength, flexibility, or muscular endurance exercise in a manner similar to actual circuit training, and continues on, jogging or running, to the next station. These courses are typically located in parks or in the country where there are many trees and hills.

Combination Programs

Dr. Per-Olof Åstrand, a world-famous exercise physiologist in Sweden, has developed his own personal conditioning program which is a combination of interval and Fartlek training (Figure 6–2). It begins with a slow warm-up of five minutes of walking and slow jogging, followed by running up a hill at top speed, walking back down the hill, and then repeating the hill run approximately five times. This is followed by a run on the level at about 80 percent of top speed for three to four minutes, resting for several minutes, and then repeating the sequence three to four times. This is followed by a good sauna (Bastu) bath and, if the athlete chooses, a jump into a cold lake. Like pure Fartlek training, this program provides variety and fun.

Most training programs do not rely purely on any one method or system of training. Each of the training methods presented in this chapter is unique and has inherent advantages or strengths not present in the other methods. Combining methods or systems gives both the coach and athlete variety in their total training program. Boredom is a real hazard of any intense training program, and variety tends to reduce the chances of the athlete becoming bored with a particular training routine.

Wilt (1968) has developed two tables to assist the coach and athlete in designing training programs for competitive runners. Tables 6–1 and 6–2 provide estimates of the training emphasis for various racing distances and the contributions of these different training systems to the major components of run-training, i.e., speed, aerobic endurance, and anaerobic endurance. On the basis of a survey of twenty to thirty top runners in each event conducted by *Runner's World* magazine, the most

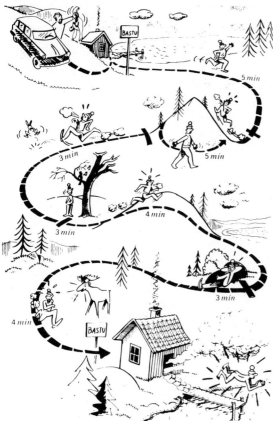

Figure 6–2 Illustration of a combined interval and Fartlek training program. (From P.-O. Åstrand and K. Rodahl, *Textbook of Work Physiology.* New York: McGraw-Hill Book Co., 1970. Reproduced by permission of the publisher.)

popular training patterns for each event were determined. A summary of this survey is presented in Table 6–3.

It appears that a total program of training should include several different systems of training. This is true not only from the stand-point of variety, but also from a physiological point of view. It has been recently theorized that a combination program is essential for the success of the runner, irrespective of the distance of competitive runs. The sprinter may benefit greatly from endurance training, since it allows one to maintain the quality of his or her repeat sprints with interval training. Likewise, the distance runner can benefit from speed work, since he or she is frequently called on to give a finishing kick which is performed at a considerably faster pace than the earlier part of the run. Undoubtedly,

Table 6–1 *Training Requirements for Various Running Distances* (Expressed Relative to the Percentage of Emphasis)*

Event	Speed	Aerobic endurance	Anaerobic endurance
Marathon	5	90	5
6 mi	5	80	15
3 mi	10	70	20
2 mi	20	40	40
1 mi	20	25	55
880 yd	30	5	65
440 yd	80	5	15
220 yd	95	3	2
100 yd	95	2	3

*From F. Wilt "Training for Competitive Running," in Exercise Physiology, *edited by H. B. Falls. (New York: Academic Press, 1968.) Reproduced by permission of the publisher.*

Table 6–2 *Components of Various Systems of Endurance and Sprint Training* (Expressed Relative to Percentage Involvement)*

Type of training	Speed	Aerobic endurance	Anaerobic endurance
Repetitions of sprints	90	4	6
Continuous slow running	2	93	5
Continuous fast running	2	90	8
Slow interval	10	60	30
Fast interval	30	20	50
Repetition running	10	40	50
Speed play	20	40	40
Interval sprinting	20	70	10
Acceleration sprinting	90	5	5

*Adapted from F. Wilt "Training for Competitive Running," in Exercise Physiology, *edited by H. B. Falls. (New York: Academic Press, 1968.) Reproduced by permission of the publisher.*

Table 6–3 Runner's World *Survey* of the Training Patterns of Top-Level Runners*

Race	Avg. Time	Days/ Week	Miles/ Day	Types of Running† (% each)					Training Site (% each)		
				S.D.	F.D.	Int.	Flk.	Race	Track	Road	C-country
100 yards	9.8	5.8	4.8	17	16	49	12	6	50	30	20
220 yards	21.9	5.9	5.0	35	12	39	10	4	37	37	26
440 yards	48.8	5.9	7.5	40	12	35	9	4	44	33	23
880 yards	1:52	6.4	9.0	55	17	17	7	4	28	50	22
1 mile	4:10	6.8	10.5	55	19	15	6	6	22	52	26
2 miles	9:00	6.8	11.0	58	18	11	7	6	17	60	23
3 miles	13:50	6.8	12.8	53	26	9	8	4	18	50	32
6 miles	29:00	6.9	13.0	59	21	10	4	6	18	63	19
9–15 miles	—	6.9	13.0	51	21	5	15	8	17	54	29
Marathon	2:26	6.9	13.1	51	25	5	13	6	13	63	24

†S.D. = slow distance; F.D. = fast distance; Int. = intervals; Flk. = Fartlek.

*From The Complete Runner, *Mountain View, Calif.: World Publications, 1974. Reproduced by permission of the publisher.*

further research in this area will bring forward even better systems of training and a better understanding of the training needs for various sports, activities, or events. However, the basic components have been identified and are probably present in the various systems presently being used.

MECHANISMS FOR GAINING CARDIOVASCULAR ENDURANCE

Cardiovascular endurance can be increased dramatically with endurance training. From previous research, it is clear that an untrained individual can expect to improve one's $\dot{V}O_2$ max between 15 and 25 percent following six months of moderate endurance training, i.e., 3 days/week, 30 min/day, at 60–80 percent of endurance capacity (Pollock, 1973). The better the condition of the athlete, the smaller will be the relative improvement for the same program of training. In fact, it appears that in fully mature athletes, the highest attainable $\dot{V}O_2$ max is reached within twelve to eighteen months of heavy endurance training, indicating that each athlete has a finite level that can be attained. This finite level is clearly influenced by genetic factors and may also be influenced by training in early childhood. The latter observation is purely conjecture, at this point in time, and needs substantiation by experimental research.

The genetic aspects of $\dot{V}O_2$ max have been clearly demonstrated by Klissouras in a series of studies conducted in the late 1960s and early 1970s. Figure 6–3 illustrates the fact that identical, or monozygous, twins have nearly identical HRmax values, while the variability for dizygous, or fraternal, twins was much greater. Similar results have been found for $\dot{V}O_2$ max, as illustrated in Figure 6–4. Åstrand (1972) has stated that the best way to become a champion Olympic athlete is to be selective when choosing one's parents. World-class athletes who have been away from endurance training for many years have been found to have high $\dot{V}O_2$ max values in this sedentary, deconditioned state. It appears that both genetic and environmental factors can influence $\dot{V}O_2$ max values, and that the genetic factors probably establish the boundaries for the athlete, but endurance training can push the $\dot{V}O_2$ max value to the upper limit of these boundaries.

Age and sex can also influence VO_2 max values. However, these values may lead to an improper interpretation of true age and sex differences. Figure 6–5 illustrates the $\dot{V}O_2$ max values of a group of older sprinters and distance runners between forty and seventy-four years old. Their $\dot{V}O_2$ max values do decrease with age, but they are considerably higher than the mean values for their particular age. Similar trends have been found in highly conditioned, female endurance athletes when compared to the normal, sedentary population of

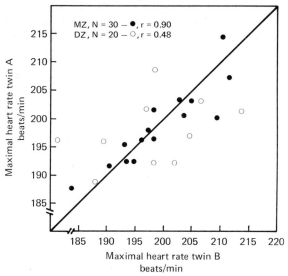

Figure 6–3 Comparison of HRmax between monozygous and dizygous twins. (From V. Klissouras, *J. Appl. Physiol.* 31 (1971): 338–344. Reproduced by permission of the publisher.)

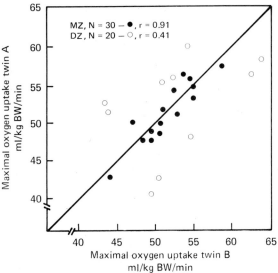

Figure 6–4 Comparison of $\dot{V}O_2$ max between monozygous and dizygous twins. (From V. Klissouras, *J. Appl. Physiol.* 33 (1971): 338–344. Reproduced by permission of the publisher.)

females. In both cases, the average $\dot{V}O_2$ max values for the older individual and for the female are lower than they should be due to the sedentary nature of the two populations.

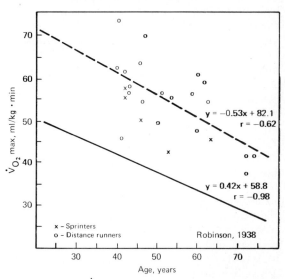

Figure 6–5 $\dot{V}O_2$ max values for a group of older sprinters and distance runners in comparison to normal values for the same age range. (Normal data from S. Robinson, "Experimental Studies of Physical Fitness in Relation to Age," *Arbeitsphysiol.* 10 (1938): 251–323. Reproduced by permission of the publisher.)

When $\dot{V}O_2$ max does improve with endurance training, what physiological factors are responsible for this improvement? As was stated in Chapter 3, Adaptations to Chronic Exercise, this is an area of great controversy at present. Two theories exist at this time. The first states that endurance performance is not limited by the supply of oxygen coming into the tissue by way of arterialized blood, but, rather, by the lack of oxidative enzymes in the mitochondria. Proponents of this theory provide impressive evidence that endurance training programs increase these oxidative enzymes, allowing the active tissue to utilize more of the available oxygen, which would also result in a higher $\dot{V}O_2$ max. In addition, endurance training results in increases in muscle mitochondria. Thus, this theory argues that it is not solely a lack of oxygen coming into the active muscles that limits endurance performance, but that it must also involve an inability of the existing mitochondria to utilize the available oxygen.

The second theory proposes that central and peripheral circulatory factors limit endurance capacity, i.e., an inability to deliver a sufficient amount of oxygen to the active tissue. In this theory, improvement in $\dot{V}O_2$ max following endurance training is believed to result from increases in blood volume, cardiac output (via stroke volume), and a better perfusion of blood in the active tissue. Again, impressive research evidence provides strong support for this theory. In one study, the subjects breathed a mixture of carbon monoxide and air during the exercise to exhaustion (Pirnay et al., 1971). The decrease in $\dot{V}O_2$ max was in direct proportion to the percentage of carbon monoxide breathed. The carbon monoxide molecules were bonded to approximately 15 percent of the total hemoglobin, exactly the same percentage as the reduction in $\dot{V}O_2$ max. In another study, approximately 15–20 percent of the total blood volume was removed, and the $\dot{V}O_2$ max decreased by approximately the same relative amount (Ekblom et al., 1972). In both of these studies, the reduction in the oxygen-carrying capacity of the blood, by either blocking hemoglobin or removing whole blood, resulted in less oxygen being delivered to the active tissues and a corresponding reduction in $\dot{V}O_2$ max. Similarly, breathing oxygen-enriched mixtures, where the partial pressure of oxygen in the inspired air is substantially increased, resulted in large increases in endurance capacity. These studies tend to indicate that it is the available oxygen supply that limits endurance performance. A 1980 review article by Saltin and Rowell confirms the theory that it is the oxygen transport to the working muscles which limits $\dot{V}O_2$ max.

Although it was stated that the highest attainable endurance capacity is usually reached within eighteen months of intense endurance conditioning, endurance performance will continue to improve for many, additional years with continued training. In Chapter 3, it was theorized that this improvement in endurance performance in the absence of improvements in $\dot{V}O_2$ max might possibly be related to being able to perform at increasingly higher percentages of $\dot{V}O_2$ max for extended periods of time (see Figure 2–9 and the text in Chapter 3). The mechanisms for this improvement are probably related to greater mechanical and metabolic efficiency, improved anaerobic metabolism, and greater utilization of fat metabolism. Research interest is starting to focus in this area, and a better understanding of the various factors involved should be possible in the near future.

The use of interval training methods is based on sound physiological principles, as was stated earlier in this chapter. Research has demonstrated that the total amount or volume of work accomplished in a given period of time is much greater if the work is broken into short, intense bouts of work with rest periods interspersed between them, as compared to continuous bouts of work without rest intervals. It should be pointed out, however, that the few studies that have compared interval training with continuous training have not found any differences in results between the two systems, but have found that both systems produce substantial gains in endurance capacity (Saltin, 1975). Additional research in this area is certainly necessary before any final conclusions can be drawn.

RELATIONSHIP OF CARDIOVASCULAR ENDURANCE TO ATHLETIC PERFORMANCE

Cardiovascular endurance is generally regarded as the most important component of physical fitness. Since all athletes should have above-average levels of physical fitness, endurance conditioning becomes an important part of their training program. Even the golfer, whose sport is considered relatively sedentary, will benefit from cardiovascular endurance conditioning. The gains in endurance from such conditioning will allow the golfer to complete a round of golf with less total fatigue, and his or her legs will be better able to withstand the long periods of walking and standing. For the sedentary, middle-aged adult, this should be the primary emphasis of the training program. This will be discussed at length in Chapter 15, Physical Activity for Health and Fitness.

For any athlete, fatigue represents a major deterrent to one's best performance. Even minor or low levels of fatigue have negative influences on the athlete's total performance. Muscular strength is decreased, the reaction and movement times are prolonged, agility and neuromuscular coordination are reduced, the speed of total body movement is slowed, and the level of concentration and alertness is reduced. This latter factor is particularly important, for the athlete may become careless and more prone to serious injury, especially in contact sports. Even though this decrease in the athlete's performance may be small, it may be just enough to cause the individual to miss the critical free-throw in the basketball game, the three-point field goal in football, or the twenty-foot putt in golf.

The extent of endurance training that is necessary will vary considerably from one athlete to the next, depending on their existing endurance capacity and the endurance demands of the sport. It is obvious that the marathon runner will use endurance training almost exclusively, with limited attention to strength, flexibility, and speed. The baseball player, however, has very limited demands placed on endurance capacity, so the training program will emphasize endurance conditioning to a much lesser extent. Nevertheless, it is felt that the baseball player could gain substantially from endurance running, even if the periods are limited to 3 mi/day for 3 days/week at a moderate intensity. He would have little or no trouble with his legs (a frequent complaint of baseball players), and he would be able to complete a double header with little or no fatigue. Many athletes in nonendurance sports, activities, or events have never incorporated even moderate endurance training into their training programs. Those that have incorporated endurance training, generally, are well aware of their improved physical condition and its impact on their athletic performance.

GENERAL SUMMARY

Cardiovascular endurance, in contrast to muscular endurance, is probably the most important component of general physical fitness. As a result, it is an important area that should be developed in the training programs of all athletes. Cardiovascular endurance is defined as the ability of the total body to sustain prolonged, rhythmical exercise. The best measure of cardiovascular endurance capacity in the laboratory is the athlete's maximal oxygen consumption ($\dot{V}O_2$ max), which is assessed by having the athlete exercise to total exhaustion on a stationary work device, such as a motor-driven treadmill or a bicycle ergometer. At higher levels of work, as the athlete approaches exhaustion, oxygen consumption values will start to plateau, or even decline, indicating that the person has attained $\dot{V}O_2$ max and that the end of the exercise bout is near. Field tests such as the 12-minute run, the 1.5-mile

run, step tests, and PWC tests have been used in the past and are presently being used to assess endurance capacity. Several of these tests provide a moderately accurate estimate of endurance capacity, but most of the submaximal tests are inaccurate for a high percentage of the population.

A number of specific training methods or systems exist for developing cardiovascular endurance. The two major classifications of training systems are interval training and continuous training. Interval training involves periods of high-intensity work with rest periods interspersed between the work bouts. In designing an interval training program, attention must be given to the rate and distance of the work interval, the number of repetitions and sets during each training session, the duration of the rest interval, the type of activity during the rest interval, and the frequency of training per week.

Continuous training involves continuous activity without rest intervals. This type of training can be of high intensity, or of moderate intensity and an extended duration (LSD). A third type of continuous activity is the Swedish Fartlek system, which consists of jogging and bursts of sprinting dictated by the will of the athlete. Interval circuit training involves an extended circuit one to five miles long, with several stations along the circuit for exercises of a strength, flexibility, or muscular endurance nature.

Most coaches and athletes develop comprehensive training programs that combine two or more of the above systems. In this manner, the athlete can have more variety in his training, as well as gain from the strengths of the additional systems.

It is known that endurance capacity is influenced by genetic factors, sex, and age. In addition, it can be greatly influenced by physical conditioning. The mechanisms by which the $\dot{V}O_2$ max is increased with endurance training are unclear at the present time, but it is probably the result of a combination of increased mitochondria and oxidative enzymes in the active tissue, as well as an increased blood volume, increased cardiac output, and better perfusion of the active tissue, i.e., increased muscle blood flow.

Cardiovascular endurance conditioning is a critical aspect of any athlete's training program. Low endurance capacity leads to fatigue, even in the more sedentary sports or activities. Such a condition can only work to lower the performance potential of the athlete, since fatigue will reduce strength, speed, reaction and movement time and will have a negative influence on agility and neuromuscular coordination. In addition, the athlete becomes more prone to serious injury, due to an inability to fully concentrate on performance, as well as to the above factors. Adequate cardiovascular conditioning must be the foundation of any athlete's general conditioning program.

STUDY QUESTIONS

1. Differentiate between muscular endurance and cardiovascular endurance.
2. What is the maximal oxygen uptake or consumption ($\dot{V}O_2$ max)?
3. Of what importance is $\dot{V}O_2$ max to endurance performance?
4. What is the best field test of $\dot{V}O_2$ max?
5. Would a two-mile run at full speed be considered an anaerobic or an aerobic activity? Why?
6. How does the concept of progressive overload apply to cardiovascular endurance training?
7. What are the major factors that must be considered when developing a cardiovascular endurance conditioning program?
8. Design an interval training program for a middle-distance runner.
9. How can work intervals be monitored when using interval training procedures?
10. How does high-intensity continuous training differ from interval training?
11. Discuss the relative merits of both interval and continuous training.
12. Explain the two theories that have been proposed to account for improvements in $\dot{V}O_2$ max.
13. How important is genetic potential in developing a young athlete?
14. Why would cardiovascular endurance conditioning be important for athletes in nonendurance sports?

REFERENCES

Åstrand, P.-O. *Journal of Physical Education* (March-April 1972): 129–136.

Åstrand, P.-O., and Rodahl, K. *Textbook of Work Physiology.* 2nd ed. New York: McGraw-Hill Book Co., 1977.

Clausen, J. P. "Effect of Physical Training on Cardiovascular Adjustments to Exercise in Man." *Physiol. Rev.* 57: (1977) 779–815.

Cooper, K. H. *Aerobics.* New York: M. Evans, 1968.

Costes, N. *Interval Training.* Mountain View, Calif.: World Publications, 1972.

Costill, D. L. *A Scientific Approach to Distance Running.* Los Altos, Calif.: Track and Field News, 1979.

deVries, H. A. *Physiology of Exercise for Physical Education and Athletics.* 2nd ed. Dubuque, Iowa: William C. Brown Co., 1974.

Edington, D. W., and Edgerton, V. R. *The Biology of Physical Activity.* Boston: Houghton Mifflin Co., 1976.

Ekblom, B.; Goldbarg, A. M.; and Gullbring, B. "Response to Exercise after Blood Loss and Reinfusion." *J. Appl. Physiol.* 33 (1972): 175–180.

Fox, E. L. *Sports Physiology.* Philadelphia: W. B. Saunders Co., 1979.

Fox, E. L., and Mathews, D. K. *Interval Training Conditioning for Sports and General Fitness.* Philadelphia: W. B. Saunders Co., 1974.

Jensen, C. R., and Fisher, A. G. *Scientific Bases of Athletic Conditioning.* 2nd ed. Philadelphia: Lea & Febiger, 1979.

Klissouras, V. "Adaptability of Genetic Variation." *J. Appl. Physiol.* 31 (1971): 338–344.

Lamb, D. R. *Physiology of Exercise: Responses and Adaptations.* New York: Macmillan Publishing Co., 1978.

Mathews, D. K., and Fox, E. L. *The Physiological Basis of Physical Education and Athletics.* 3rd ed. Philadelphia: W. B. Saunders Co., 1981.

Pirnay, F.; Dujardin, J.; Deroanne, R.; and Petit, J. M. "Muscular Exercise during Intoxication by Carbon Monoxide." *J. Appl. Physiol.* 31 (1971): 573–575.

Pollock, M. L. "Quantification of Endurance Training Programs." In *Exercise and Sport Sciences Reviews,* vol. 1, edited by J. H. Wilmore. New York: Academic Press, 1973.

Runner's World. The Complete Runner. Mountain View, Calif.: World Publications, 1974.

Saltin, B. *Intermittent Exercise: Its Physiology and Practical Applications.* Muncie, Ind.: Ball State University, 1975.

Saltin, B., and Rowell, L. B. "Functional Adaptations to Physical Activity and Inactivity." *Fed. Proc.* 39 (1980): 1506–1513.

Sharkey, B. J. *Physiology of Fitness,* Champaign, Ill.: Human Kinetics Publishers, 1979.

Shephard, R. J. *Endurance Fitness.* Toronto: University of Toronto Press, 1971.

Vodak, P. A., and Wilmore, J. H. "Validity of the 6-Minute Jog-Walk and the 600-Yard Run-Walk in Estimating Endurance Capacity in Boys, 9–12 Years of Age." *Res. Quart.* 46 (1975): 230–234.

Wilt, F. "Training for Competitive Running." In *Exercise Physiology,* edited by H. B. Falls. New York: Academic Press, 1968.

7

Body Build and Composition

INTRODUCTION

The appropriate size, shape, build and composition of the athlete's body is of major importance to success in almost all athletic endeavors. It is obvious that the 7-foot 1-inch center in basketball could never have developed into a proficient jockey. Similarly, the 130-pound marathon runner would not be the ideal candidate for a starting assignment on the defensive line of a professional football team. As was discussed earlier in regard to other components of physical training, each athlete has a genetic profile that largely dictates limits for both body build and composition. Muscle training will develop increased muscle mass to varying degrees, and diet and vigorous exercise, when combined, will lead to substantial losses in body fat. However, when compared to the broad range of body sizes and builds in the total world of athletics, from the small gymnast to the gigantic Sumo wrestler, the range of variability within any one individual is small and quite restricted. Athlete's are then limited by what was given to them by their parents. This does not imply that athletes should dismiss this aspect of their physical profile with the feeling that nothing can be done to improve themselves. While body type or build can be altered only slightly, substantial alterations can occur in body composition that can be of major importance for the athlete's performance.

What is the difference between body build, body size, and body composition? Body build refers to the morphology, or the form and structure, of the body.

Somatotyping is a procedure used in science to describe the morphology of the body in a quantitative manner. Most somatotyping systems utilize the concept that the body has three major components or dimensions: muscularity, linearity, and fatness. The three components have been termed *mesomorphy* for muscularity, *ectomorphy* for linearity, and *endomorphy* for fatness. Since almost everyone has some degree of each of these components, a rating procedure was developed in which each person could be given a rating in each of these three major areas. The original system developed by Sheldon used a rating scale of 1 to 7 to designate, on an increasing basis, the absence of the component to the preponderance of the component, respectively. As an example, a rating of 2–7–2 (endomorphy-mesomorphy-ectomorphy) would indicate an individual who would be described as having a preponderance of muscle, very little fat, and a stocky frame (lack of linearity).

Body size simply refers to the height and mass, or weight, of the individual, e.g., short and small or tall and large. The distinctions of being short or tall, large or small, heavy or light depend entirely on the sport, position within a sport, or a particular event. A height of 6 feet 3 inches would be relatively short for a professional basketball player, but tall for a long-distance runner. Similarly, a weight of 230 pounds would be heavy for a quarterback, but light for a defensive end in football. Body size, therefore, must be considered relative to the sport, position, or event.

Body composition adds a new dimension to the athlete's self-understanding. To know that the athlete weighs 200 pounds means very little to either the athlete or the coach. To know that only 10 pounds is fat and the remaining 190 pounds is lean provides considerably more information that can be of use in assisting that athlete to reach performance potential. With this distribution, the athlete knows that only 5 percent of his body weight [(10 lb/200 lb) × 100] is fat, which is about as low as any athlete should go. He would realize that his weight was not a problem, and that he should not be concerned about a weight loss. However, an athlete of the same weight, 200 pounds, who had 50 pounds of fat and 150 pounds of lean weight would be 25 percent fat, which would constitute a serious weight problem. If the amount of fat in proportion to an individual's total weight is high, it will have a negative influence on athletic performance, i.e., the higher the fat percentage, the poorer the performance. Thus, an accurate assessment of the athlete's body composition will provide one with valuable insight into the most efficient weight for a particular sport or event. As was stated in Chapter 3, Adaptations to Chronic Exercise, total weight is composed of the fat weight and the lean weight. The lean weight is merely a convenient term to account for all of the body tissue that is not fat, e.g., muscle, bone, skin, and weight of the organs. Fortunately, when working with athletes and weight gains and losses, it is primarily the fat and muscle mass that change, therefore, any changes in lean weight are generally reflective of changes in muscle mass.

ASSESSMENT OF BODY BUILD AND COMPOSITION

Somatotype

As was mentioned in the previous section, body build is usually assessed by one of the standard systems of somatotyping. Somatotyping dates back to the time of Hippocrates, who used two basic body types: phthisic habitus, or a long, thin body, and apoplectic habitus, or a short, thick body. Several somatotype systems were developed in the 1800s and early 1900s. In the 1930s, Sheldon revolutionized the science of somatotyping by assigning ratings to each of three categories, endomorphy, mesomorphy and ectomorphy. Prior to this time, somatotyping systems attempted to classify each individual into one of the only two or three broad categories. Sheldon's system allowed for the extreme variability between individuals.

In Sheldon's system, endomorphy is characterized by roundness and softness, as typified by the grossly obese individual. Mesomorphy is characterized by a square body with prominent musculature, as illustrated by the middle-weight weight lifter. The ectomorph is linear and fragile with small muscles and prominent bones, as illustrated by the long-distance runner.

The Sheldon system of somatotyping is quite complex and requires the assistance of a highly skilled, trained technician. First, photographs of the athlete are taken showing the front, rear, and side views. Figure 7–1 illustrates the somatotype photograph of former world-record holder and Olympic champion Peter Snell, a middle-distance runner from New Zealand. Snell, regarded by many as the best all-around track athlete of the twentieth century, was rated 2–6–2, which is predominently mesomorphy, with very little endomorphy or ectomorphy. Once the photograph has been taken, a history of the athlete's height and weight is recorded with special attention to one's maximal achieved weight throughout his or her lifetime. Two indices are calculated: the inverse *ponderal index* (height/$\sqrt[3]{\text{weight}}$) and the trunk index. The trunk index is the ratio of the photographic area of the thoracic trunk to that of the abdominal trunk. It is a measure of the relative degree of endomorphy and mesomorphy, while the inverse ponderal index provides an index of ectomorphy. A series of tables is then used to derive the final somatotype values for the three categories.

A somatogram is used for plotting the various somatotypes of different athletes. This is illustrated in Figure 7–2. A distribution of somatotypes for 4,000 American college students is shown in Figure 7–3 and can be compared with those for Olympic track and field athletes (Figure 7–4). It is interesting to note the absence of any athletes in the endomorphic section of the somatogram.

More recently, several individuals have attempted to simplify the Sheldon system of somatotyping. Probably the most widely used system was intro-

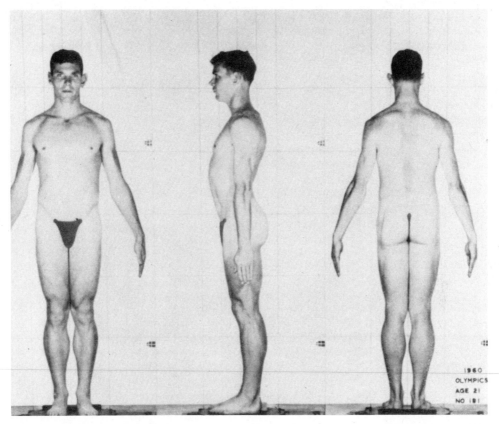

Figure 7–1 Somatotype photograph of former world-record holder and Olympic-champion, middle-distance runner Peter Snell. Somatotype was rated as a 2–6–2. (From J. M. Tanner, *The Physique of the Olympic Athlete*. London: George Allen and Unwin, Ltd., 1964. Reproduced by permission of the publisher.)

duced by Heath and Carter in 1967. Their technique can be effectively utilized by anyone trained in anthropometry, i.e., the study of human body measurements, and it does not require a somatotype photograph. For the first component, similar to endomorphy, the triceps, subscapular, and suprailiac skinfolds are measured; the resulting values are added together; and the total compared with a scale of values to obtain the component rating (Figure 7–5). For the second component, similar to mesomorphy, measurements are taken of height in centimeters, the width of the upper arm bone (humerus) at the elbow joint, the width of the upper leg, or thigh bone (femur), at the knee joint, the girth or circumference of the upper arm and calf,

and the skinfold at the triceps and calf. Again, using a series of scales, the appropriate component rating is obtained. The third component, similar to ectomorphy, is determined by calculating the inverse ponderal index, i.e., height/$\sqrt[3]{\text{weight}}$, and comparing this value with a scale to obtain the rating component. The resulting somatotype is similar to a Sheldon somatotype, as the athlete is rated in all three components. However, the rating scale is open-ended, instead of varying between only 1 and 7. The scale allows an individual to have a rating that exceeds 7 for any one component, but realistically, this seldom happens. The primary advantage of the Heath-Carter system is the ease with which a somatotype can be obtained.

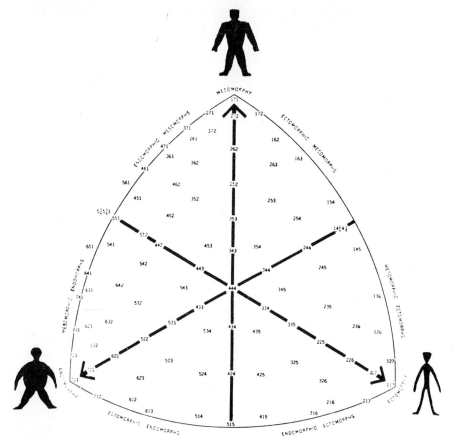

Figure 7–2 Illustration of a somatogram.

Body Composition

Few body composition assessments have ever been conducted directly. A direct analysis can only be performed on a dead body, or cadaver, where the different body tissues can be carefully dissected. This requires a tremendous amount of time and effort, and cadavers are not easy to obtain. Furthermore, of what value is the assessment to the cadaver? Because of the problems associated with direct analysis and the relatively limited use of the resulting data, a number of indirect techniques have been developed to provide an estimate of the body's composition in the living human. The majority of these techniques fractionate the body into only two components, or compartments: the lean body weight and the fat weight. These indirect techniques can be divided into either laboratory or field assessment techniques.

Laboratory Assessment. Probably the most widely used and most accurate laboratory method for assessing body composition is the body density assessment (Behnke and Wilmore, 1974). As was explained in Chapter 3, Adaptations to Chronic Exercise, body density = (body weight/body volume). Body weight is easily determined. The determination of body volume presents a slight problem, but it can be determined rather easily in the laboratory. While there are several ways of determining body volume, the easiest and least expensive way is to measure the athlete's loss of weight in water, which Archimedes discovered was equivalent to the volume of the body. The athlete is

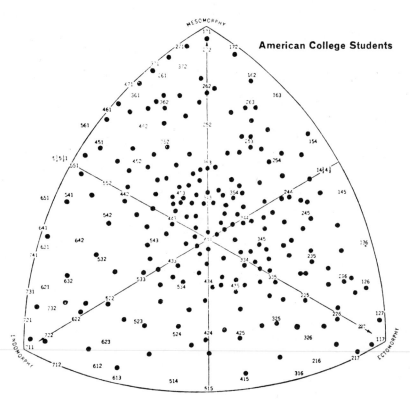

Figure 7–3 Somatogram illustrating the distribution of somatotypes of 4,000 American male, college students. (From J. M. Tanner, *The Physique of the Olympic Athlete.* London: George Allen and Unwin, Ltd., 1964. Reproduced by permission of the publisher.)

weighed while totally submerged under water (refer to Figure 3–3), and this weight subtracted from the athlete's body weight provides an estimate of his or her volume. A correction must be made for the volume of air trapped in the lungs. This is not difficult and can even be estimated in young athletes. An example for two athletes was presented in Chapter 3.

Body volume can also be determined by other methods (Behnke and Wilmore, 1974). One method determines the actual volume of water displaced by the athlete when totally submerged under water. This can be done by having the athlete climb into a large cylinder filled to the top with water. As one lowers oneself into the water, his or her volume will displace an equivalent volume of water. The volume of water that spills over, or the volume of water

necessary to refill the cylinder to the top once the athlete is out of the cylinder, will give approximations of the athlete's body volume when corrected for the air trapped in the lungs. Another technique uses an air-tight booth, similar in appearance to a telephone booth. A small known volume of helium is introduced into the booth where the athlete is sitting relaxed in a chair. The athlete's body volume is determined by the degree of dilution of the helium within the chamber. With a small athlete of low volume, the air space in the booth is quite large and the helium concentration is low due to the dilution by the large volume of air surrounding the athlete. A large athlete has a large body volume, filling most of the booth, leaving a small volume of surrounding air. Introducing the same volume of helium will result in a higher concentration of

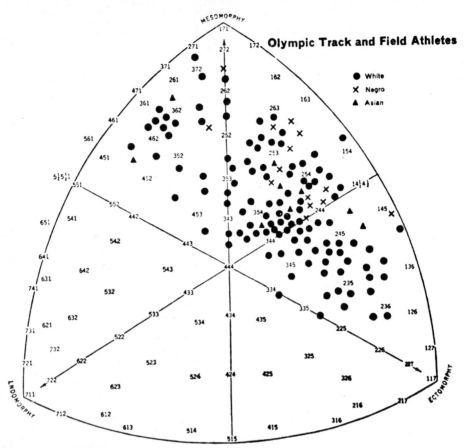

Figure 7–4   Somatogram showing the distribution of the somatotypes of 137 male Olympic track-and-field athletes. (From J. M. Tanner, *The Physique of the Olympic Athlete*. London: George Allen and Unwin, Ltd., 1964. Reproduced by permission of the publisher.)

helium in the chamber, since the air volume is so small. This technique is relatively complex, requiring a rather elaborate engineering design, but it does provide a comparatively comfortable experience for the subject.

Additional methods are available for determining the composition of the body. Radiography is an excellent way to assess local areas of the body, such as the calf, thigh, or upper arm (Behnke and Wilmore, 1974). Soft tissue X-ray differentiates between the various layers of skin, fat, bone, and muscle. An example of this technique is shown in Figure 7–6, illustrating the X-ray of a world-class shotputter. Measurements of bone, muscle, and fat are taken at three specific sites and combined to pro-

vide an estimate of the individual's total body composition. While this technique allows a direct quantification of all three major components, it does present the problem that all areas of the body are not similarly developed. Thus, the estimation of the total body composition could be considerably in error.

Another method that is frequently used in the body composition assessment of athletes is the whole-body counter, which measures the amount of gamma radiation emitted by the body from its naturally occurring potassium-40 (Behnke and Wilmore, 1974). There is a rather constant relationship between the total amount of potassium-40 in the body and the lean body mass. Again,

HEATH-CARTER SOMATOTYPE RATING FORM

NAME .... AGE .... SEX: M F NO: ....

OCCUPATION .... ETHNIC GROUP .... DATE ....

PROJECT: .... MEASURED BY: ....

Skinfolds mm		TOTAL SKINFOLDS (mm)
Triceps =	Upper Limit	10.9 14.9 18.9 22.9 26.9 31.2 35.8 40.7 46.2 52.2 58.7 65.7 73.2 81.2 89.7 98.9 108.9 119.7 131.2 143.7 157.2 171.9 187.9 204.0
Subcapular =	Mid-point	9.0 13.0 17.0 21.0 25.0 29.0 33.5 38.0 43.5 49.0 55.5 62.0 69.5 77.0 85.5 94.0 104.0 114.0 125.5 137.0 150.5 164.0 180.0 196.0
Supraliac =	Lower Limit	7.0 11.0 15.0 19.0 23.0 27.0 31.3 35.9 40.8 46.3 52.3 58.8 65.8 73.3 81.3 89.8 99.0 109.0 119.8 131.3 143.8 157.3 172.0 188.0
TOTAL SKINFOLDS = [ ]		
Calf =		

FIRST COMPONENT ½ 1 1½ 2 2½ 3 3½ 4 4½ 5 5½ 6 6½ 7 7½ 8 8½ 9 9½ 10 10½ 11 11½ 12

Height cm [ ]	139.7 143.5 147.3 151.1 154.9 158.8 162.6 166.4 170.2 174.0 177.8 181.6 185.4 189.2 193.0 196.9 200.7 204.5 208.3 212.1 215.9 219.7 223.5 227.3
Humerus width cm [ ]	5.19 5.34 5.49 5.64 5.78 5.93 6.07 6.22 6.37 6.51 6.65 6.80 6.95 7.09 7.24 7.38 7.53 7.67 7.82 7.97 8.11 8.25 8.40 8.55
Femur width cm [ ]	7.41 7.62 7.83 8.04 8.24 8.45 8.66 8.87 9.08 9.28 9.49 9.70 9.91 10.12 10.33 10.53 10.74 10.95 11.16 11.36 11.57 11.78 11.99 12.21
Biceps girth [ ] -T*	23.7 24.4 25.0 25.7 26.3 27.0 27.7 28.3 29.0 29.7 30.3 31.0 31.6 32.2 33.0 33.6 34.3 35.0 35.6 36.3 37.0 37.6 38.3 39.0
Calf girth [ ] -C▲	27.7 28.5 29.3 30.1 30.8 31.6 32.4 33.2 33.9 34.7 35.5 36.3 37.1 37.8 38.6 39.4 40.2 41.0 41.7 42.5 43.3 44.1 44.9 45.6

SECOND COMPONENT ½ 1 1½ 2 2½ 3 3½ 4 4½ 5 5½ 6 6½ 7 7½ 8 8½ 9

Weight kg =	Upper limit	39.65 40.74 41.43 42.13 42.82 43.48 44.18 44.84 45.53 46.23 46.92 47.58 48.25 48.94 49.63 50.33 50.99 51.68
Ht. / ∛Wt. = [ ]	Mid-point and	40.20 41.09 41.79 42.48 43.14 43.84 44.50 45.19 45.89 46.32 47.24 47.94 48.60 49.29 49.99 50.68 51.34
	Lower limit below	39.66 40.75 41.44 42.14 42.83 43.49 44.19 44.85 45.54 46.24 46.93 47.59 48.26 48.95 49.64 50.34 51.00

THIRD COMPONENT ½ 1 1½ 2 2½ 3 3½ 4 4½ 5 5½ 6 6½ 7 7½ 8 8½ 9

	FIRST COMPONENT	SECOND COMPONENT	THIRD COMPONENT	
Anthropometric Somatotype				BY: ....
Anthropometric plus Photoscopic Somatotype				RATER: ....

*Biceps girth in cm corrected for fat by subtracting triceps skinfold value expressed in cm.
▲Calf girth in cm corrected for fat by subtracting medial calf skinfold cm.

Figure 7–5 Heath-Carter somatotype form.

the technique is complex and requires expensive equipment, but the analyses are accurate and the subject discomfort is minimal.

One last method, which has been used in the past, employs ultrasound (Behnke and Wilmore, 1974). Muscle, bone, and fat have different densities and accoustical properties, so it is possible to use high-frequency sound waves to differentiate between tissue types. A special transducer generates sound waves, which pass into the tissue. When a change in density is encountered, some of these waves are reflected, received by a pickup device, and converted to an electrical impulse. The impulse is passed to a detecting device for amplification and recording. The thickness of the fat, muscle, and bone of any one particular segment can be calculated from the recording.

Field Assessment. A number of techniques have been devised for assessing body composition outside of the laboratory. One of the most accurate is the underwater weighing technique. While this is normally a laboratory technique, it can also be easily performed outside of the laboratory, if a swimming pool, or smaller body of water, and a hanging scale are available. Figure 7–7 illustrates a system used to assess the body composition of an entire professional football team while at their summer, pre-

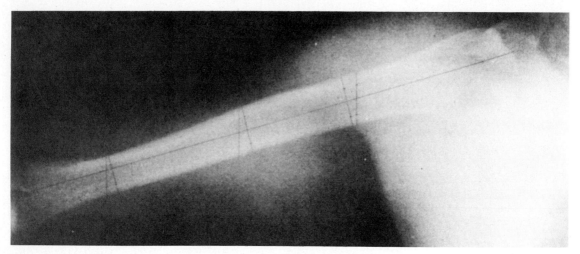

Figure 7–6 Radiographic analyses of body composition, using the upper arm of a world-class, male shot-putter. (From Albert R. Behnke and Jack H. Wilmore, *Evaluation and Regulation of Body Build and Composition,* © 1974, p. 28. Reprinted by permission of Prentice-Hall, Inc., Englewood Cliffs, New Jersey.)

season training camp. The technique is simple, fast, and accurate. The air remaining in the lungs at the time the underwater weight is determined can be estimated from normal population values for the same age, height, and sex as the athlete. A comprehensive description of how to conduct a complete assesssent using this technique, is presented in Appendix C, Field Tests for Assessing Physical Fitness.

Over the years, a number of different anthropometric techniques have been derived to estimate various components of body composition. As stated earlier, anthropometry is the study of human body measurements and usually includes girths or circumferences of limbs or segments, e.g., girth of the calf; breadths or diameters of bones, e.g., width of the hips or pelvis; and skinfold estimates of the thickness of subcutaneous fat, e.g., triceps skinfold. By using girths, breadths, or skinfolds, or a combination, equations have been derived to predict body density, relative and absolute body fat, lean body weight, and ideal weight. The majority of these equations have been found to be population-specific, i.e., they provide an accurate assessment only for groups or populations that are similar in age, sex, nationality, and general physical fitness. This simply implies that it is necessary to select an equation that was derived from a group of subjects as similar as possible to the group of

athletes or individuals to be studied. It would not be appropriate to use an equation derived from a group of middle-aged males for the evaluation of a group of young, adolescent males. Several recent studies have reported more generalized equations (Jackson and Pollock, 1978, 1980).

Anthropometric techniques are simple to apply and require little in the way of equipment. Most of the equations that have been derived are reasonably accurate. However, almost all existing equations have been derived from normal, nonathletic populations. Their applicability to athletic populations, particularly to extremely lean athletes or athletes with highly developed musculature, is unknown at the present time. It has been assumed that these equations are equally accurate for all athletes, but this requires confirmation by additional research. Another area of uncertainty in using anthropometric equations is the question of their ability to accurately estimate changes in body composition. While most equations predict, with reasonable accuracy, the individual's body composition at any one point in time, there is some doubt as to how accurately these equations can predict those changes in body composition that occur with either weight gains or weight losses through diet and exercise. Again, further research will be necessary to determine the ability of these equations to estimate change. Several anthropometric techniques for es-

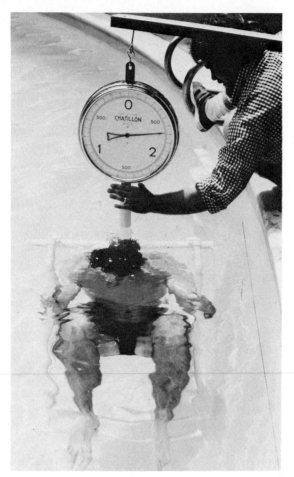

Figure 7–7 Underwater weighing technique conducted outside of the laboratory.

timating body composition are outlined in Appendix C, Field Tests for Assessing Physical Fitness.

ALTERATIONS IN BODY BUILD AND COMPOSITION WITH PHYSICAL TRAINING

Body build can be altered to a limited extent with physical training. However, previous research has suggested that somatotypes change very little within the individual's total life span. In fact, one study has shown that adult somatotypes can be predicted with a high degree of accuracy during the period of preadolescence. It is apparent that muscle

mass can be both lost and gained with physical inactivity and strength training, respectively, and that body fat can be gained or lost with manipulations in both diet and exercise patterns. These changes are usually of a limited nature, resulting in little or no change in the somatotype. This inability to substantially alter somatotype is largely the result of the inherited, or genetic, nature of body type.

Body composition can undergo substantial alterations with physical training (Oscai, 1973). In the past, it has been frequently stated that physical activity has only a limited influence in changing body composition. It was argued that even exercise of a vigorous nature required the expenditure of too few calories to result in substantial reductions in body fat. To illustrate, it has been estimated that a 150-pound woman would have to climb up and down a 10-foot flight of stairs approximately 1,000 times at a moderate pace in order to loose 1 pound of fat. Chopping wood for eight hours at a moderate pace would cause the same weight loss. These examples tend to discourage the use of exercise for weight loss and weight control. Yet, exercise has been found to be very effective in the past in promoting major alterations in body composition. How is this apparent conflict in results accounted for?

When estimating the energy cost of an activity, it is customary to use the steady-state, energy-expenditure value during the exercise. If, for example, it requires 7.5 Kcals/min to shovel snow, i.e., steady-state value during exercise, it would require a total of only 450 Kcals for one hour of work, or a loss of approximately 0.13 pound of fat. As was explained in Chapter 2, Responses to Acute Exercise, the metabolism remains elevated during the period immediately following exercise. This was referred to as the "period of oxygen debt." This recovery back to pre-exercise levels can require several minutes for light exercise, up to several hours for heavy exercise, and up to twelve to twenty-four hours for prolonged, exhaustive exercise. The elevation of the metabolism above normal levels during the recovery period from heavy to prolonged exhaustive exercise can total a substantial number of Kcals. If the oxygen consumption following exercise remains elevated by only 100 ml or 0.1 liter/min, this will amount to approximately 0.5 Kcal/min or 30 Kcal/hr. If the metabolism remains elevated for ten hours, this would amount to an additional 300 Kcal expended that would not normally be included in the calculated total energy expenditure for that particular activity. Therefore, this major source of energy expenditure, which occurs as a result of the exercise bout, is frequently ignored in most calculations of the energy cost of various activities. If the individual in this example exercised five days per week, he or she would have expended 1,500 Kcal, or approximately 0.4 pound, in one week just from the recovery period alone.

Among those who accept the fact that exercise can substantially alter body composition, there are many who feel that the process is too slow. The average jogger who jogs three days a week for 30 minutes a day at a seven-mph pace, or slightly over 8 1/2 minutes a mile, will use approximately 14.5 Kcal/min, or 435 Kcal, for the total run/day, resulting in a total expenditure per week of approximately 1,305 Kcal, or slightly over 1/3 pound of fat loss each week. Why even bother for that small amount? Individuals who are short sighted might conclude that there are better and easier ways, and that exercise is a painfully slow way to significantly reduce fat. What if the jogger were stubborn and stayed with his or her routine? In fifty-two weeks, providing energy intake remained constant, he or she would lose a total of seventeen pounds, a figure that looks more impressive.

Generally, present society is time oriented and has to have what it wants immediately, if not sooner. Consider the twenty-five-year-old professional athlete who finds that his weight is fifteen to twenty pounds more than it was at twenty-one years. He finally decides to lose his excess poundage but wants to accomplish this by the start of the pre-season training, which is less than three weeks away. Obviously, exercise is of no value to him, for he would need nine to twelve months to lose this much weight through exercise alone. He needs to lose more than five pounds per week, so he relies on a "crash" diet, selecting whichever diet is in vogue at that time. Everyone knows that it is possible to lose six to eight pounds per week with these diets. What kind of success might this athlete have?

This example is not unique. Many athletes find themselves out of shape and overweight as a result of overeating and inactivity during the off-season. Also, they typically will wait until the last few weeks prior to reporting for their sport before they attempt to attack the problem. In this example, the athlete may be able to shed fifteen pounds in less than three weeks as a result of a crash diet. However, much of this weight loss will be from the body's water compartment and very little from stored fat. Several studies have reported that substantial weight losses will occur with starvation and semi-starvation (500 Kcal/day or less) diets, but of the weight lost, over 60 percent comes from the body's lean weight and less than 40 percent from the fat weight. Much of the lean weight lost is in the form of water. Most of these crash diets require a very low carbohydrate intake. As a result, the carbohydrate stores of the body become depleted. With every 1 gram of carbohydrate used, approximately 3 grams of water are lost. With a total body glycogen content of 800 grams, a depletion of the stored glycogen would result in a loss of approximately 2,400 grams of water, or slightly more than 5 pounds of the weight lost. Water is also lost as a result of ketosis, which accompanies most of these diets. Much of this loss will occur during the first week of the diet.

It is literally impossible to lose more than 4 pounds of fat per week, even if on a total starvation diet. This can be demonstrated quite easily. Assuming that it requires a 3,500 Kcal deficit to lose 1 pound of fat, the athlete could lose no more than 0.7 pound per day on a total starvation diet. His maintenance level would be approximately 2,500 Kcal/day, so he would have a 2,500 Kcal deficit per day if he abstained completely from food. However, during a starvation diet, research indicates that the total body metabolism is reduced by 20–25 percent. A 20-percent reduction in the athlete's metabolism would lower his total deficit to only 2,000 Kcal per day, or approximately 0.57 pound of fat loss per day. In one week this would result in a loss of only 4 pounds of fat. And this is on a total starvation diet! Few people would be able to tolerate the discomfort associated with prolonged periods of starvation.

The sensible approach to weight reduction is to combine moderate dietary restriction with increased levels of exercise. The appetite is delicately balanced with the actual caloric needs of the body. Simply removing one buttered slice of bread from the diet each day and keeping the activity levels and diet constant will result in a weight loss of 10 pounds per year (100 Kcal/day × 364 days), which is not an insignificant amount. Combined with a modest 0.25–0.30-pound weight loss per week from a three-day per week jogging program, the total weight lost would amount to 25–30 pounds in a single year. Patience is a virtue, for this form of weight loss has been found to be more permanent. The rapid weight losses experienced with crash diets are quickly regained, probably due to the fact that when a balanced diet is substituted for the low-carbohydrate diet, the water that was lost is quickly regained. In addition, research evidence suggests that combining exercise with diet reduces the proportion of the weight lost from the lean tissue to an insignificant level. Since the purpose of the weight-loss program is to lose body fat, and not lean tissue, the combination diet and exercise program is the preferred approach.

When combining diet and exercise, the exercise should be performed a minimum of 3 days per week. The greater the frequency, intensity, and duration of training, the greater will be the resulting weight loss. With respect to dietary modifications, a reduction of 200–500 Kcal/day from the athlete's normal diet will add up to a substantial weight loss over time. Weight losses of approximately one pound per week, which represents a more realistic goal, can be achieved with such a combination. It should be added that a balanced diet is essential to assure the necessary vitamins and minerals that the athlete needs. Vitamin supplementation may or may not be essential. Results of research at this time conflict. This topic will receive additional coverage in Chapter 12, Ergogenic Aids.

The diet should be consumed over at least three meals per day. Many athletes make the mistake of eating only one or two meals per day, skipping either breakfast or lunch, or both, and then consuming a very large dinner. Research in animals has demonstrated that, given the same number of total calories, the animals that ate their daily food ration in one or two hours gained more weight than those that nibbled their ration throughout the day (Mayer, 1968).

Another misconception that has been used frequently to discount the benefits of exercise in weight control is the contention that the exercise itself will stimulate the appetite to such an extent that voluntary food intake will be increased to account for the additional expenditure of energy through exercise. Jean Mayer (1954), world-famous

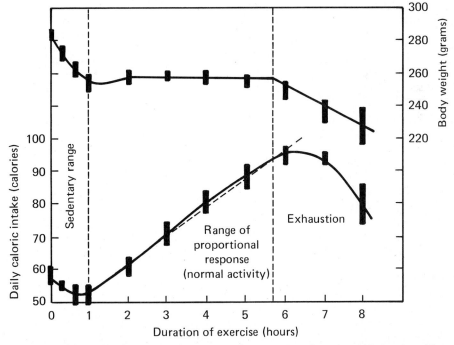

Figure 7–8   Food intake and body weight changes with increasing durations of exercise. (From J. Mayer, *Amer. J. Physiol.* 177 (1954): 544–548. Reproduced by permission of the publisher.)

Table 7–1   *Caloric Expenditure of Running and Jogging at Different Paces on the Basis of Body Weight* *

	Calories/hour Pace per mile							
Weight	5:20	6:00	6:40	7:20	8:00	8:40	9:20	10:00
120	936	828	726	654	594	540	498	456
130	1,014	888	792	708	642	582	534	492
140	1,086	954	846	756	690	630	576	528
150	1,164	1,020	906	810	738	672	612	564
160	1,236	1,086	966	870	780	708	654	600
170	1,314	1,152	1,020	918	828	762	690	636
180	1,386	1,212	1,080	972	876	798	732	672
190	1,464	1,278	1,140	1,020	924	840	774	708
200	1,536	1,344	1,194	1,074	972	888	810	744
210	1,614	1,416	1,230	1,122	1,020	930	846	780
220	1,686	1,482	1,314	1,176	1,068	972	888	816

Adapted from J. Henderson, "Planning High-Calorie Workouts." Runner's World 9 (1974): 24–25. Reproduced by permission of the publisher.

nutritionist at Harvard University, reported many years ago that in animals exercising for up to one hour, there is actually a decrease in appetite when compared to the appetites of sedentary animals (Figure 7–8). Similar results have been reported for humans. Exercise does appear to be a mild, appetite suppressant.

From this discussion, it can be concluded that exercise plays an important role in weight-loss and weight-control programs. The exercise does not have to be of an extended and exhaustive nature to be effective. The athlete should select an endurance-type of activity that is enjoyable, and participate in this activity for 30–40 min/day, 4–5 days/week, at an intensity of from 60 to 75 percent of his or her endurance capacity. Over time, this exercise program will produce the desired results. Table 7–1 provides an example of the caloric expenditure of running on the basis of the pace of running and body weight.

The role of exercise in spot weight reduction is a controversial area. Many individuals, including athletes, believe that by exercising a specific area the fat in that localized area will be utilized, thus reducing the locally stored fat. Several research studies have reported results that tend to support the concept of spot reduction. However, recent work suggests that spot reduction is a myth and that

exercise, even when localized, draws from all of the fat stores of the body, not just from the local depots. A study by Gwinup et al. (1971) utilized outstanding tennis players to investigate this phenomenon. The researchers theorized that the tennis players would be ideal subjects for studying spot reduction since they could act as their own controls, i.e., the dominant arm exercises vigorously every day for several hours, while the nondominant arm is relatively sedentary. They postulated that if spot reduction were a reality, the nondominant (inactive) arm should have substantially more fat than the dominant (active) arm. In fact, while the arm girths were substantially greater in the dominant arm, due to exercise hypertrophy, there were absolutely no differences in the fat contents of the two arms, as assessed by subcutaneous skinfold fat thicknesses. The general impression among researchers at the present time is that fat is mobilized from those areas of highest concentration and not from specific localized areas, thus negating the spot reduction theory.

The effectiveness of spot reduction has been promoted by many health studios with the claim that they can take off several inches from the customer's waist in a few short weeks. Substantial reductions of the abdominal girth can result from localized exercise, e.g., bent-knee sit-ups, but this is not due to localized fat losses. A loss of three to four inches in the abdominal girth can occur from sit-up exercises alone, without any loss at all in either total or localized fat. This is due to a strengthening of the abdominal muscles, which pulls the abdominal contents back into their normal position. Progressive abdominal weakness leads to a spilling-out of the abdominal contents, which results in a "pot belly" appearance. Strengthening these abdominal muscles pulls everything back into place but does little if anything to alter the fat content of that area.

Exercise can also lead to substantial weight gains. These gains, however, appear to be predominantly, if not totally, increases in lean body weight. Strength and power training programs lead to the largest gains in lean weight, as a result of their relationship with muscle hypertrophy. Even limited muscle hypertrophy will result from endurance training programs. It is somewhat ironic that in previously sedentary, middle-aged men, an endurance training program will frequently lead to little or no change in total body weight, but that body composition will undergo a marked change. Typically, there is a substantial loss in body fat, but also an increase in lean tissue of about the same magnitude. This phenomenon can be deceiving, since there is no change in scale weight even after months of hard work. Although it is natural to become quite angry over the apparent inability to lose weight, individuals, when questioned, admit that their clothes do not fit as well as they once did. Usually their clothes are tight in the arms and legs and loose in the abdominal area, which illustrates both the gain in muscle as well as the loss in fat. As was mentioned earlier, with regard to body composition, the scale weight of the individual is not an accurate indication of body composition, nor does it accurately reflect the changes that result from chronic exercise.

MECHANISMS OF CHANGE

It would appear that weight losses and weight gains are a simple matter of either energy input, energy expenditure, or both. To lose weight, one can reduce the caloric intake, increase the caloric expenditure, or combine the two. Likewise, with weight gains, one can increase the caloric intake, reduce the energy expenditure, or combine the two. Unfortunately, common observation and recent research suggests that energy balance is not that simple. Nearly everyone has known of individuals who can literally gorge themselves daily, yet remain lean, or conversely, of individuals who continue gaining body fat even though they eat only limited amounts, well below what would be expected to be their maintenance levels. Individuals do metabolize food differently, some being more efficient than others. Also, some individuals are more efficient in their expenditure of energy for fixed work tasks. These phenomena are not well understood at the present time, and considerably more research will be necessary to determine which factors are involved and their relative importance.

With specific reference to exercise, it would appear that the reduction in fat by exercise is solely the result of an added expenditure of calories. Yet, the body might be expected to adapt to this additional expenditure by increasing the appetite to compensate for the deficit. This is a difficult problem that defies a simple solution. Several research studies have pointed to the possible role of human growth hormone as being responsible for the increased fatty acid mobilization during exercise (Oscai, 1973). Growth hormone levels do increase sharply with exercise and remain elevated for up to several hours in the recovery period. Other research has suggested that the adipose tissue is more sensitive to the sympathetic nervous system or to the levels of circulating catecholamines, which would result in increased lipid mobilization (Oscai, 1973). More recent research suggests that a specific fat-mobilizing substance, which is highly responsive to elevated levels of activity, is responsible. At the present time, it is impossible to state with certainty which factors are of greatest importance in mediating this response.

It was demonstrated in the previous section that exercise tends to suppress the appetite. While this is true for male laboratory animals, it has been shown that exercise actually increases the appetites of female laboratory animals (Oscai, 1973). The reason for this sex difference is not presently known. In humans, most of the research has been conducted on males, and the results indicate either no change in appetite with increased levels of exercise or slight decreases. It is possible that the decrease in appetite occurs only with intense levels of work in which the increased catecholamine levels suppress the appetite.

The gains in lean weight with exercise are undoubtedly due to increases in protein anabolism, or synthesis, which leads to muscle hypertrophy. In Chapter 3, Adaptations to Chronic Exercise, the potential cause of muscle hypertrophy was explored and found to be the result of increases in muscle fiber size, possibly due to an increased number of myofibrils. The possibility of fiber splitting was also discussed. Without knowing the specific changes that occur within the muscle, it is difficult to postulate the possible mechanisms that trigger these changes. Again, since human growth hormone has anabolic properties, its rise with exercise and its continued elevation during recovery have led several investigators to suggest that this might explain the gains in lean tissue. Obviously, further research is needed before the actual mechanisms for these changes can be adequately defined.

RELATIONSHIP OF BODY BUILD AND COMPOSITION TO ATHLETIC PERFORMANCE

The body build of an individual is determined largely through genetics. Characteristics that are inherited from parents establish rather narrow limits of variation in an athlete's body build. Size is also largely determined genetically. With this in mind, it is important to understand that most sports require a certain body type for success. This is illustrated in Figure 7–4, which presents somatotype data from a large number of participants in the 1960 Olympic Games. Within any one sport, there is considerable variation, as is illustrated in Figure 7–9. From this information, it is obvious that to be successful, the athlete should select a sport in which his or her somatotype will be an asset. With few exceptions, almost all sports require a moderate to high rating in mesomorphy. On the other hand, extreme endomorphs and extreme ectomorphs do very poorly in most sports.

A number of studies have related somatotype and body size to athletic performance in various sports. These have typically been associated with the Olympic Games in a particular year. Cureton (1951) studied the structural and functional capacities of 21 male members of the 1948 United States Olympic Team and 24 national- and international-caliber track and field athletes. He found considerable differences between sports and between events in the same sport. Correnti and Zauli (1964) studied 166 Olympic track and field athletes and 8 swimmers at the 1960 Olympics in Rome. They observed differences in age, height, and weight for athletes in different events, but they found that the body shapes were similar within the same event.

Tanner (1964) studied 137 track and field athletes at the 1960 Olympics in Rome. He found that there were racial differences between athletes within the same event, that the somatotypes tended to cluster in specific areas, depending on the event, and that athletes can be separated by certain body dimensions according to their events. deGaray et al. (1974) conducted an exhaustive study on the athletes participating in the 1968 Olympic Games in Mexico City. From all of these studies, it is apparent that body size and somatotype are important in determining success within any one sport, activity, or event. Since somatotype is largely genetically determined, this points to the importance of placing athletes in sports in which they can achieve, at least, a modest degree of success.

Body composition must be considered equally important to body build when attempting to maximize the athlete's performance potential. Several studies have found a high, negative relationship between performance in various activities and the relative amount of body fat (Wilmore and Haskell, 1972). The higher the percentage of body fat, the poorer the performance of the individual. This was true of all activities in which the body weight had to be moved either vertically or horizontally through space, e.g., sprinting and long jumping. Many athletes are under the impression that they must be big to be good in their sport. Size has been associated with the quality of the athlete's performance; the bigger the athlete, the better the performance. It is now recognized that this is true only if the size increase is due to an increase in the lean tissue. To add additional fat to the body just to increase the weight and overall size is detrimental to performance, with the possible exception of the heavyweight weight lifter. These individuals may put on large amounts of fat weight under the pretense that

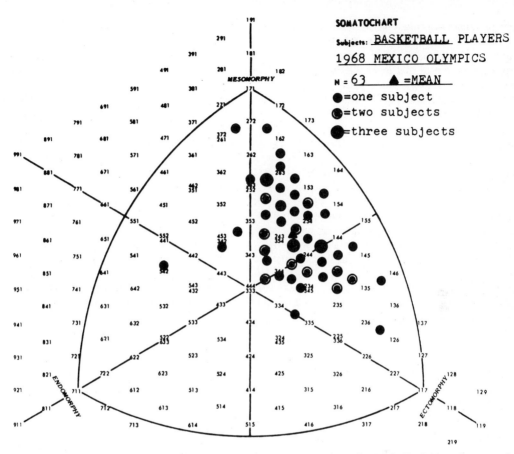

Figure 7-9 Somatogram illustrating the variation in somatotype for basketball players from various countries participating in the 1968 Olympic Games. (From A. L. deGaray et al., eds., *Genetic and Anthropological Studies of Olympic Athletes*. New York: Academic Press, 1974. Reproduced by permission of the publisher.)

the additional weight will help to lower their center of gravity and give them a greater mechanical advantage in lifting. To the best of the author's knowledge, the value of this has yet to be confirmed through research. Another notable exception to the theory that overall size is not the major determinant of athletic success is the Sumo wrestler. The larger individual does have a decided advantage, but the wrestler with the higher lean weight should have the greatest, overall success.

Rather than being concerned with overall weight, most athletes should be specifically concerned with their lean body weight. Eventually, techniques will be available that will allow a young athlete to undergo an extensive evaluation to provide an estimate of fat weight, lean weight, and a projected estimate of one's potential for increasing lean body weight. In this way, the athlete could design a training program that would develop lean tissue to this projected maximum, while maintaining fat content at relatively low levels. While this would be a desirable approach for the athlete dependent on strength, power, and muscular endurance, it would be counterproductive for the endurance athlete who is forced to move his or her total body mass horizontally for extended periods of time. Increased lean weight may prove to be a major detriment to successful performance for this athlete since it is an additional load that must be carried. The same may also be true for the high jumper, long jumper, and triple jumper who depend on maximizing their vertical and horizontal distances. Additional weight, even though it is active lean tissue, may decrease rather than facilitate performance potential for these athletes.

An accurate assessment, or estimate, of the athlete's body composition is essential. Use of standard height-weight tables does not provide an accurate estimate of what the athlete should weigh. This fact was established in the original classic study relating body composition to athletics. Welham and Behnke studied the body compositions of twenty-five professional football players in 1942. Of these twenty-five professional athletes, seventeen were physically unqualified for military duty or first-class insurance on the basis of their weight. Of the seventeen "overweight" players, eleven were found to have very low levels of body fat, indicating that the overweight condition was the result of an excess of lean tissue and not excess fat. Wilmore and

Haskell (1972) investigated the body composition of forty-four professional football players according to the positions that they played. The defensive backs were the leanest, lightest, and shortest of the five groups analyzed, while the defensive linemen were the fattest, heaviest, and nearly the tallest. The offensive backs and receivers were similar to the defensive backs, and the offensive linemen were comparable to the defensive linemen. The linebackers were unique and fell approximately between the linemen and backs relative to the observed variables. In comparison with the Welham and Behnke data for the 1942-era ball players, the linemen studied in 1969 through 1971 were taller and considerably heavier, but there were no substantial differences between the backs. The increased weight of the players studied recently was due to an increase in both the lean and fat weights of the linemen. These results, combined with additional results from 1972–1976, are summarized in Tables 7–2 and 7–3.

Body composition values tend to vary with the

Table 7–2 *Body Composition Characteristics of Professional Football Players Grouped by Position.*

Position	Number	Height (in.)	Weight (lb)	Fat (%)	Fat (lb)	Lean Weight (lb)
Defensive backs	26	71.9	187.0	9.6	18.1	168.9
Offensive backs and wide receivers	40	72.4	200.0	9.4	19.2	180.8
Linebackers	28	74.3	225.3	14.0	32.0	193.3
Offensive linemen and tight ends	38	76.0	248.3	15.6	38.7	209.0
Defensive linemen	32	75.8	258.2	18.2	47.0	211.2
Quarterbacks and kickers	16	72.8	198.7	14.4	28.7	170.0

Table 7–3 *Comparison of the Body Composition of Professional Football Players of the Early 1940s with those of the Late 1960s and Early 1970s.*

Position	Number	Height (in.)	Weight (lb)	Fat (%)	Fat (lb)	Lean Weight (lb)
Backs						
1940–41	13	71.3	189.0	7.1	13.5	175.6
Present	66	72.2	194.9	9.5	18.8	176.1
Linemen						
1940–41	12	73.1	214.1	14.0	30.0	184.1
Present	70	75.9	252.8	16.8	42.5	210.0

sport. Those sports or activities that have a high endurance component will typically have athletes who have low relative body fats. Long-distance runners generally have less than 10 percent body fat. By contrast, the male and female of college age will average 15 percent and 25 percent fat, respectively. However, even the better women endurance runners have body fat levels below 10 percent. Is this the result of natural selection of lean individuals for distance running, or is this the result of running sixty to one hundred miles or more per week as a part of their training program? Information is not available to answer this question at the present time, although it undoubtedly is a combination of both.

Of great concern to the medical and scientific community, as well as the involved coach and athlete, is the area of "making weight." While the major concern has been with the sport of wrestling, many schools, districts, or state-level organizations have organized their athletic programs on the basis of size, including weight as the predominant factor. The athlete attempts to get down to the lowest weight possible in order to gain an advantage over the opponent. In so doing, many athletes have jeopardized their health. In a manner similar to using crash diets as mentioned earlier in this chapter, these athletes will lose large amounts of weight predominantly through dehydration. They will exercise in rubberized sweat suits, sit in steam and sauna baths, chew on towels to lose saliva, and keep their food and fluid intake minimal. Such severe water losses compromise kidney and general cardiovascular function and are potentially dangerous. Weight losses of 2 to 4 percent of the athlete's weight due to dehydration can even impair performance. Standards should be established on the basis of the athlete's lean body weight. For males, total body weight should consist of not less than 5 percent fat.* This would imply that 95 percent of the athlete's weight should be lean. Knowing lean weight, competition weight should not drop below the following weight:

Minimal Competitive Weight = Lean Weight/0.95

*T. K. Tcheng and C. M. Tipton, "Iowa Wrestling Study; Anthropometric Measurements and The Prediction of a 'Minimal' Body Weight for High School Wrestlers." *Med. Sci. Sport* 5 (1973): 1–10.

Of course, as the lean weight is increased, the minimal competitive weight will increase.

GENERAL SUMMARY

It has become increasingly more evident that the athlete's body build and composition play a major role in determining athletic success. Body build refers to the form and structure of the body and is quantified by determining the athlete's somatotype. In somatotyping, the body is rated for each of three different components: endomorphy, mesomorphy and ectomorphy, which reflect adiposity, muscularity, and linearity, respectively. Body size simply refers to the height and body mass or weight of the individual. Body composition refers to the individual components that constitute the total body mass. Of primary concern to the athlete is the distinction between fat weight and lean weight; the latter refers to the fat-free weight of the body, which includes the weight of muscle, bone, skin, and organs among others. Body composition can be measured in the laboratory or estimated in the field. The underwater weighing technique is one of the more accurate and reliable techniques and can be used both inside and outside the laboratory. This technique provides an estimate of the body's volume. Body density is then calculated by the ratio of body mass or weight to body volume. From the body density, accurate estimates can be made of the body's lean and fat components. Anthropometric techniques, using girths of body segments, breadths of bones, and thicknesses of subcutaneous fat, provide fairly accurate estimates of the lean and fat components of the total body weight.

Physical training has only a modest influence on the athlete's body build. The somatotype is established early in life and is primarily determined by the genetic constitution of the individual athlete. Body composition is changed markedly with physical training. With chronic exercise, the lean body weight is increased and the fat weight is decreased. The magnitude of these changes is largely dependent on the type of exercise used in the training program, with strength training facilitating gains in lean weight and endurance training facilitating losses in fat weight. For purposes of losing body fat, the athlete should combine a moderate endurance training program with a modest reduction in total caloric intake of 200–500 Kcal/day. A goal of one pound of weight loss per week is attainable and much more desirable than more rigid goals of three to four pounds of weight loss per week.

Exercise up to one hour in duration does not markedly increase the appetite of the individual, and, in fact, may tend to suppress it. This could be the result of the increased levels of circulating catecholamines, which accompany moderate to heavy levels of exercise. These catecholamines may also have a fat-mobilizing effect on the adipose tissue, which may explain the fat loss normally experienced with chronic exercise. Human growth hormone may also play a significant role in the mobilization of fat and it may possibly be responsible for the increase of lean tissue with chronic exercise, due to its known anabolic action.

Spot reduction has been investigated in a number of studies and is now generally regarded as a myth. The body apparently mobilizes fat from the general body stores, calling first on those areas of highest concentration. Selective utilization of fat from isolated areas undergoing vigorous exercise has not been confirmed in recent research and is probably not possible.

Body build and composition are extremely important to the athlete. A certain body type is necessary for almost all sports, and each sport appears to require a different type. While mesomorphy is a predominant component for all athletes, few athletes are extreme endomorphs or ectomorphs. Body composition is of primary importance where the athlete must move his body vertically or horizontally through space. Many studies have found substantial negative correlations between athletic performance and relative fat; the higher the percentage of body fat, the poorer the athletic performance. While there is considerable variation between athletes in different sports with regard to relative fat values, it is generally felt that the lower the relative body fat, the greater the performance potential of the athlete, with only a few possible exceptions.

STUDY QUESTIONS

1. Differentiate between body build, body size, and body composition.
2. What is somatotyping? What are the three basic components of the somatotype and what do they represent?
3. How much will somatotype change with endurance training? Strength training?
4. What body tissues constitute the lean body weight?
5. Describe the appearance of a football player who is 22 percent fat and has a somatotype rating of 5–5–1.
6. What is a major problem associated with most equations that predict body composition from anthropometric measurements?
7. How important is regular exercise in a weight reduction program? In a weight control program?
8. How much weight should an overweight athlete lose per week in order to maximize fat loss and minimize lean weight loss?
9. Why is there substantial water loss with most "crash" diets?
10. What effect does exercise have on the appetite?
11. Defend the use of spot-reducing techniques.
12. How important is somatotype and body composition to athletic performance?
13. What is the lowest weight an athlete should be allowed to attain?

REFERENCES

Behnke, A. R., and Wilmore, J. H. *Evaluation and Regulation of Body Build and Composition.* Englewood Cliffs, N.J.: Prentice-Hall, 1974.

Bray, G. A., and Bethune, J. E. *Treatment and Management of Obesity.* New York: Harper and Row, Publishers, 1974.

Correnti, V., and Zauli, B. *Olimpionici 1960.* Rome: Marves, 1964.

Cureton, T. K., Jr. *Physical Fitness of Champion Athletes.* Urbana, Ill.: University of Illinois Press, 1951.

deGaray, A. L.; Levine, L.; and Carter, J. E. L., eds. *Genetic and Anthropological Studies of Olympic Athletes.* New York: Academic Press, 1974.

deVries, H. A. *Physiology of Exercise for Physical Education and Athletics.* 2nd ed. Dubuque, Iowa: William C. Brown Co., 1974.

Fox, E. L. *Sport Physiology.* Philadelphia: W. B. Saunders Co., 1979.

Gwinup, G.; Chelvam, R.; and Steinberg, T. "Thickness of Subcutaneous Fat and Activity of Underlying Muscles." *Annals Int. Med.* 74 (1971): 408–411.

Heath, B. H., and Carter, J. E. L. "A Modified Somatotype Method." *Am. J. Phys. Anthro.* 27 (1967): 57–74.

Jackson, A. S., and Pollock, M. L. "Generalized Equations for Predicting Body Density of Men." *Br. J. Nutr.* 40 (1978): 497–504.

Jackson, A. S., and Pollock, M. L. "Generalized Equations for Predicting Body Density of Women." *Med. Sci. Sports Exercise* 12 (1980): 175–182.

Karpovich, P. V., and Sinning, W. E. *Physiology of Muscular Activity.* 7th ed. Philadelphia: W. B. Saunders Co. 1971.

Katch, F. I., and McArdle, W. D. *Nutrition, Weight Control, and Exercise.* Boston: Houghton Mifflin Company, 1977.

Kuntzleman, C. T. *Activetics.* New York: Peter H. Wyden Publisher, 1975.

Mayer, J. *Overweight Causes, Cost, and Control.* Englewood Cliffs, N.J.: Prentice-Hall, 1968.

Mayer, J.; Marshall, H. B.; Vitale, J. J.; Christensen, J. H.; Mashayekhi, M. B.; and Stare, F. J. "Exercise, Food Intake, and Body Weight in Normal Rats and Genetically Obese Adult Mice." *Amer. J. Physiol.* 177 (1954): 544–548.

Oscai, L. B. "The Role of Exercise in Weight Control." In *Exercise and Sport Sciences Reviews,* vol. 1, edited by J. H. Wilmore. New York: Academic Press, 1973.

Pařízková, J. *Body Fat and Physical Fitness.* The Hague: Martinus Nijhoff B. V., 1977.

Pařízková, J., and Rogozkin, V. A. *Nutrition, Physical Fitness, and Health.* Baltimore: University Park Press, 1978.

Stuart, R. B., and Davis, B. *Slim Chance in a Fat World: Behavioral Control of Obesity.* Champaign, Ill.: Research Press, 1972.

Stunkard, A. J., ed. *Obesity.* Philadelphia: W. B. Saunders, 1980.

Tanner, J. M. *The Physique of the Olympic Athlete.* London: George Allen and Unwin, 1964.

Welham, W. C., and Behnke, A. R. "The Specific Gravity of Healthy Men." *J.A.M.A.* 118 (1942): 498–501.

Wilmore, J. H., and Haskell, W. L. "Body Composition and Endurance Capacity of Professional Football Players." *J. Appl. Physiol.* 33 (1972): 564–567.

Wilson, N. L., ed. *Obesity.* Philadelphia: F. A. Davis, 1969.

Winick, M. *Childhood Obesity.* New York: John Wiley & Sons, 1975.

8

Detraining and Off-Season Training Programs

INTRODUCTION

The preceding chapters have been concerned with the actual process of physical training and the physiological adaptations that result, which allow athletes to improve their athletic ability and performance in competitive situations. An area that is equally important, but one that has been given considerably less attention by both athletes and coaches and has practically been ignored by the researcher in the exercise and sport sciences, is the area of detraining and off-season conditioning programs. What happens to highly conditioned athletes who have fine tuned their performance potential to its peak when the competitive season comes to a sudden end and the mandatory, daily training program is no longer required? Most athletes in team sports go into physical hibernation following the completion of their competitive season. Many have been working two to five hours per day in perfecting their skills and improving their levels of physical condition, and welcome the opportunity to completely relax, purposely avoiding any strenuous physical activity. How does total physical inactivity affect the highly trained and conditioned athlete? Does the body need this period of rest, or will it undergo rapid, physical deterioration? Are physical training programs necessary during the off-season to maintain the athlete's general physical condition? These and other related questions will be discussed in the first section of this chapter. The last section is devoted to a discussion of off-season, physical training programs.

PHYSICAL DETRAINING

Much of our knowledge about physical detraining comes from research by the National Aeronautics and Space Administration to improve the safety of astronauts on missions requiring extended periods of weightlessness in a relatively confined living environment. In addition to forced inactivity, the lack of gravity also imposes a number of physiological stresses on the human body. Humans have successfully adapted to the earth's environment and have extreme difficulty in adapting to the weightless state. Physical detraining has been investigated through two major approaches: by observing changes following total bed rest for extended periods of time, and by observing changes in trained individuals as they cease formal physical training and become physically inactive. The results of these various studies will be discussed individually, according to the specific components of physical training.

Strength, Power, and Muscular Endurance

When an individual breaks an arm or a leg and the broken limb is placed in a rigid cast to render it completely immobile, changes immediately start taking place in both the bone and surrounding muscles. Within a period of only a few days, the cast, which was applied very tightly around the injured segment, becomes quite loose. By the end of several weeks, there is a large space between the cast and the limb. Is this the result of the cast expanding

138

with use or of the limb decreasing in size with a lack of use? It is now clearly understood that skeletal muscles will undergo a substantial decrease in size with inactivity. Accompanying this decrease in size is a considerable loss in strength, power, and muscular endurance (Clarke, 1973). While total inactivity will lead to very rapid losses in each of these areas, even periods of decreased activity will lead to gradual losses that become sizeable as the losses accumulate over long periods of time.

Research confirms that levels of strength, power, and muscular endurance are reduced once the athlete stops training (Clarke, 1973). However, these reductions are not very large during the first few months following the cessation of training. In one study, no loss in strength was noted six weeks after a three-week training program. In another study, 45 percent of the original strength gained from a twelve-week training program was lost by the time the subjects were reevaluated one year later. Similar results have been found for muscular endurance. Thus, for the trained athlete, it appears that the strength and muscular endurance gained during the training period will be fully retained for periods up to six weeks, and approximately 50 percent of the strength gained will be retained for up to a year following the end of the training program. Also, studies have shown that it takes far less effort than originally required to regain the strength which was lost (Clarke, 1973). In addition, it appears that by working out once every ten to fourteen days, the athlete will be able to maintain the strength, power, and muscular endurance that was gained through more vigorous and frequent training.

These findings tend to conflict with the observations, noted earlier, that rather sizeable losses in strength, power, and muscular endurance, in addition to losses in muscle mass (atrophy), result from periods of inactivity when a limb is totally immobilized. Apparently, the average individual gets sufficient exercise through walking, climbing stairs, pushing, pulling, and lifting to allow a substantial retention of the strength previously gained through strength training. With immobilization, there is almost no activity at all within the muscle. Evidently, it requires only a minimal stimulus to retain the strength, power, endurance, and size of a muscle or muscle group. This has extremely important implications for the injured athlete. There will be a great savings in time and effort during the

period of rehabilitation if the athlete can perform even a very low level of exercise in the injured segment, starting in the first few days of the recovery period. Simple, isometric contractions have been found to be very effective in this respect, since they can be graded in intensity and do not require movement at the joint. Any program of rehabilitation, however, must be worked out in cooperation with the supervising physician.

Speed, Agility, and Flexibility

As was stated in Chapter 5, physical training can influence speed and agility, but the degree of improvement will be far less than in the areas of strength, power, muscular endurance, flexibility, and cardiovascular endurance. Consequently, the loss of speed and agility with physical inactivity is relatively small, and peak levels can be maintained with only a limited amount of training. This does not imply that the sprinter in track can get by with training only a few days a week. Success in actual competition relies on factors other than basic speed, such as timing and the finishing kick. It takes many hours of practice during the week to tune performance to its optimal level, but most of this time is spent in developing aspects of one's performance other than speed.

Flexibility, on the other hand, is lost rather quickly and must be worked on throughout the year. Stretching exercises, such as those outlined in Appendix B, Warm-Up and Flexibility Exercises, should be incorporated into both the in-season and off-season training programs. While flexibility can be attained in a relatively short period of time, it is in the best interests of the athlete to maintain the desired levels of flexibility on a year-round basis. Many athletes, however, tend to ignore flexibility training during the off-season, since it can be regained so rapidly. Reduced flexibility leaves the athlete more susceptible to serious injury; this could be a major factor in determining the longevity of his athletic career.

Cardiovascular Endurance

It is now well understood that periods of inactivity lead to substantial, cardiovascular deconditioning. Astronauts returning from extended periods of weightlessness have been found to have severe cardiovascular deterioration, resulting from the combination of inactivity and weightlessness. Even limited activity on earth provides considerable work for the heart, since the heart must contract forcefully enough to circulate the blood throughout the body against the forces of gravity. In the weightless state, this is no longer necessary, and the work of the heart is reduced considerably. The result is a decrease in heart function. For this reason, astronauts in the series of Skylab flights during the early 1970s were required to perform daily bouts of exercise on a stationary bicycle ergometer or on an ingeniously designed "space treadmill." This exercise was found to be essential in preventing serious cardiovascular deterioration.

These same types of results have been observed in studies conducted on subjects undergoing long periods of total bed rest. In these studies, the subject is not allowed to leave the bed, and physical activity while in bed is kept to an absolute minimum. Many of these studies attempted to use total bed rest to simulate weightlessness. Figure 3–1 (Chapter 3) illustrates the heart rate at a constant metabolic

load before and following a twenty-day period of bed rest, and at varying times during a subsequent fifty-day period of physical reconditioning, in a study conducted by Saltin et al. (1968). The considerable increase in the working heart rate was indicative of the 25-percent decrease observed in the stroke volume at this level of work. In addition, at maximal levels of work, the period of bed rest resulted in a 25-percent reduction in maximal cardiac output and a 27-percent decrease in maximal oxygen uptake (Figure 8–1). This reduction in cardiac output and $\dot{V}O_2$ max was due primarily to a reduction in stroke volume, which was probably the result of a decrease in heart volume, a decrease in total blood volume and plasma volume, and a decrease in ventricular contractility.

It is interesting to note in Figure 8–1 the relatively large decrease in $\dot{V}O_2$ max in the two more highly conditioned subjects in this study, compared to lesser decreases in the remaining three subjects who were considered sedentary. Furthermore, the three relatively sedentary subjects regained their

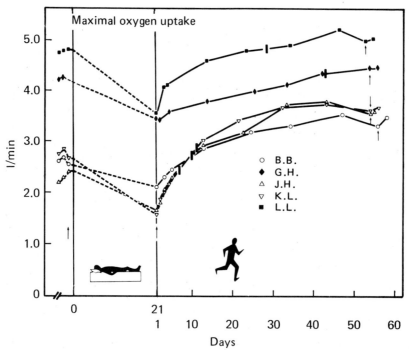

Figure 8–1   Reduction in maximal oxygen uptake with a twenty-day period of physical inactivity (bed rest). (From B. Saltin et al., "Response to Submaximal and Maximal Exercise after Bed Rest and after Training," Circulation 38 (Suppl. 7) (1968). By permission of the American Heart Association, Inc.)

initial, or pre-bedrest, level of conditioning within the first ten days of reconditioning, while the two physically active subjects needed about forty days to regain their initial levels. This would tend to suggest that the more highly trained individuals will not be able to afford long periods of inactivity away from endurance training activities. The athlete who goes into total hibernation at the completion of the season will experience a great deal of difficulty in getting back into physical condition when the new season begins.

Studies have also observed changes in the cardiovascular endurance capacity of trained subjects during periods of inactivity following intensive endurance conditioning. Most of these studies have shown rather marked decreases in endurance capacity with detraining or periods of inactivity. This reduction is of considerably greater magnitude than that observed in the areas of strength, power, and muscular endurance for the same period of inactivity. Drinkwater and Horvath (1972) observed seven female track athletes at the end of the competitive season and again three months after the cessation of formal training. During the three-month period following formal training, the girls participated in physical activities normal for their age group, including required physical education. They observed a 15.5-percent decrease in $\dot{V}O_2$ max over the three-month period, and noted that the new $\dot{V}O_2$ max levels were similar to those found in nonathletic girls of the same age.

Michael et al. (1972) observed ten female runners, fifteen to eighteen years of age, during twenty-three weeks of inactivity following a three to four month training program for competitive track. They found that by the third week of detraining, the heart rate response to standardized submaximal levels of work was considerably higher than those values found at the beginning of the study when the girls were still in training. These results are nearly identical to those illustrated in Figure 3–1 for five men undergoing complete bedrest.

Brynteson and Sinning (1973) attempted to determine the amount of exercise necessary for the maintenance of those gains attained from a formal training program. The subjects exercised five days per week for five weeks to develop their initial training levels. They were then divided into four groups, exercising either one, two, three, or four times per week, to determine the minimal frequency that would maintain the initial training level. They found that cardiovascular fitness was maintained by exercising three times per week, and that there were significant losses in conditioning in the two groups that exercised only once or twice per week. Siegel et al. (1970) found an increase in $\dot{V}O_2$ max of 19 percent following fifteen weeks of training in nine men who trained twelve minutes a day, three days per week. At the end of training, five subjects continued to train once a week for an additional fourteen weeks, at which time their $\dot{V}O_2$ max had decreased to only 6 percent above their initial control level. The remaining four subjects stopped training altogether, and their $\dot{V}O_2$ max values, following fourteen weeks of detraining, dropped below their original control values.

Pate et al. (1978) examined the effects of arm training on the retention of training effects produced by leg training. Initially, the subjects trained on bicycle ergometers for eight weeks. The subjects were then divided into one of three groups: arm training, continued leg training, and no training. After four weeks in one of the three subgroups, the subjects were retested. $\dot{V}O_2$ max continued to increase in the group that continued leg training (+3.7 percent), while the arm training group and the group that discontinued training decreased −2.6 percent and −6.8 percent respectively. The authors concluded that arm training does not significantly affect the deterioration in metabolic response to leg work which occurs with the cessation of leg training.

From these studies, and other studies of a similar design, it is apparent that cardiovascular endurance capacity is lost very rapidly following the cessation of formal endurance training. While complete bedrest provides the most dramatic decreases, even periods of light activity or formal endurance training once or twice a week, are not sufficient to prevent the loss of cardiovascular conditioning. Thus, the athlete must consciously work on maintaining his or her endurance capacity during the off-season, for once it is lost, it takes a considerable period of time to regain the peak levels. The sooner the injured athlete can get back into some modified form of endurance exercise, the smaller will be the loss in cardiovascular endurance capacity. While it may be impossible to return to a running or swimming type of activity, stationary or regular bicycling are excellent cardiovascular conditioning exercises that will place little stress on the joints or muscles.

Body Composition

Changes in body composition with decreased physical activity are similar to those found for increased physical activity, except that they are in the opposite direction. With inactivity, the lean body weight tends to decrease and total body fat tends to increase. This is illustrated in Figure 8–2 by changes in subcutaneous fat as measured by skinfold thicknesses in a group of female gymnasts over a period of several years, with indicated periods of total inactivity, moderate training, and intense training. A substantial variation in skinfold thickness occurred over this period of time, reflecting the influence of marked changes in activity patterns. The degree of change in lean and fat weight will depend to a large extent on the initial size and composition of the individual and on the eating and activity habits of the athlete during the period of detraining. The athlete who has developed considerable muscle bulk from strength training activities during the season will lose a considerable amount of lean weight once training is stopped. Losses of ten to twenty pounds or more are not uncommon. The extremely lean athlete, such as the long-distance runner who trains one hundred miles or more per week, will gain a considerable amount of fat if he becomes totally inactive.

Optimal body composition levels can be maintained during the off-season with a modest level of physical training and a conscious effort to control the diet. Although most athletes who work hard

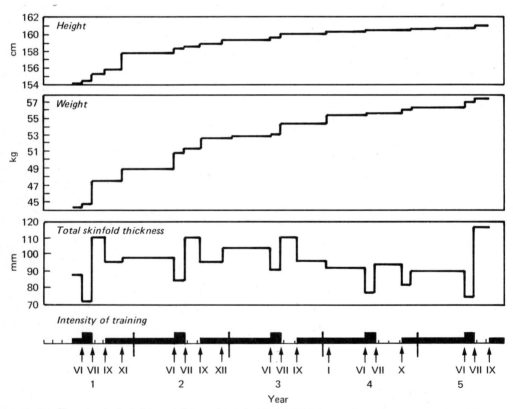

Figure 8–2 Changes in height, weight, and total skinfold thickness in young gymnasts as they progress from periods of limited, moderate, and heavy activity. (From Parízková, *Annals N. Y. Acad. Sci.* 110: 666, 1963).

during the season can eat almost anything and as much as they want to, they must watch their weight carefully during the off-season and regulate their diet accordingly.

OFF-SEASON TRAINING PROGRAMS

From the data in the previous section, it is obvious that the athlete undergoes considerable change as a result of periods of inactivity or detraining. Is this necessarily bad? The athlete can always start the reconditioning process several weeks before beginning a new season. Maybe the athlete needs several months of total inactivity to help pull things back together! While a definite answer to this question is not presently available, it appears that the athlete can receive great benefits from a comprehensive off-season conditioning program that is individually designed to meet personal needs and interests. The highly conditioned athlete who becomes totally inactive loses a considerable amount of that conditioning. Regaining this takes a considerable amount of time and effort, which could mean that the athlete might not regain peak form or performance potential until well into the competitive season. The inability to perform at optimal levels early in the season may prove costly, both in success and in potential serious injury. In addition, extreme cyclic variations in body composition and physiological condition may reduce the athlete's longevity. Observations of a number of professional athletes suggest that those who maintain themselves in reasonable condition throughout the year are able to continue their sport longer and more successfully than those who go into hibernation during the off-season.

In the previous discussion, it was demonstrated that peak levels of conditioning can be maintained by training at frequencies considerably less than those required during the season. Strength can be maintained by one full workout every ten to fourteen days. Cardiovascular endurance, however, is maintained by training a minimum of three times per week. Therefore, an off-season program can be designed that requires no more than three days of activity per week. In addition, the workout periods need not exceed one to two hours in length. This totals only three to six hours of training per week,

which is a minimum investment in time for the resulting benefits.

The athlete and coach must give considerable thought to the design of the off-season conditioning program. All too frequently this is left strictly to chance. One of the most important factors is that it must be fun and enjoyable for the athlete. The activities that are selected should differ somewhat from those used during the season to prevent boredom. Occasional or frequent competition is suggested, since this provides additional motivation to participate. Several professional football teams have organized formal competition in basketball for their athletes in the off-season as a part of the off-season training program. This activity is physically demanding, has components of training that are similar to those for football, and the stimulus of competition maintains interest and enthusiasm.

The period of training during the off-season also allows the athlete to concentrate on the development of areas in which he or she is weak. The swimmer who lacks upper body strength can use this time to concentrate on the development of strength in this area in a way that will be applicable to performance in the pool. The wrestler who lacks cardiovascular endurance can use this time to develop endurance through running or bicycling. The off-season presents the athlete with a relatively free, unstructured period of time in which all aspects of performance can be worked on. As the athlete gets older, this off-season time becomes even more critical. He or she will notice that aging will gradually decrease peak levels of performance, and may find that it becomes increasingly more difficult to regain peak levels if his or her condition is allowed to deteriorate with periods of inactivity.

With this in mind, it is important that off-season conditioning programs be designed for the individual as much as possible. Every off-season program must also attend to the areas of strength, power, muscular endurance, flexibility, cardiovascular endurance, and body composition. An activity such as circuit training (refer to the section on circuit training in Chapter 4) meets almost every need in each of these areas. An hour of circuit training, three days per week, combined with two to three hours of vigorous, game-type activities each week, e.g., basketball, handball, squash, or badminton, should provide a balanced off-season program for most athletes. If the athlete has a particular weakness, an additional hour or two can be devoted to developing this specific area. Another approach would be to combine running three to five miles per day, three days per week, with strength, power, and muscular endurance training exercises and selected flexibility exercises. Specific exercises should be selected on the basis of the needs of the individual and the demands of the sport.

Last, the athlete should receive sound nutritional counseling to assure a properly balanced diet which will provide the essential vitamins and minerals and assist in controlling weight. This is an area of considerable ignorance, lack of knowledge, and many myths. Nutrition will be discussed in greater detail in Chapter 10.

In conclusion, it should be realized that the off-season training program is an extremely important aspect of the athlete's total training program, although it is frequently given little thought or attention and is left strictly to chance. The coach and athlete should work closely together to design a program that will meet the needs of the athlete and provide him some variation from his typical or traditional approach to training. The off-season provides an excellent opportunity to develop a basic foundation for each of the various components of physical training. For example, each program should devote at least some time to each of the following areas.

- Strength
- Power
- Muscular endurance
- Flexibility
- Speed
- Agility and neuromuscular coordination
- Cardiovascular endurance
- Body composition
- Nutrition

Ideally, athletes would be provided with an individualized program to follow on their own, which would provide them with the opportunity to report at the beginning of the new season in peak physical condition.

IN-SEASON TRAINING PROGRAMS

Coaches and athletes have recently become concerned about the physical condition of the athlete during the season. Many athletes feel that they become deconditioned as the season progresses. In analyzing training programs in many, if not most, sports, it is evident that once the competition begins, very little attention is given to physical conditioning. It is assumed that the competition alone will maintain the high level of conditioning that was developed in the pre-season conditioning program. While there has been no research to determine if, in fact, one does become deconditioned as the season progresses, it would seem reasonable to initiate in-season training programs to insure the maintenance of the athlete's fitness. Since so much time is needed during the season for skill and technique development, in-season conditioning programs must not require a great deal of time. These programs should, however, be designed to give attention to each of those areas previously listed.

Professional baseball and basketball provide examples of such a concern. For the athlete who is playing every day, there is reason to believe that the competition itself allows the athlete to maintain his or her physical condition, although this would certainly be questionable for the sport of baseball. For the eighth player on the basketball team, or the reserve catcher on the baseball team, games mean little more than riding the bench for several hours. Those individuals who are not playing regularly are most certainly undergoing deconditioning during the course of the season. It would seem wise to institute an in-season conditioning or maintenance program for all athletes, whether they are playing regularly or not. There will be a maximum return for a minimum investment.

GENERAL SUMMARY

Most athletes regard the conclusion of a long season of intense physical training and competition as the beginning of a welcomed and necessary period of rest and relaxation. While this rest and relaxation are certainly necessary and well-deserved, unfortunately many interpret this as a time to go into physical hibernation. However, physical conditioning cannot simply be put into storage and recalled at will when needed. *If you don't use it, you lose it.* Research evidence abundantly demonstrates that periods of physical inactivity will lead to losses in strength, power, muscular endurance, flexibility, and cardiovascular endurance. While the losses in strength and power are somewhat gradual, the loss in cardiovascular endurance capacity occurs very rapidly. Body composition will also change with inactivity, particularly without concomitant changes in diet. These changes would include a loss in the lean body weight and an increase in fat weight, which would result in a substantial increase in relative fat.

To prevent or minimize the physiological changes that result from periods of physical inactivity, the athlete is strongly advised to participate in an off-season program of physical training. The off-season program should be varied so it includes activities that are enjoyable, but it should be sufficiently structured so each of the major components of physical training are stressed. The off-season program is also an opportune time to work on areas of weakness where supplemental training would be of considerable value. Circuit training provides one of the more versatile approaches to off-season conditioning, since it stresses each of the major components in a relatively brief workout. This type of activity performed three times per week and coupled with a vigorous game-type of activity several days each week would provide the athlete with an interesting, challenging, and physiologically rewarding program that would fully prepare him for the start of the new season.

STUDY QUESTIONS

1. What alterations occur in strength, power, and muscular endurance with physical detraining?
2. What alterations occur in speed, agility, and flexibility with physical detraining?
3. What changes occur in the cardiovascular system as one becomes deconditioned?
4. How important is an off-season conditioning program for a football player? A swimmer? A gymnast?
5. Design an off-season conditioning program for a professional baseball player.
6. As one becomes inactive, what are the resulting changes in body composition?

REFERENCES

Åstrand, P.-O., and Rodahl, K. *Textbook of Work Physiology.* 2nd ed. New York: McGraw-Hill Book Co., 1977.

Brynteson, P., and Sinning, W. E. "The Effects of Training Frequencies on the Retention of Cardiovascular Fitness." *Med. Sci. Sports* 5 (1973): 29–33.

Clarke, D. H. "Adaptations in Strength and Muscular Endurance Resulting from Exercise." In *Exercise and Sport Sciences Reviews,* vol. 1, edited by J. H. Wilmore. New York: Academic Press, 1973.

Drinkwater, B. L., and Horvath, S. M. "Detraining Effects in Young Women." *Med. Sci. Sports* 4 (1972): 91–95.

Fox, E. L. *Sports Physiology.* Philadelphia: W. B. Saunders Co., 1979.

Gettman, L. R., and Pollock, M. L. "Circuit Weight Training: A Critical Review of its Physiological Benefits." *Physician Sportsmed.* in press, 1981.

Jensen, C. R., and Fisher, A. G. *Scientific Basis of Athletic Conditioning.* 2nd ed. Philadelphia: Lea & Febiger, 1979.

Mathews, D. K., and Fox, E. L. *The Physiological Basis of Physical Education and Athletics.* 2nd. ed. Philadelphia: W. B. Saunders Co., 1976.

Michael, E.; Evert, J.; and Jeffers, K. "Physiological Changes of Teenage Girls during Five Months of Detraining." *Med. Sci. Sports* 4 (1972): 214–218.

Pate, R. R.; Hughes, R. D.; Chandler, J. V.; and Ratliffe, J. L. "Effects of Arm Training on Retention of Training Effects Derived from Leg Training." *Med. Sci. Sports* 10 (1978): 71–74.

Pollock, M. L. "Quantification of Endurance Training Programs." *Exercise and Sport Sciences Reviews,* vol. 1, edited by J. H. Wilmore. New York: Academic Press, 1973.

Saltin, B.; Blomqvist, G.; Mitchell, J. H.; Johnson, Jr., R. L.; Wildenthal, K.; and Chapman, C. B. "Response to Submaximal and Maximal Exercise after Bed Rest and Training." *Circulation* 38 (Suppl. 7) (1968).

Siegel, W.; Blomqvist, G.; and Mitchell, J. H. "Effects of a Quantified Physical Training Program on Middle-Aged Sedentary Men." *Circulation* 41 (1970): 19–29.

Thorstensson, A. "Observations on Strength Training and Detraining." *Acta Physiol. Scand.* 100 (1977): 491–493.

SECTION C

Special Considerations in Physical Training

Considerable variation exists both within and among athletes relative to their performance potential. This results from a number of factors, some of which are outside the control of either the coach or the athlete, e.g., genetic constitution, but many can be either controlled, e.g., taking water to prevent dehydration, or adaptations can be made to reduce or enhance the potential influencing factor, e.g., acclimatization to altitude or thermal stress.

First, profiles of elite athletes in selected sports will be presented in Chapter 9. Chapter 10 will discuss the importance of nutrition to athletic performance. The various environmental factors that can influence athletic performance will be discussed in Chapter 11. How does the athlete contend with extreme variations in temperature, both hot and cold? How does humidity interact with temperature to influence the performance of the athlete? Can the athlete perform at moderate or even high altitudes without experiencing decrements in performance potential? What performance limitations does the athlete experience when exercising under increased atmospheric pressures, as in underwater diving? Chapter 12 discusses how performance can be improved by the use of various ergogenic or work-producing aids and how other agents that are thought to be ergogenic in nature have a relative small influence on the athlete's performance. This will include a discussion of drugs, oxygen, diet, warm-up, and social facilitation, among other topics. Chapters 13 and 14 will deal with the special problems of the female athlete and with the growing and aging athlete. In addition to the special considerations of the aging athlete, Chapter 15 will discuss the role of exercise in preventive medicine, with particular reference to coronary artery disease and obesity.

9

Profiles of Elite Athletes

INTRODUCTION

Recent advances in sports physiology have led to an interest in the development of physiological profiles to describe the qualities and characteristics of elite athletes in their various sports. Detailed profiles have been established for athletes in track and field, rowing, gymnastics, swimming, orienteering, speed skating, wrestling, weight lifting, body building, horse racing, skiing, basketball, baseball, football, ice hockey, tennis, racketball, and volleyball. These profiles have considerable application in developing a better understanding of the sport, and in providing data on elite athletes against which data from aspiring athletes can be compared. With respect to better understanding the sport, the profile of the elite athlete provides insights into those areas of training that should be emphasized, and also those areas that would need little, if any, attention. Middle-distance runners and cross-country skiiers have exceptionally high $\dot{V}O_2$ max values, but the upper body strength of the middle-distance runner is low to average, while the cross-country skiier has relatively high upper body strength. Thus, the middle-distance runner needs to spend relatively little training time and effort on upper body development, but a considerable amount on aerobic training. The cross-country skiier needs to emphasize both areas. While this example may seem very obvious, the next example is not. In a comprehensive profile of elite jockeys, it was discovered that strength and cardiorespiratory endurance capacity were extremely important components, while relative body fat was not as important as had been anticipated. The better jockies had their body composition under control and had developed excellent strength and cardiorespiratory endurance capacity.

Obviously, the natural or genetic endowment of the athlete is going to greatly influence the profiles of the elite athletes. It is specifically for this reason that some coaches and sport scientists have joined forces to develop profiles of the elite for a specific sport, and then go out into the world attempting to identify athletes who match that profile. As was mentioned in Chapter 5, Borzov, the great Russian sprinter who won gold medals in the 1972 Olympic Games, was selected in this manner. The profile of the young, developing athlete can be compared with the profile of the elite athlete to determine one's potential for that sport. In addition, the physical conditioning needs become apparent. Where the young athlete is deficient, the training program can be modified to help develop or strengthen the areas of weakness. This provides for an accurate individualization in the prescription of both in-season and off-season conditioning programs.

Profiling of athletes is not a new twist in sports physiology. Dr. Thomas K. Cureton, Professor emeritus at the University of Illinois, pioneered much of the early work in this area. His book, *Physical Fitness of Champion Athletes*, published in 1951, is still considered a classic and contains a great deal of valuable information on swimmers,

149

divers, skaters, wrestlers, gymnasts, and participants in track and field. More recently, the Russians and East Germans have placed a great deal of emphasis on athletic profiling, and the subsequent results have been obvious from the performances of these two countries in international competition over the last ten years. In 1976, the United States Olympic Committee opened an Olympic Training Center in Squaw Valley, California, and opened a second center in Colorado Springs, Colorado, in 1978. The Squaw Valley Center was closed in September, 1980, and all of the resources were transferred to the Colorado Springs Center. While called a "training center," these centers have also been involved in the testing of athletes, with the intent of developing and refining athletic profiles for a number of different sports. Data from these two centers are just now finding their way into the literature.

While many physiological aspects of performance have been quantified for selected or small groups of athletes, the largest volume of data exist in the areas of body composition and physique, muscle fiber characteristics, strength, and cardiovascular endurance capacity. The remainder of this chapter will be devoted to presenting those data published in the literature in each of these areas, with a very brief discussion of each area. The emphasis will be on the presentation of the data.

BODY COMPOSITION AND PHYSIQUE

Height, weight, and relative body fat values for athletes in various sports are presented in Table 9–1. From this table, it is apparent that the female athlete is typically fatter than her male counterpart, and that athletes who are involved in endurance activities, or who must control their weight to meet a certain competitive weight classification, have very low relative body fats. It is generally felt that a low relative body fat is desirable for successful competition in almost any sport. There is a high negative correlation between percentage of body fat and performance in those activities where the body mass must be moved through space, either vertically, as in jumping, or horizontally, as in running.

Figure 9–1 illustrates the relative body fat values for a number of national and international class track and field female athletes. This figure illus-

trates several very important points. First, although not obvious from the figure, the better runners generally had low relative body fat values, usually below 12 percent body fat. However, one of the best runners, who held most of the American middle-distance records, was over 17 percent body fat. She was training very intensely, with both a great volume of high intensity training and long-distance running. It is unlikely that this athlete could have reduced her relative body fat to levels below 12 percent without having a negative influence on her subsequent performance. This points to the importance of treating each athlete as an individual, and not only as a member of a group where all athletes in the same sport, or event within a sport, have to achieve the same level of body fat. It is appropriate to establish guidelines for each sport, e.g., female distance runners should be less than 12 percent fat, but consideration must be given to these exceptions!

Another point that must be emphasized from Figure 9–1 relates to the very high body fat percentages observed in discus throwers and shot putters. This figure might leave one with the impression that to be a national-class shot putter or discus thrower, one needs to be fat, i.e., greater than 30 percent fat. This is very misleading. First, many of these women were shot put and discus athletes because of their size, not because of their high level of body fat. Most people associate strength and power with body size, so the bigger the athlete the better. Unfortunately, much of the size increase is from increases in fat weight, not in lean body weight. This points to the importance of monitoring ath-

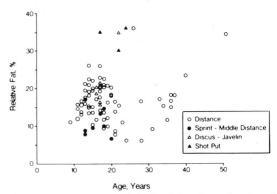

Figure 9–1 Relative body fat values for female track and field athletes.

Table 9–1 *Body Composition Values in Male and Female Athletes**

Athletic Group or Sport	Sex	Age, yr.	Height, cm	Weight, kg	Relative Fat %	Reference
Baseball	male	20.8	182.7	83.3	14.2	Novak et al., 1968
	male	—	—	—	11.8	Forsyth and Sinning, 1973
	male	27.4	183.1	88.0	12.6	Wilmore, unpublished
Basketball	female	19.1	169.1	62.6	20.8	Sinning, 1973
	female	19.4	167.0	63.9	26.9	Conger and Macnab, 1967
Centers	male	27.7	214.0	109.2	7.1	Parr et al., 1978
Forwards	male	25.3	200.6	96.9	9.0	Parr et al., 1978
Guards	male	25.2	188.0	83.6	10.6	Parr et al., 1978
Canoeing	male	23.7	182.0	79.6	12.4	Rusko et al., 1978
Football	male	20.3	184.9	96.4	13.8	Novak et al., 1968
	male	—	—	—	13.9	Forsyth and Sinning, 1973
Defensive backs	male	17–23	178.3	77.3	11.5	Wickkiser and Kelly, 1975
	male	24.5	182.5	84.8	9.6	Wilmore et al., 1976
Offensive backs	male	17–23	179.7	79.8	12.4	Wickkiser and Kelly, 1975
	male	24.7	183.8	90.7	9.4	Wilmore et al., 1976
Linebackers	male	17–23	180.1	87.2	13.4	Wickkiser and Kelly, 1975
	male	24.2	188.6	102.2	14.0	Wilmore et al., 1976
Offensive linemen	male	17–23	186.0	99.2	19.1	Wickkiser and Kelly, 1975
	male	24.7	193.0	112.6	15.6	Wilmore et al., 1976
Defensive linemen	male	17–23	186.6	97.8	18.5	Wickkiser and Kelly, 1975
	male	25.7	192.4	117.1	18.2	Wilmore et al., 1976
Quarterbacks, kickers	male	24.1	185.0	90.1	14.4	Wilmore et al., 1976
Gymnastics	male	20.3	178.5	69.2	4.6	Novak et al., 1968
	female	19.4	163.0	57.9	23.8	Conger and MacNab, 1967
	female	20.0	158.5	51.5	15.5	Sinning and Lindberg, 1972
	female	14.0	—	—	17.0	Parízková, 1973
	female	23.0	—	—	11.0	Parízková, 1973
	female	23.0	—	—	9.6	Parízková and Poupa, 1963
Ice hockey	male	26.3	180.3	86.7	15.1	Wilmore, unpublished
	male	22.5	179.0	77.3	13.0	Rusko et al., 1978
Jockeys	male	30.9	158.2	50.3	14.1	Wilmore, unpublished
Orienteering	male	31.2	—	72.2	16.3	Knowlton et al., 1980
	female	29.0	—	58.1	18.7	Knowlton et al., 1980
Pentathalon	female	21.5	175.4	65.4	11.0	Krahenbuhl et al., 1979
Racketball	male	25.0	181.7	80.3	8.1	Pipes, 1978b

Table 9-1 *(continued)*

Athletic Group or Sport	Sex	Age, yr.	Height, cm	Weight, kg	Relative Fat %	Reference
Rowing						
Heavyweight	male	23.0	192.0	88.0	11.0	Hagerman et al., 1979
Lightweight	male	21.0	186.0	71.0	8.5	Hagerman et al., 1979
	female	23.0	173.0	68.0	14.0	Hagerman et al., 1979
Skiing						
Alpine	male[a]	25.9	176.6	74.8	7.4	Sprynarová and Parízková, 1971
	male	21.2	176.0	70.1	14.1	Rusko et al., 1978
	male	21.8	177.8	75.5	10.2	Haymes and Dickinson, 1980
	female	19.5	165.1	58.8	20.6	Haymes and Dickinson, 1980
Cross-country	male	21.2	176.0	66.6	12.5	Niinimaa et al., 1978
	male	25.6	174.0	69.3	10.2	Rusko et al., 1978
	male	22.7	176.2	73.2	7.9	Haymes and Dickinson, 1980
	female	24.3	163.0	59.1	21.8	Rusko et al., 1978
	female	20.2	163.4	55.9	15.7	Haymes and Dickinson, 1980
Nordic combination	male	22.9	176.0	70.4	11.2	Rusko et al., 1978
	male	21.7	181.7	70.4	8.9	Haymes and Dickinson, 1980
Skijumping	male	22.2	174.0	69.9	14.3	Rusko et al., 1978
Soccer	male	26.0	176.0	75.5	9.6	Raven et al., 1976
Speed skating	male	21.0	181.0	76.5	11.4	Rusko et al., 1978
Swimming	male[a]	21.8	182.3	79.1	8.5	Sprynarová and Parízková, 1971
	male[a]	20.6	182.9	78.9	5.0	Novak et al., 1968
	female[a]	19.4	168.0	63.8	26.3	Conger and Macnab, 1968
Sprint	female	—	165.1	57.1	14.6	Wilmore et al., 1977
Middle distance	female	—	166.6	66.8	24.1	Wilmore et al., 1977
Distance	female	—	166.3	60.9	17.1	Wilmore et al., 1977
Tennis	male	—	—	—	15.2	Forsyth and Sinning, 1973
	male	42.0	179.6	77.1	16.3	Vodak et al., 1980
	female	39.0	163.3	55.7	20.3	Vodak et al., 1980
Track and field	male[a]	21.3	180.6	71.6	3.7	Novak et al., 1968
	male[a]	—	—	—	8.8	Forsyth and Sinning, 1973
Runners	male	22.5	177.4	64.5	6.3	Sprynarová and Parízková, 1971
Distance	male	26.1	175.7	64.2	7.5	Costill et al., 1970
	male	26.2	177.0	66.2	8.4	Rusko et al., 1978
	male	40–49	180.7	71.6	11.2	Pollock et al., 1974
	male	55.3	174.5	63.4	18.0	Barnard et al., 1979
	male	50–59	174.7	67.2	10.9	Pollock et al., 1974
	male	60–69	175.7	67.1	11.3	Pollock et al., 1974

Table 9-1 *(continued)*

Athletic Group or Sport	Sex	Age, yr.	Height, cm	Weight, kg	Relative Fat %	Reference
	male	70–75	175.6	66.8	13.6	Pollock et al., 1974
	male	47.2	176.5	70.7	13.2	Lewis et al., 1975
	female	19.9	161.3	52.9	19.2	Malina et al., 1971
	female	32.4	169.4	57.2	15.2	Wilmore and Brown, 1974
Middle distance	male	24.6	179.0	72.3	12.4	Rusko et al., 1978
Sprint	female	20.1	164.9	56.7	19.3	Malina et al., 1971
	male	46.5	177.0	74.1	16.5	Barnard et al., 1979
Discus	male	28.3	186.1	104.7	16.4	Fahey et al., 1975
	male	26.4	190.8	110.5	16.3	Wilmore, unpublished
Jumpers & hurdlers	female	21.1	168.1	71.0	25.0	Malina et al., 1971
Shot Put	female	20.3	165.9	59.0	20.7	Malina et al., 1971
	male	27.0	188.2	112.5	16.5	Fahey et al., 1975
	male	22.0	191.6	126.2	19.6	Behnke and Wilmore, 1974
Volleyball	female	21.5	167.6	78.1	28.0	Malina et al., 1971
	female	19.4	166.0	59.8	25.3	Conger and Macnab, 1968
Weight lifting	female	19.9	172.2	64.1	21.3	Kovaleski et al., 1980
Power	male	24.9	166.4	77.2	9.8	Sprynarová and Parízková, 1971
Olympic	male	26.3	176.1	92.0	15.6	Fahey et al., 1975
Body builders	male	25.3	177.1	88.2	12.2	Fahey et al., 1975
	male	29.0	172.4	83.1	8.4	Fahey et al., 1975
Wrestling	male	27.6	178.8	88.1	8.3	Pipes, 1979a
	male	26.0	177.8	81.8	9.8	Fahey et al., 1975
	male	27.0	176.0	75.7	10.7	Gale and Flynn, 1974
	male	22.0	—	—	5.0	Parízková, 1973
	male	23.0	—	79.3	14.3	Taylor et al., 1979
	male	19.6	174.6	74.8	8.8	Sinning, 1974
	male	15–18	172.3	66.3	6.9	Katch and Michael, 1971
	male	20.6	174.8	67.3	4.0	Stine et al., 1979

[a]Specific events were not specified.

*Adapted from J. H. Wilmore et al., "Body Physique and Composition of the Female Distance Runner," Ann. New York Acad. Sci. 301 (1977).

letes who are on weight gain or weight loss programs, to determine if the gains or losses are in the desired compartments, i.e., lean weight gains and fat weight losses. One of these shot putters, who went on to shatter the American record, lost a considerable amount of body fat and gained lean body weight through a combination weight training and dietary program. As she continued to lose fat and gain lean weight, her performances continued to improve.

Somatotypes of athletes in various sports are presented in Table 9–2. Unfortunately, there have not been as many athletes somatotyped as there have been athletes who have had body composition assessments. Dr. J. E. Lindsay Carter, Professor at San Diego State University, has conducted most of the studies presently available in the literature, and conducted all of the somatotypes listed in Table

9–2 under the deGaray reference. Dr. Carter is continuing to collect data on elite athletes in a number of different sports, and these data should be available in the very near future. From the data in Table 9–2 and Figures 9–2 and 9–3, it is obvious that athletes are generally low in endomorphy, with the exception of the throwers in track and field. Mesomorphy values range from moderate in runners to high in activities dependent on strength. Ectomorphy ranges from low in strength athletes to moderate in distance runners and jumpers.

MUSCLE FIBER CHARACTERISTICS

At present, few athletes have undergone muscle biopsies to determine their relative distribution of fast- and slow-twitch fibers. Since this is a compara-

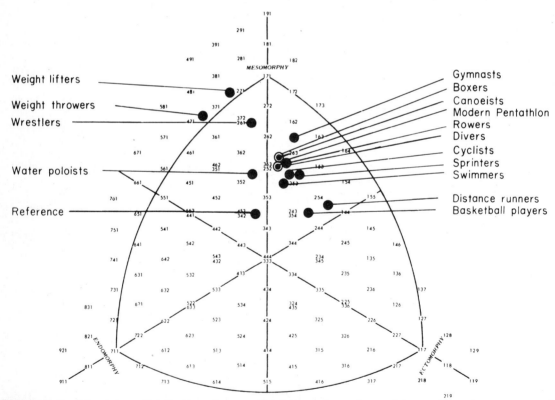

Figure 9–2 Somatotype distribution of mean somatotypes for male participants in various sports at the 1968 Olympic Games. (From A. L. deGaray et al., eds., *Genetic and Anthropological Studies of Olympic Athletes.* New York: Academic Press, 1974. Reproduced by permission of the publisher.)

Table 9–2 *Somatotype Values for Male and Female Athletes**

Athletic Group or Sport	Sex	Age, yrs.	Height, cm	Weight, kg	Somatotype Endo	Meso	Ecto	Reference
Orienteers	male	31	—	72.2	2.3	3.6	2.9	Knowlton et al., 1980
	female	29	—	58.1	3.9	3.7	2.5	Knowlton et al., 1980
Racketball	male	25	181.7	80.3	3.1	3.6	2.8	Pipes, 1979b
Swimming	male	19	179.3	72.1	2.1	5.0	2.9	deGaray, 1974
	female	16	164.4	56.9	3.4	4.0	3.0	deGaray, 1974
Track and Field Runners								
Marathon	male	26	168.7	56.6	1.4	4.3	3.5	deGaray, 1974
Long distance	male	—	171.1	59.9	2.6	4.4	3.9	Tanner, 1964
	male	25	171.9	59.8	1.4	4.1	3.6	deGaray, 1974
Middle distance	male	—	174.4	60.8	2.7	4.2	4.3	Tanner, 1964
	male	23	177.3	65.0	1.5	4.2	3.6	deGaray, 1974
	female	20	166.9	54.3	2.0	3.3	3.7	deGaray, 1974
Sprint	male	24	175.4	68.4	1.7	5.0	2.8	deGaray, 1974
	female	21	165.0	56.8	2.7	3.9	2.9	deGaray, 1974
Jumpers	male	24	182.8	73.2	1.7	4.4	3.4	deGaray, 1974
Throwers	female	22	169.4	56.4	2.2	3.3	3.7	deGaray, 1974
	male	27	186.1	102.3	3.5	7.1	1.0	deGaray, 1974
Volleyball	female	20	170.9	73.5	5.3	5.2	1.7	deGaray, 1974
	female	20	172.2	64.1	4.2	3.7	3.3	Kovaleski et al., 1980
Weight lifting	male	27	168.0	76.6	2.4	7.1	1.0	deGaray, 1974
Body building	male	27	178.8	88.1	3.9	6.8	1.5	Pipes, 1979a
Wrestling	male	26	169.3	70.6	2.2	6.3	1.6	deGaray, 1974
	male	—	172.4	72.0	2.7	5.6	2.5	Tanner, 1964
	male	23	—	79.2	2.9	6.4	1.2	Taylor et al., 1979

*Adapted from J. H. Wilmore et al., "Body Physique and Composition of the Female Distance Runner," Ann. New York Acad. Sci. 301 (1977).

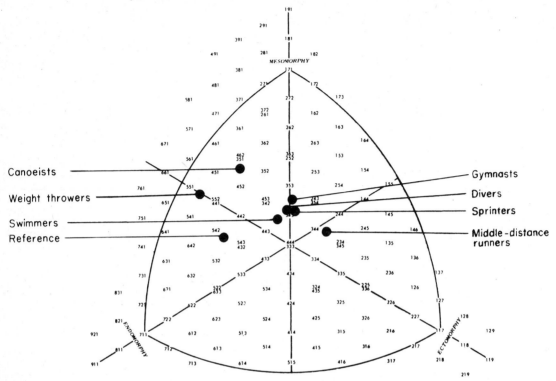

Figure 9–3 Somatotype distribution of mean somatotypes for female participants in various sports at the 1968 Olympic Games. (From A. L. deGaray et al., eds., *Genetic and Anthropological Studies of Olympic Athletes.* New York: Academic Press, 1974. Reproduced by permission of the publisher.)

tively new technique, and has not been widely used due to the inherent complexity of the subsequent analyses, few athletic populations have been studied. Table 9–3 provides data for those few athletic populations that have been studied. From these data, it is clear that there is a direct linear relationship between the endurance nature of the activity and the percentage of slow-twitch fibers. Bergh et al. (1978) reported a correlation of $r = 0.72$ between $\dot{V}O_2$ max and percentage of slow-twitch fibers in endurance and strength trained athletes, while Rusko et al. (1978) reported a correlation of $r = 0.56$ in athletes representing various sports and events. Where data are available for both males and females in similar sports or events, there does appear to be little difference between the sexes relative to the percentage of slow-twitch fibers, although males appear to have larger fiber areas.

STRENGTH

Strength, power, and muscular endurance are critical factors for most athletes. However, only limited data are available for a few athletic populations, and these are primarily in the area of strength. Power and muscular endurance are very difficult to assess accurately; the most complete data available exist only for professional football players (Wilmore et al., 1976) and professional basketball players (Parr et al., 1978). Table 9–4 lists selected strength values for various male athletic populations. At the present, similar data do not exist for females. It is obvious that strength is highly correlated to size, and that in those sports where strength is not a major prerequisite for success, strength values are considerably lower for athletes of similar body size.

Table 9–3   *Muscle Fiber Characteristics of Athletes**

Athletic Group or Sport	Sex	Age, yrs.	Height, cm	Weight, kg	Slow-Twitch Fibers, %	Slow-Twitch Fiber Area μ^2	Slow-Twitch Fiber Area %	Reference
Bicyclists	male	24	182	74.5	61.4[a]	—	—	Gollnick et al., 1972
	male	25	180	72.8	56.8[a]	6,333	59.7	Burke et al., 1977
	female	20	165	55.0	50.5[a]	5,487	47.6	Burke et al., 1977
Canoeists	male	26	181	74.0	61.4[a]	—	—	Gollnick et al., 1972
	male	24	182	79.6	58.0[a]	—	—	Rusko et al., 1978
Field hockey	female	23	161	57.7	48.2[a]	4,305	27.5	Prince et al., 1977
Ice hockey	male	22	179	77.3	61.0[a]	—	—	Rusko et al., 1978
Orienteers	male	52	176	72.7	68.8[a]	—	—	Gollnick et al., 1972
	male	25	181	68.5	67.0[a]	—	—	Thorstensson et al., 1977
Skiers								
Alpine	male	21	178	69.4	48.0[a]	—	—	Thorstensson et al., 1977
	male	21	176	70.1	63.0[a]	—	—	Rusko et al., 1978
Cross-country	male	26	174	69.3	63.0[a]/72.0[c]	—	—	Rusko et al., 1978
	female	24	163	59.1	60.0[a]/61.0[c]	—	—	Rusko et al., 1978
Nordic combination	male	23	176	70.4	63.0[a]/74.0[c]	—	—	Rusko et al., 1978
Skijumping	male	22	174	69.9	55.0[a]	—	—	Rusko et al., 1978
Speed skating	male	21	181	76.5	69.0[a]/63.0[c]	—	—	Rusko et al., 1978
Swimmers	male	21	181	78.3	57.7[a]/74.3[b]	—	—	Gollnick et al., 1972
Track and field								
Sprint runners	male	19	181	71.5	24.0[c]	5,878	23.5	Costill et al., 1976a
	female	19	168	55.6	27.4[c]	3,752	26.8	Costill et al., 1976a
Middle-distance runners	male	23	179	65.7	51.9[c]	6,099	46.5	Costill et al., 1976a
	male	25	179	72.3	45.0[a]	—	—	Rusko et al., 1978
	female	20	166	52.5	60.6[c]	6,069	60.4	Costill et al., 1976a
	male	25	180	67.8	61.8[c]	6,378	62.1	Costill et al., 1976b
Long-distance runners	male	24	180	70.8	69.4[c]	6,613	62.3	Costill et al., 1976a
	male	26	179	63.9	79.0[c]	8,342	82.9	Costill et al., 1976b
Runners	male	26	177	66.2	78.0[a]/88.0[b]	—	—	Rusko et al., 1978
	male	23	177	69.5	58.9[a]	—	—	Gollnick et al., 1972
	male	27	178	64.5	59.0[a]	—	—	Thorstensson et al., 1977

Table 9–3 *(continued)*

Athletic Group or Sport	Sex	Age, yrs.	Height, cm	Weight, kg	Slow-Twitch Fibers, %	Slow-Twitch Fiber Area μ_2	Slow-Twitch Fiber Area %	Reference
Sprinters, jumpers	male	24	187	77.6	38.0[a]	—	—	Thorstensson et al., 1977
Long/high jumpers	male	29	183	77.3	46.7[c]	4,718	38.8	Costill et al., 1976a
	female	22	177	61.1	48.7[c]	4,163	44.0	Costill et al., 1976a
Javelin throwers	male	25	176	83.6	50.4[c]	5,585	47.7	Costill et al., 1976a
	female	21	169	65.3	41.6[c]	4,864	42.9	Costill et al., 1976a
Shotput, discus throwers	male	27	198	129.0	37.7[c]	7,702	34.0	Costill et al., 1976a
Weightlifters	female	24	171	77.0	51.2[c]	5,192	46.9	Costill et al., 1976a
	male	25	171	81.3	46.1[a]/52.6[b]	—	—	Gollnick et al., 1972
	male	20	—	72.8	44.0	4,550	—	Edström and Ekblom, 1972
Wrestlers	male	23	—	79.2	48.7[a]	4,998	45.4	Taylor et al., 1979

[a]biopsy from vastus lateralis
[b]biopsy from deltoid
[c]biopsy from gastrocnemius

Adapted from J. H. Wilmore and J. A. Bergfield, "A Comparison of Sports: Physiological and Medical Aspects." In Sports Medicine and Physiology, edited by R. H. Strauss. Philadelphia: W. B. Saunders, 1979.

Table 9–4   *Selected Strength Measurements of Male Athletes**

Athletic Group or Sport	Age, yrs.	Height, cm	Weight, kg	One-Repetition Maximum Values			
				Bench Press, lbs.	Standing Press, lbs.	Curl, lbs.	Leg Press, lbs.
Baseball	28	183.6	88.1	202	144	113	720
Basketball	26	196.6	91.2	207	161	—	576
Football							
Defensive backs	25	182.5	84.8	276	181	132	—
Offensive backs							
and wide							
receivers	25	183.8	90.7	285	203	156	—
Linebackers	24	188.6	102.2	343	215	174	—
Offensive linemen							
and tight ends	25	193.0	112.6	333	214	177	—
Defensive linemen	26	192.4	117.1	325	224	189	—
Quarterbacks,							
kickers	24	185.0	90.1	258	205	146	—
Ice hockey	26	180.1	86.4	240	155	111	699
Jockeys	31	158.2	50.3	134	92	57	501
Racketball	25	181.7	80.3	144	102	78	392
Weightlifting,							
body builders	27	178.8	88.1	407	275	197	392

*Adapted from J. H. Wilmore and J. A. Bergfield, "A Comparison of Sports: Physiological and Medical Aspects." In Sports Medicine and Physiology, *edited by R. H. Strauss. Philadelphia: W. B. Saunders, 1979.*

CARDIOVASCULAR ENDURANCE CAPACITY

Table 9–5 presents $\dot{V}O_2$ max values for male and female athletes in a variety of sports. It is apparent that in those sports having a low aerobic or cardiovascular endurance requirement, the respective athletes have relatively low $\dot{V}O_2$ max values. While their values range from the high 30s into the low 40s, the highly conditioned endurance athlete will have values in the high 60s to low 80s. The distance runner and cross-country skier typically have the highest values.

While elite athletes generally are as well trained as any athlete in a given sport, there sometimes are notable exceptions. In the mid-1970s, we had the opportunity to test two members of the Pittsburgh Pirates professional baseball team. Both were outstanding players, and had made major contributions to their team's World Series victory the previous season. The testing was conducted in mid-season, when most athletes are supposed to be at the peak of their physical condition. Both of these players had very low $\dot{V}O_2$ max values, i.e., less than 40 ml/kg •min. When asked about what they did to condition themselves, both responded that they played their way into condition. When pressed further to elaborate on this, the outfielder described his conditioning program as running out to his position at the start of the inning and back to the dugout at the end of the inning. He then suddenly came up with the explanation for his poor showing on the treadmill—they had moved him to first base! Subsequent work with the Los Angeles Dodger professional baseball team produced totally different results. Four of their pitchers were running as many as ten miles per day on days when they were not pitching. Most of the other players were also in-

Table 9-5 *Cardiovascular Endurance Capacity of Male and Female Athletes**

Athletic Group or Sport	Sex	Age, yrs.	Height, cm	Weight, kg	V̇O₂ max ml/kg·min	Reference
Baseball	male	21	182.7	83.3	52.3[a]	Novak et al., 1968
	male	28	183.6	88.1	52.0[a]	Wilmore, unpublished
Basketball	female	19	167.0	63.9	42.3[b]	Conger and Macnab, 1968
	female	19	169.1	62.6	42.9[b]	Sinning, 1973
Centers	male	28	214.0	109.2	41.9[a]	Parr et al., 1978
Forwards	male	25	200.6	96.9	45.9[a]	Parr et al., 1978
Guards	male	25	188.0	83.6	50.0[a]	Parr et al., 1978
Bicycling (competitive)	male	24	182.0	74.5	68.2[b]	Gollnick et al., 1972
	male	25	180.0	72.8	67.1[b]	Burke et al., 1977
	female	20	165.0	55.0	50.2[b]	Burke et al., 1977
Canoeing	male	26	181.0	74.0	56.8[b]	Gollnick et al., 1972
	male	24	182.0	79.6	66.1[a]	Rusko et al., 1978
Football	male	20	184.9	96.4	51.3	Novak et al., 1968
	male	25	182.5	84.8	53.1[a]	Wilmore et al., 1976
Defensive backs	male	25	183.8	90.7	52.2[a]	Wilmore et al., 1976
Offensive backs, wide receivers Linebackers	male	24	188.6	102.2	52.1[a]	Wilmore et al., 1976
Offensive linemen, tight ends	male	25	193.0	112.6	49.9[a]	Wilmore et al., 1976
Defensive linemen	male	26	192.4	117.1	44.9[a]	Wilmore et al., 1976
Quarterbacks, kickers	male	24	185.0	90.1	49.0[a]	Wilmore et al., 1976
Gymnastics	male	20	178.5	69.2	55.5[a]	Novak et al., 1968
	female	19	163.0	57.9	36.3[b]	Conger and Macnab, 1968
Ice hockey	male	11	140.5	35.5	56.6[b]	Cunningham et al., 1976
	male	22	179.0	77.3	61.5[a]	Rusko et al., 1978
	male	24	179.3	81.8	54.6	Seliger et al., 1972
	male	26	180.1	86.4	53.6[a]	Wilmore, unpublished
Jockey	male	31	158.2	50.3	53.8[a]	Wilmore, unpublished
Orienteering	male	52	176.0	72.7	50.7[a]	Gollnick et al., 1972
	male	31	—	72.2	61.6[a]	Knowlton et al., 1980
	female	29	—	58.1	46.1[a]	Knowlton et al., 1980
Pentathalon	female	21	175.4	65.4	45.9	Krahenbuhl et al., 1979

Table 9-5 *(continued)*

Athletic Group or Sport	Sex	Age yrs.	Height, cm	Weight, kg	VO₂ max ml/kg·min	Reference
Racketball	male	25	181.7	80.3	58.3	Pipes, 1979b
Rowing						
Heavyweight	male	23	192.0	88.0	68.9[d]	Hagerman et al., 1979
Lightweight	male	21	186.0	71.0	71.1[d]	Hagerman, et al., 1979
	female	23	173.0	68.0	60.3[d]	Hagerman, et al., 1979
Skiing						
Alpine	male	26	176.6	74.8	62.3[a]	Sprynarová and Parízková, 1971
	male	21	176.0	70.1	63.8[a]	Rusko et al., 1978
	male	22	177.8	75.5	66.6	Haymes and Dickinson, 1980
	female	19	165.1	58.8	52.7[a]	Haymes and Dickinson, 1980
Cross-country	male	21	176.0	66.6	63.9[a]	Niinimaa et al., 1978
	male	26	174.0	69.3	78.3	Rusko et al., 1978
	male	23	176.2	73.2	73.0[a]	Haymes and Dickinson, 1980
	female	24	163.0	59.1	68.2[a]	Rusko et al., 1978
	female	20	163.4	55.9	61.5[a]	Haymes and Dickinson, 1980
Nordic combination	male	23	176.0	70.4	72.8[a]	Rusko et al., 1978
	male	22	181.7	70.4	67.4[a]	Haymes and Dickinson, 1980
Skijumping	male	22	174.0	69.9	61.3[a]	Rusko et al., 1978
Soccer	male	26	176.0	75.5	58.4[a]	Raven et al., 1976
Speed Skating	male	20	175.5	73.9	56.1[a]	Maksud et al., 1970
	male	21	181.0	76.5	72.9[a]	Rusko et al., 1978
	female	21	164.5	60.8	46.1[a]	Maksud et al., 1970
Swimming	male	12	150.4	41.2	52.5[b]	Cunningham and Eynon, 1973
	female	12	154.8	43.3	46.2[b]	Cunningham and Eynon, 1973
	male	13	164.8	52.1	52.9[b]	Cunningham and Eynon, 1973
	female	13	160.0	52.1	43.4[b]	Cunningham and Eynon, 1973
	male	15	169.6	59.8	56.6[b]	Cunningham and Eynon, 1973
	female	15	164.8	53.7	40.5[b]	Cunningham and Eynon, 1973
	male	22	182.3	79.7	55.9[b]	Cunningham and Eynon, 1973
	male	20	181.4	76.7	55.7[a]/54.6[c]	Magel and Faulkner, 1967
	male	20	181.0	73.0	50.4[b]	Charbonnier et al., 1975
	male	21	182.9	78.9	62.1[a]	Novak et al., 1968
	male	21	181.0	78.3	69.9[b]	Gollnick et al., 1972
	male	22	182.3	79.1	56.9[a]	Sprynarová and Parízková, 1971

Table 9-5 *(continued)*

Athletic Group or Sport	Sex	Age, yrs.	Height, cm	Weight, kg	$\dot{V}O_2$ max ml/kg·min	Reference
Sprint	male	19	181.1	75.0	58.3[a]	Shephard et al., 1974
Middle-distance	male	22	178.0	74.6	55.4[a]	Shephard et al., 1974
Long-distance	male	21	179.0	74.9	65.4[a]	Shephard et al., 1974
Tennis	female	19	168.0	63.8	37.6[b]	Conger and Macnab, 1968
	male	42	179.6	77.1	50.2[a]	Vodak et al., 1980
	female	39	163.3	55.7	44.2[a]	Vodak et al., 1980
Track and field	male	21	180.6	71.6	66.1[a]	Novak et al., 1968
Runners	male	22	177.4	64.5	64.0[a]	Sprynarová and Parízková, 1971
	male	23	177.0	69.5	72.4[a]	Gollnick et al., 1972
Sprint	male	46	177.0	74.1	47.2[a]	Barnard et al., 1979
Middle-distance	male	25	180.1	67.8	70.1[a]	Costill et al., 1976b
	male	25	179.0	72.3	69.8[a]	Rusko et al., 1978
Distance	male	10	144.3	31.9	56.6	Mayers and Gutin, 1979
	male	26	178.9	63.9	77.4[a]	Costill et al., 1976b
	male	26	177.0	66.2	78.1[a]	Rusko et al., 1978
	male	27	178.7	64.9	73.2	Costill, 1970
	male	32	177.3	64.3	70.3[a]	Costill and Winrow, 1970
	male	35	174.0	63.1	66.6[a]	Costill et al., 1976b
	male	40–49	180.7	71.6	57.5[a]	Pollock et al., 1974
	male	55.3	174.5	63.4	54.4[a]	Barnard et al., 1979
	male	50–59	174.7	67.2	54.4[a]	Pollock et al., 1974
	male	60–69	175.7	67.1	51.4[a]	Pollock et al., 1974
	male	70–75	175.6	66.8	40.0[a]	Pollock et al., 1974
	female	16.2	162.2	48.6	63.2[a]	Burke and Brush, 1979
	female	32	169.4	57.2	59.1	Wilmore and Brown, 1974
Discus	male	28	186.1	104.7	47.5[b]	Fahey et al., 1975
	male	26	190.8	110.5	42.8[a]	Wilmore, unpublished
Shot Put	male	27	188.2	112.5	42.6[b]	Fahey et al., 1975
Volleyball	female	19	166.0	59.8	43.5[a]	Conger and Macnab, 1968
	female	20	172.2	64.1	56.0[a]	Kovaleski et al., 1980
Weightlifting	male	25	171.0	81.3	40.1[b]	Gollnick et al., 1972
	male	25	166.4	77.2	42.6[a]	Sprynarová and Parízková, 1971

Table 9–5 *(continued)*

Athletic Group or Sport	Sex	Age, yrs.	Height, cm	Weight, kg	VO$_2$ max ml/kg·min	Reference
Power	male	26	176.1	92.0	49.5[b]	Fahey et al., 1975
Olympic	male	25	177.1	88.2	50.7[b]	Fahey et al., 1975
Body builders	male	29	172.4	83.1	41.5[b]	Fahey et al., 1975
	male	27	178.8	88.1	46.3[b]	Pipes, 1979a
	male	24	175.6	77.7	60.9[a]	Nagel et al., 1975
Wrestling	male	23	—	79.2	50.4[a]	Taylor et al., 1979
	male	26	177.0	81.8	64.0[b]	Fahey et al., 1975
	male	27	176.0	75.7	54.3[a]	Gale and Flynn, 1974
	male	21	174.8	67.3	58.3[a]	Stine et al., 1979

[a]Treadmill
[b]Bicycle ergometer
[c]Tethered swimming
[d]Rowing ergometer

Adapted from J. H. Wilmore and J. A. Bergfield, "A Comparison of Sports: Physiological and Medical Aspects." In Sports Medicine and Physiology, edited by R. H. Strauss. Philadelphia: W. B. Saunders, 1979.

volved in running programs. The Dodger players had considerably higher $\dot{V}O_2$ max values, most of them above 50 ml/kg·min.

GENERAL SUMMARY

This chapter has attempted to present the rationale for developing athletic performance profiles. Profiles on elite athletes allow a better understanding of the performance requirements of that sport. In addition, the performance profile of elite athletes in any one sport, or event within a sport, provides a template against which the younger, developing athletes can measure themselves. This provides an estimate of athletic potential in that young athlete, and also provides information that is then used in individualizing that athlete's conditioning program. Data were then presented in the areas of body composition and physique, muscle fiber type, strength, and cardiovascular endurance capacity ($\dot{V}O_2$ max) for males and females in various sports.

It is important to mention at this point that the data presented in this chapter do not include all of the data available in the literature, nor do the areas selected for discussion constitute all of the areas that have been included in performance test batteries. It is becoming more obvious that profile test batteries should be designed specifically for each sport, with the unique characteristics of that sport kept in mind. From what is known with respect to the area of specificity, it would be a mistake to give all athletes in every sport the same test battery. The batteries must be individualized for each sport. This will require considerable time and effort on the part of the sport scientist, but it will greatly improve the final product.

STUDY QUESTIONS

1. What are the purposes of performance profiles of athletes?
2. What components should be included in a performance profile?
3. Which athletes are the leanest athletes? The fatest?
4. What standards should be established for relative body fat for football? Basketball? Swimming?
5. How do somatotypes vary from one sport, or event within a sport, to another?
6. What is the relationship between $\dot{V}O_2$ max and muscle fiber type?
7. Why do some power athletes such as shot putters and discus throwers have about an equal distribution of fast-twitch and slow-twitch fibers, when sprinters predominantly have fast-twitch fibers?
8. How does strength vary from one sport to the next? Why?
9. Could a strong case be made for endurance conditioning in those athletes that have been identified as having low $\dot{V}O_2$ max values in sports that have little aerobic involvement?
10. What value is all of this testing to the athlete?

REFERENCES

Åstrand, P.-O. and Rodahl, K. Textbook of Work Physiology. 2nd ed. New York: McGraw-Hill Publishing Co., 1977.

Barnard, R. J.; Grimditch, G. K.; and Wilmore, J. H. "Physiological Characteristics of Sprint and Endurance Masters Runners." *Med. Sci. Sports.* 11 (1979):167–171.

Behnke, A. R., and Wilmore, J. H. *Evaluation and Regulation of Body Build and Composition.* Englewood Cliffs, N. J.: Prentice-Hall, 1974.

Bergh, U.; Thorstensson, A.; Sjöden, B.; Hulten, B.; Piehl, K.; and Karlsson, J. "Maximal Oxygen Uptake and Muscle Fiber Types in Trained and Untrained Humans." *Med. Sci. Sports.* 10 (1978):151–154.

Brown, C. H., and Wilmore, J. H. "The Effects of Maximal Resistance Training on the Strength and Body Composition of Women Athletes. *Med. Sci. Sports.* 6 (1974):174–177.

Burke, E. R., and Brush, F. C. "Physiological and Anthropometric Assessment of Successful Teenage Female Distance Runners." *Res. Quart.* 50 (1979):180–187.

Burke, E. R.; Cerny, F.; Costill, D. L.; and Fink, W. "Characteristics of Skeletal Muscle in Competitive Cyclists." *Med. Sci. Sports.* 9 (1977):109–112.

Charbonnier, J. P.; Lacour, J. R.; Riffat, J.; and Flandrois, R. "Experimental Study of the Performance of Competition Swimmers." *Europ. J. Appl. Physiol.* 34 (1975):157–167.

Conger, P. R., and Macnab, R. B. J. "Strength, Body Composition and Work Capacity of Participants and Nonparticipants in Women's Intercollegiate Sports." *Res. Quart.* 38 (1967):184–192.

Costill, D. L. "The Relationship between Selected Physiological Variables and Distance Running Performance." *J. Sports Med.* 7 (1967):61–66.

Costill, D. L. "Metabolic Responses during Distance Running." *J. Appl. Physiol.* 28 (1970):251–255.

Costill, D. L.; Bowers, R.; and Kammer, W. F. Skinfold Estimates of Body Fat among Marathon Runners. *Med. Sci. Sports.* 2 (1970):93–95.

Costill, D. L.; Daniels, J.; Evans, W.; Fink, W.; Krahenbuhl, G.; and Saltin, B. "Skeletal Muscle Enzymes and Fiber Composition in Male and Female Track Athletes." *J. Appl. Physiol.* 40 (1976a):149–154.

Costill, D. L.; Fink, W. J.; and Pollock, M. L. "Muscle Fiber Composition and Enzyme Activities of Elite Distance Runners." *Med. Sci. Sports.* 8 (1976b):96–100.

Costill, D. L.; Thomason, H.; and Roberts, E. "Fractional Utilization of the Aerobic Capacity during Distance Running." *Med. Sci. Sports.* 5 (1973):248–252.

Costill, D. L., and Winrow, E. "Maximal Oxygen Consumption among Marathon Runners." *Arch. Phys. Med.* 51 (1970):317–320.

Cunningham, D. A., and Eynon, R. B. "The Working Capacity of Young Competitive Swimmers, 10–16 Years of Age." *Med. Sci. Sports.* 5 (1973):227–231.

Cunningham, D. A.; Telford, P.; and Swart, G. T. "The Cardio-Pulmonary Capacities of Young Hockey Players: Age 10." *Med. Sci. Sports.* 8 (1976):23–25.

Cureton, T. K. *Physical Fitness of Champion Athletes.* Urbana, Ill.: University of Illinois Press, 1951.

Davies, C. T. M. "Body Composition in Children: A Reference Standard for Maximum Aerobic Power Output on a Stationary Bicycle Ergometer, in Proceedings of the III International Symposium on Pediatric Work Physiology." *Acta Paediatr. Scand. Suppl.* 217 (1971).

deGaray, A. L.; Levine, L.; and Carter, J. E. L. *Genetic and Anthropological Studies of Olympic Athletes.* New York: Academic Press, 1974.

Drinkwater, B. L. "Physiological Responses of Women to Exercise." In *Exercise and Sport Sciences Reviews,* vol. 1, edited by J. H. Wilmore. New York: Academic Press, 1973.

Edström, L., and Ekblom, B. "Differences in Sizes of Red and White Muscle Fibers in Vastus Lateralis of Musculus Quadriceps Femoris of Normal Individuals and Athletes: Relation to Physical Performance." *Scand. J. Clin. Lab. Invest.* 30 (1972):175–181.

Fahey, T. D.; Akka, L.; and Rolph, R. "Body Composition and $\dot{V}O_2$ max of Exceptional Weight-Trained Athletes." *J. Appl. Physiol.* 39 (1975):559–561.

Forsyth, H. L., and Sinning, W. E. "The Anthropometric Estimation of Body Density and Lean Body Weight of Male Athletes." *Med. Sci. Sport.* 5 (1973):174–180.

Gale, J. B., and Flynn, K. W. "Maximal Oxygen Consumption and Relative Body Fat of High-Ability Wrestlers." *Med. Sci. Sports.* 6 (1974):232–234.

Gollnick, P. D.; Armstrong, R. B.; Saubert IV, C. W.; Piehl, K.; and Saltin, B. "Enzyme Activity and Fiber Composition in Skeletal Muscle of Untrained and Trained Men." *J. Appl. Physiol.* 33 (1972):312–319.

Hagerman, F. C.; Hagerman, G. R.; and Mickelson, T. C. "Physiological Profiles of Elite Rowers." *Physician Sportsmed.* 7 (1979):74–83.

Haymes, E. M., and Dickinson, A. L. Characteristics of Elite Male and Female Ski Racers. *Med. Sci. Sports Exercise* 12 (1980):153–158.

Hermansen, L., and Andersen, K. L. "Aerobic Work Capacity in Young Norwegian Men and Women." *J. Appl. Physiol.* 20 (1965):425–431.

Katch, F. I., and Michael, E. D. "Body Composition of High School Wrestlers According to Age and Wrestling Weight Category." *Med. Sci. Sports.* 3 (1971):190–194.

Knowlton, R. G.; Ackerman, K. J.; Fitzgerald, P. I.; Wilde, S. W.; and Tahamont, M. V. "Physiological and Performance Characteristics of United States Championship Class Orienteers." *Med. Sci. Sports Exercise.* 12 (1980):164–169.

Kovaleski, J. E.; Parr, R. B.; Hornak, J. E.; and Roitman, J. L. "Athletic Profile of Women College Volleyball Players." *Physician Sportsmed.* 8 (1980):112–118.

Krahenbuhl, G. S.; Wells, C. L.; Brown, C. H.; and Ward, P. E. "Characteristics of National and World Class Female Pentathletes." *Med. Sci. Sports.* 11 (1979):20–23.

Lewis, S.; Haskell, W. L.; Klein, H.; Halpern, J.; and Wood, P. D. "Prediction of Body Composition in Habitually Active Middle-Aged Men." *J. Appl. Physiol.* 39 (1975):221–225.

Magel, J. R., and Faulkner, J. A. "Maximum Oxygen Uptakes of College Swimmers." *J. Appl. Physiol.* 22 (1967):929–938.

Maksud, M. G.; Wiley, R. L.; Hamilton, L. H.; and Lockhart, B. "Maximal VO_2, Ventilation, and Heart Rate of Olympic Speed Skating Candidates." *J. Appl. Physiol.* 29 (1970):186–190.

Malina, R. M.; Harper, A. B.; Avent, H. H.; and Campbell, D. E. "Physique of Female Track and Field Athletes." *Med. Sci. Sports* 3 (1971):32–38.

Malina, R. M., and Rarick, G. L. "Growth, Physique and Motor Performance." In *Physical Activity Human Growth and Development,* edited by G. L. Rarick. New York: Academic Press, 1973, pp. 125–153.

Mayers, N., and Gutin, B. "Physiological Characteristics of Elite Pre-Pubertal Cross-Country Runners." *Med. Sci. Sports* 11 (1979):172–176.

Nagle, F. J.; Morgan, W. P.; Hellickson, R. O.; Serfass, R. C.; and Alexander, J. F. "Spotting Success Traits in Olympic Contenders." *Physician and Sports Med.* 3 (1975):31–36.

Niinimaa, V.; Dyon, M.; and Shepard, R. J. "Performance and Efficiency of Intercollegiate Cross-Country Skiers." *Med. Sci. Sports* 10 (1978):91–93.

Novak, L. P.; Hyatt, R. E.; and Alexander, J. F. "Body Composition and Physiologic Function of Athletes." *J. Amer. Med. Assoc.* 205 (1968):764–770.

Pařizková, J. "Body Composition and Exercise during Growth and Development." In *Physical Activity Human Growth and Development,* edited by G. L. Rarick. New York: Academic Press, 1973, pp. 97–124.

Pařizková, J., and Poupa, D. "Some Metabolic Consequences of Adaptation to Muscular Work." *Brit. J. Nutr.* 17 (1963):341–345.

Parr, R. B.; Wilmore, J. H.; Hoover, R.; Bachman, D.; and Kerlan, R. "Professional Basketball Players: Athletic Profiles." *Physician Sportsmed.* 6 (1978):77–84.

Pipes, T. V. "Physiological Characteristics of Elite Body Builders." *Physician Sportsmed.* 7 (1979a):116–122.

Pipes, T. V. "The Racquetball Pro: A Physiological Profile." *Physician Sportsmed.* 7 (1976b):91–94.

Pollock, M. L. "The Quantification of Endurance Training Programs." In *Exercise and Sport Sciences Reviews,* vol. 1, edited by J. H. Wilmore. New York: Academic Press, 1973.

Pollock, M. L.; Miller, H. S.; and Wilmore, J. "Physiological Characteristics of Champion American Track Athletes 40 to 75 Years of Age." *J. Gerontology* 29 (1974):645–649.

Prince, F. P.; Hikida, R. S.; and Hagerman, F. C. "Muscle Fiber Types in Women Athletes and Non-Athletes." *Pflügers Arch.* 371 (1977):161–165.

Raven, P. B.; Gettman, L. R.; Pollock, M. L.; and Cooper, K. H. "A Physiological Evaluation of Professional Soccer Players." *British J. Sports Med.* 10 (1976):209–216.

Rusko, H.; Hara, M.; and Karvinen, E. "Aerobic Performance Capacity in Athletes." *Europ. J. Appl. Physiol.* 38 (1978):151–159.

Seliger, V.; Kostaka, V.; Grusová, D.; Kovac, J.; Machovcova, J.; Pauer M.; Pribylová, A.; and Urbankova, R. "Energy Expenditure and Physical Fitness of Ice Hockey Players." *Int. Z. Angew. Physiol.* 30 (1972):283–291.

Shephard, R. J.; Godin, G.; and Campbell, R. "Characteristics of Sprint, Medium and Long-Distance Swimmers." *Europ. J. Appl. Physiol.* 32 (1974):99–103.

Sinning, W. E. "Body Composition, Cardiovascular Function, and Rule Changes in Women's Basketball." *Res. Quart.* 44 (1973):313–321.

Sinning, W. E. "Body Composition Assessment of College Wrestlers." *Med. Sci. Sports.* 6 (1974):139–145.

Sinning, W. E., and Lindberg, G. D. "Physical Characteristics of College Age Women Gymnasts." *Res. Quart.* 43 (1972):226–234.

Sprynarová, S., and Pařizková, J. "Functional Capacity and Body Composition in Top Weight-Lifters, Swimmers, Runners and Skiers." *Int. Z. Angew. Physiol.* 29 (1971):184–194.

Stine, G.; Ratliff, R.; Shierman, G.; and Grana, W. A. "Physical Profile of the Wrestlers at the 1977 NCAA Championships." *Physician Sportsmed.* 7 (1979):98–105.

Tanner, J. M. *The Physique of the Olympic Athlete.* London: George Allen and Unwin Ltd., 1964.

Taylor, A. W.; Brassard, L.; Proteau, L.; and Robin, D. "A Physiological Profile of Canadian Greco-Roman Wrestlers." *Can. J. Appl. Sport Sci.* 4 (1979):131-134.

Thorstensson, A.; Larsson, L.; Tesch, P.; and Karlsson, J. "Muscle Strength and Fiber Composition in Athletes and Sedentary Men." *Med. Sci. Sports.* 9 (1977):26–30.

Vodak, P. A.; Savin, W. M.; Haskell, W. L.; and Wood, P. D. "Physiological Profile of Middle-aged Male and Female Tennis Players." *Med. Sci. Sports Exercise.* 12 (1980):159–163.

Wickkiser, J. D., and Kelly, J. M. "The Body Composition of a College Football Team." *Med. Sci. Sports.* 7 (1975):199–202.

Wilmore, J. H. "Alterations in Strength, Body Composition and Anthropometric Measurements Consequent to a 10-Week Weight Training Program." *Med. Sci. Sports.* 6 (1974).133–138.

Wilmore, J. H., and Bergfield, J. A. "A Comparison of Sports: Physiological and Medical Aspects." In *Sports Medicine and Physiology,* edited by R. H. Strauss. Philadelphia: W. B. Saunders, 1979.

Wilmore, J. H., and Brown, C. H. "Physiological Profiles of Women Distance Runners." *Med. Sci. Sports.* 6 (1974):178–181.

Wilmore, J. H.; Brown, C. H.; and Davis, J. A. "Body Physique and Composition of the Female Distance Runner." *Ann. New York Acad. Sci.* 301 (1977):764–776.

Wilmore, J. H.; Parr, R. B.; Haskell, W. L.; Costill, D. L.; Milburn, L. J.; and Kerlan, R. K. "Athletic Profile of Professional Football Players." *Physician Sportsmed.* 4 (1976): 45–54.

10

Nutrition and Athletic Performance

INTRODUCTION

The specific role that nutrition plays in athletic performance is not yet well-defined. Unfortunately, there are many self-proclaimed experts in the field of nutrition, and the athletic arena provides an excellent "laboratory" for self-experimentation by athletes. The net results are confusion and many claims that are not only unsound, but potentially dangerous. As an example, many elite athletes have attributed their athletic success to various nutritional manipulations or rituals. One of baseball's leading home run hitters in the early 1970s was relatively small in stature and did not appear overly muscular. When asked how he was able to generate the power necessary to hit the ball over the fence, he responded by attributing his power to eating honey just prior to game time. Other athletes have advocated buffalo meat, dessicated liver, vitamins A, C, E, and B_{15}, bee's pollen, fructose, amino acid supplements, and various minerals, to name but a few. The American public, as a whole, is hungry for information on nutrition, spending billions of dollars each year on nutrition-related services or items. During 1973, over ten billion dollars were spent on the diet industry alone, with over a billion dollars spent on special diet food. It is important that more effort be placed on consumer education, making the public aware of the tremendous potential for fraud, misrepresentation, and misguided zeal.

This chapter will first concentrate on providing basic nutritional information. This will include a definition and brief discussion of the six classes of nutrients. Next, the specific contents of the athlete's diet will be discussed, including a discussion of variations from the "normal" diet, and the pre-contest meal. Finally, the last section will focus on the various nutritional manipulations that have been proposed for increasing one's athletic performance potential, i.e., nutrition as an ergogenic aid, attempting to determine which, if any, of the nutritional supplements or manipulations improve performance.

BASIC CONCEPTS IN NUTRITION

Simply defined, food includes all the solid and liquid materials taken into the digestive tract that are utilized to maintain and build body tissues, regulate body processes, and supply body heat. Food can be categorized into six classes of nutrients, each with a unique chemical structure and a specific function within the body. The six categories include water, minerals, vitamins, proteins, fats, and carbohydrates. Each of these will be briefly discussed relative to their importance in general body function.

Water

Seldom is water thought of as a food. While it has no caloric value, and does not provide any of the other nutrients, it is second in importance only to oxygen in maintaining life. Water constitutes between 55 and 70 percent of the total body weight. However, while we can survive for weeks, or even months, without food, we can go without water for only a few days. It has been estimated that we can lose up to 40 percent of our body weight in fats, carbohydrates, and proteins and still survive, while a 20-percent loss in body water will likely lead to death.

Water is necessary for digestion, absorption, circulation, and excretion. With respect to exercise, water plays two critical roles. First, it is important in maintaining the electrolyte balance in the body. Second, it is important in controlling body temperature. This second function will be clearly outlined in the following chapter on environmental considerations.

Water intake is controlled largely by thirst sensations received by a regulatory center in the hypothalamus. These sensations are activated by the osmotic pressure of the body fluids, i.e., as the osmotic pressure increases, thirst sensations are activated. It should be mentioned, however, that the body's thirst mechanisms do not always keep up with its need for water. This has been referred to as *voluntary dehydration.* This phenomenon is not well-understood, but it does occur when working or exercising in hot climates. While this voluntary dehydration will not usually have serious consequences over a period of a single day of exercise, when faced with repeated exposures to exercise in the heat, it will be cumulative and can have serious, if not fatal, consequences. Evidently, such tremendous volumes of water are lost via sweating to maintain body temperature, that the body finds it difficult to consume and absorb an equivalent volume of water over a twenty-four-hour period. Thus, it is always important to drink more fluid than the thirst mechanisms dictate in an attempt to avoid voluntary dehydration. If too much water is ingested, the body can adapt readily by passing off the excess in the urine.

Water is normally ingested directly, in other fluids, or as a part of ingested food. The normal water intake of the average adult in a moderate climate will be approximately two liters per day. This will obviously increase in direct proportion to the fluid loss experienced by the individual through exercise and increased environmental temperature. With respect to foods, water constitutes 96

percent of the total content of lettuce, 88 percent of an orange, 87 percent of milk, 74 percent of eggs, 60 percent of lean beef, and only 4 percent of dry cereals and soda crackers. In addition to the water contained in the ingested food, water is also a by-product of the metabolism of stored food. The oxidation of 100 grams of fat, carbohydrate, and protein yields 107, 55, and 41 grams of water, respectively, which is referred to as *metabolic water.*

Ingested water is rapidly absorbed by the intestines, but it must first be emptied from the stomach. Considerable research has shown that the glucose content of the ingested solution largely dictates the speed of gastric emptying. Thus, to increase water absorption in the intestines, it is important to ingest either water, or solutions that have a very low glucose content. This will be discussed in much greater detail in the following chapter.

Minerals

Minerals refer to the elements in their simple inorganic form. While there are more than twenty mineral elements in the body, approximately seventeen have been proven to be essential in the diet. Approximately 4 percent of one's body weight is in the form of minerals, and most of this is in bone. Minerals such as calcium, phosphorus, and magnesium are needed in relatively large amounts, and are referred to as *macrominerals.* Potassium, sulfur, sodium, and chlorine also fall into this category. Macrominerals, by definition, are minerals that are needed by the body in amounts of more than one hundred milligrams per day. *Microminerals,* or trace elements, are those needed in amounts of less than one hundred milligrams per day, and include iron, zinc, selenium, manganese, copper, iodine, molybdenum, cobalt, fluorine, and chromium. Several of the more important macrominerals will be briefly discussed. In addition, Table 10–1 provides a list of the seventeen essential minerals, their location in the body, their major function, the best food source, and the 1980 recommended dietary allowance for each.

Calcium is the most abundant mineral in the body, constituting 1.5 to 2.0 percent of the total body weight, and approximately 40 percent of the total minerals present in the body. Of the total calcium in the body, 99 percent is found in the bones and teeth. The major function of calcium is to build and main-

Table 10–1   *Mineral Elements in the Body*

Mineral	Primary Location in Body	Primary Function	Food Sources	1980 Recommended Dietary Allowance
Calcium	bone and teeth	blood clotting, bone formation, transportation of fluids, muscle contraction	milk and milk products, broccoli, sardines, clams, and oysters	1200 milligrams/day for ages 11–18 years, and 800 milligrams/day for adults
Phosphorus	bone and teeth	bone formation, body's energy system, pH regulation	cheese, egg yolk, milk, meat, fish, poultry, whole grain cereals, legumes, and nuts	1200 milligrams/day for ages 11–18 years, and 800 milligrams/day for adults
Magnesium	bone and inside cells	activates enzymes	whole-grain cereals, nuts, meat, milk, green vegetables, and legumes	300–400 milligrams/day for teens and adults
Sodium	bone and extra cellular fluid	regulation of body fluid osmolarity, pH, and body fluid volume	table salt, seafood, milk and eggs, although abundant in most food except fruits	900–3,300 milligrams/day for teens and adults
Chloride	extracellular fluid	buffer and enzyme activation	table salt, seafood, milk, meat, and eggs	1,400–5,100 milligrams/day for teens and adults
Potassium	intracellular fluid	regulation of body fluid osmolarity, pH, and cell membrane transfer	fruits, meat, milk, cereals, vegetables, and legumes	1,525–5,625 milligrams/day for teens and adults
Sulfur	amino acids	oxidation-reduction reactions	protein foods including meat, fish, poultry, eggs, milk, cheese, legumes, and nuts	none
Iron	hemoglobin, liver, spleen, and bone	oxygen transportation	liver, meat, egg yolk, legumes, whole or enriched grains, dark green vegetables, shrimp, oysters	10–18 milligrams/day for teens and adults
Zinc	most tissues, with higher amounts in liver, muscle, and bone	constituent of essential enzymes and insulin	milk, liver, shellfish, herring, and wheat bran	15 milligrams/day for teens and adults

Table 10–1 *(continued)*

Mineral	Primary Location in Body	Primary Function	Food Sources	1980 Recommended Dietary Allowance
Copper	all tissues, with larger amounts in the liver, brain, heart, and kidney	constituent of enzymes	liver, shellfish, whole grains, cherries, legumes, kidney, poultry, oysters, chocolate, and nuts	2.0–3.0 milligrams/day for teens and adults
Iodine	thyroid gland	essential constituent of thyroxin	iodized table salt, sea-food, water, and vegetables	150 micrograms/day for teens and adults
Manganese	bone, pituitary, liver, pancreas, and gastro-intestinal tissue	constituent of essential enzymes	grains, nuts, legumes, fruit, and tea	2.5–5.0 milligrams/day for teens and adults
Fluoride	bone	reduces dental caries and may reduce bone loss	drinking water, tea, coffee, soybeans, spinach, gelatin, onions, and lettuce	1.5–2.5 milligrams/day for teens, and 1.5–4.0 milligrams/day for adults
Molybdenum	enzymes	constituent of essential enzymes	legumes, cereal grains, dark green leafy vegetables, and organs	0.15–0.5 milligram/day for teens and adults
Cobalt	in all cells	essential to normal function of all cells	liver, kidney, oysters, clams, poultry, and milk	none
Selenium	the cell	fat metabolism	grains, onions, meats, milk, and vegetables	0.05–0.2 milligram/day for teens and adults
Chromium	the cell	glucose metabolism	corn oil, clams, whole-grain cereals, meats, and drinking water	0.05–0.2 milligram/day for teens and adults

tain bones and teeth. It is essential for muscle contraction, blood clotting, control of cell membrane permeability, and nervous control of the heart. Milk and milk products are the best sources of calcium.

Phosphorus is closely linked to calcium, and constitutes approximately 22 percent of the total mineral content of the body. About 80 percent of phosphorus is found in combination with calcium in the form of calcium phosphate, which provides strength and rigidity to the bones and teeth. It is also an essential part of metabolism, cell membrane structure, and the buffering system to maintain the blood at a constant pH. Meat, poultry, fish, eggs, and milk are the sources of phosphorus.

Iron is present in the body in relatively small amounts, i.e., thirty-five to fifty milligrams per kilogram of body weight. Iron plays an extremely critical role in the transportation of oxygen throughout the body. As was mentioned in earlier chapters, oxygen is carried in the blood primarily by its attachment to hemoglobin, an iron-containing protein. The iron combines with oxygen in the lungs, and releases the oxygen at the level of the tissues. The myoglobin found in muscle, similar to hemoglobin, is also an iron-containing protein.

Iron deficiency is considered to be very prevalent throughout the world, with some estimates as high as 25 percent of the world's population. The major problem associated with iron deficiency is *iron deficiency anemia,* where there is a reduction in the oxygen-carrying capacity of the blood, and a resulting feeling of general tiredness and lack of energy. The major dietary source of iron is liver. However, oysters, shellfish, lean meat, and other organ meats provide good sources, as do leafy green vegetables and egg yolks.

Sodium, potassium, and chloride are classified as electrolytes and are found distributed throughout all body fluids and tissues, with sodium and chloride found predominantly extra-cellularly and potassium intra-cellularly. These electrolytes function to maintain normal water balance and distribution, normal osmotic equilibrium, normal acid-base balance, and normal muscular irritability. The major sources of sodium chloride are table salt, seafood, milk, and meat. Potassium is found most readily in fruits, milk, meat, cereals, and vegetables.

Vitamins

Vitamins are defined as a group of unrelated organic compounds. They are needed in relatively small quantities, but they are essential for specific metabolic reactions within the cell, and for normal growth and maintenance of health. Vitamins function primarily as catalysts in chemical reactions within the body. They are essential for the release of energy, for tissue building, and for controlling the body's use of food. Vitamins can be classified into one of two major categories: soluble in fat or water. Fat-soluble vitamins, A, D, E, and K, are stored by the body in lipids. Because they are stored by the body, there is the possibility that they could be taken in doses that would lead to vitamin toxicity. Vitamin C and the B-complex vitamins are water soluble, and when taken in excess will be excreted, mainly in the urine. The major vitamins of interest in sport, and their functions will be briefly discussed. Refer to Table 10–2 for a more complete list of each vitamin, its sources and functions, and the 1980 recommended dietary allowance.

Vitamin A, or Retinol, was the first fat-soluble vitamin to be discovered (1913). Natural vitamin A is usually found esterified with a fatty acid. It is essential for night vision, as an integral part of the visual purple of the retina. It is also essential for maintaining normal epithelial structure, and is thus important in the prevention of infection. It is also important for normal bone development and tooth formation. The major dietary sources of vitamin A are liver, kidney, butter, egg yolk, whole milk, and leafy dark green and yellow vegetables. Approximately 90 percent of the stored vitamin A is found in the liver. Toxicity results in bone fragility and stunted growth, loss of appetite, coarsening and loss of hair, scaly skin eruptions, enlargements of the liver and spleen, irritability, double vision, and skin rashes.

Vitamin D was discovered in 1930. It is absorbed with fats from the intestine in its ingested state, but it can also be absorbed from the skin directly into the blood. It is stored in the liver, skin, brain, and bones. It is essential for normal growth and development, and for normal bone and tooth formation. Rickets results from vitamin D deficiency, and

Table 10-2 *Vitamins and their Functions, Sources, and Associated Deficiency States*

Vitamin	Primary Function	Sources	1980 Recommended Dietary Allowance units/day
FAT-SOLUBLE VITAMINS			
A	adaptation to dim light, resistance to infection, prevents eye and skin disorders, bone and tooth development	liver, kidney, milk, butter, egg yolk, yellow vegetables, apricots, cantaloupe, and peaches	800 and 1,000 micrograms for females and males, respectively—teens and adults
D	facilitates absorption of calcium, bone, and tooth development	sunlight, fish, eggs, fortified dairy products, and liver	10 micrograms for 11–18 years of age; 5–7.5 micrograms for adults
E	prevents oxidation of essential vitamins and fatty acids and protects red blood cells from hemolysis	wheatgerm, vegetable oils, green vegetables, milk fat, egg yolk, and nuts	8–10 milligrams for teens and adults
K	blood clotting	liver, soybean oil, vegetable oil, green vegetables, tomatoes, cauliflower, and wheat bran	70–140 micrograms for teens and adults
WATER-SOLUBLE VITAMINS			
B₁ (thiamine)	energy metabolism, growth, appetite, and digestion	pork, liver, organs, meats, legumes, whole-grain and enriched cereals and breads, wheatgerm, and potatoes	1.0–1.5 milligrams for teens and adults
B₂ (riboflavin)	growth, health of eyes, and energy metabolism	milk and dairy foods, organ meats, green vegetables, eggs, fish, and enriched cereals and breads	1.2–1.7 milligrams for teens and adults
Niacin	energy metabolism and fatty acid synthesis	fish, liver, meat, poultry, grains, eggs, peanuts, milk, and legumes	13–19 milligrams for teens and adults
B₆ (pyridoxine)	protein metabolism and growth	pork, glandular meats, cereal bran and germ, milk, egg yolk, oatmeal, and legumes	1.8–2.2 milligrams for teens and adults

Table 10-2 *(continued)*

Vitamin	Primary Function	Sources	1980 Recommended Dietary Allowance *units/day*
Pantothenic acid	hemoglobin formation, and carbohydrate, protein, and fat metabolism	whole-grain cereals, organ meats, and eggs	4–7 milligrams for teens and adults
Biotin	carbohydrate, fat, and protein metabolism	liver, peanuts, yeast, milk, meat, egg yolk, cereal, nuts, legumes, bananas, grapefruit, tomatoes, watermelon, and strawberries	100–200 micrograms for teens and adults
Folic acid (folacin)	growth, fat metabolism, maturation of red blood cells	green vegetables, organ meats, lean beef, wheat, eggs, fish, dry beans, lentils, asparagus, broccoli, and yeast	400 micrograms for teens and adults
B$_{12}$ (cobalamin)	red blood cell production, nervous system metabolism, and fat metabolism	liver, kidney, milk and dairy foods, and meat	3.0 micrograms for teens and adults
C (ascorbic acid)	growth, tissue repair, tooth and bone formation	citrus fruits, tomatoes, strawberries, potatoes, melons, peppers, and pineapple	50–60 milligrams for teens and adults

toxicity leads to excessive calcification of bone, kidney stones, headache, nausea, and diarrhea.

Vitamin E was discovered in 1922, and consists of four different tocopherols: alpha, beta, gamma, and delta. Alpha tocopherol is biologically more active than the other three, and delta tocopherol is the most potent antioxidant. Vitamin E functions in metabolism, and helps to enhance the activity of vitamins A and C. Vitamin E deficiency in humans is rare, and no toxic effects have been identified. Many claims have been made for vitamin E with respect to rheumatic fever, muscular dystrophy, coronary artery disease, sterility, menstrual disorders, and spontaneous abortion, among others, but the claims for cures or benefits for any of these areas lacks supporting scientific evidence.

The B-complex vitamins were at one time considered to be a single vitamin important in the prevention of the disease beriberi. At the present time, however, more than a dozen B-complex vitamins have been identified which have very specific functions within the body. B-complex vitamins play an essential role in the metabolism of all living cells, serving as co-factors in the various enzyme systems involved in the oxidation of food and the production of energy. The B-complex vitamins have such a close interrelationship, that a deficiency in one may impair the utilization of the others. Dry yeast is the single best source of the B-complex vitamins.

Vitamin C, or ascorbic acid, was isolated in 1928, and is both the prevention and cure for scurvy. Vitamin C functions as either a co-enzyme or co-factor in metabolism. It is required for the production and maintenance of collagen, and has been postulated to assist in wound healing, combat fever and infection, and prevent or cure the common cold. Vitamin C deficiency is characterized by general weakness, poor appetite, anemia, swollen and inflamed gums and loosened teeth, shortness of breath, swollen joints, and neurotic disturbances.

Proteins

Proteins are nitrogen-containing compounds formed by amino acids, and they constitute the major structural component of the cell, antibodies, enzymes, and many hormones. Protein is necessary for growth, but it is also necessary for the repair and maintenance of body tissues; the production of hemoglobin (iron + protein); the production of en-

zymes, hormones, mucus, milk, and sperm; the maintenance of normal osmotic balance; and protection from disease through antibodies. Proteins are also potential sources of energy, but they are generally spared when fat and carbohydrate are available in ample supply. Over twenty amino acids have been identified, and of these, nine are considered to be essential as a part of the daily food intake. While many of the amino acids can be manufactured or synthesized by the body, these nine essential or indispensable amino acids either cannot be synthesized by the body or cannot be synthesized at a rate sufficient to meet the body needs, and thus become a necessary part of the diet. If any one of these nine is absent from the diet, protein cannot be synthesized or body tissue maintained. Protein sources in the diet that contain all of the essential amino acids in the proper ratio and in sufficient quantity are referred to as *complete proteins*. Meat, fish, and poultry are the three primary complete proteins. The proteins in vegetables and grains are referred to as *incomplete proteins*, as they do not supply all of the essential amino acids in appropriate amounts. This concept becomes important for individuals on vegetarian diets. This will be discussed in much greater detail in the next section of this chapter.

Approximately 5 to 15 percent of the total calories consumed per day in the United States are in the form of protein. This is considered by many to be two to three times the actual amount of protein necessary for proper body function. The daily recommended allowance published in 1980 by the National Research Council, is 45 and 56 grams per day for the teenage and adult male, respectively, and 44 to 46 grams per day for the teenage and adult female. Since the allowance is dependent on the individual's body weight, an allowance of 0.8 gram per kilogram of body weight is considered appropriate for the adult. These recommendations are substantially lower than the 1968 recommendations.

Fats

Fats, or lipids, are composed of about 98 percent triglycerides, with the remainder including traces of mono- and diglycerides, free fatty acids, phospholipids, and sterols. Triglycerides are composed of three molecules of fatty acids and one molecule of glycerol. While fat has generally been thought of in negative terms, i.e., a person is too fat, or the blood fats are elevated placing the person at risk for coronary artery disease, fat provides many useful functions in the body. It is an essential component of cell walls and nerve fibers; a primary energy source, providing up to 70 percent of the total energy when the body is in the resting state; a support and cushion for vital organs; involved in the absorption and transport of the fat-soluble vitamins; and an insulative layer subcutaneously for the preservation of body heat.

There are two types of fatty acids: saturated and unsaturated. The difference between the two is in the bonding between carbon and hydrogen atoms. Unsaturated fats contain one (monounsaturated) or more (polyunsaturated) double bonds between carbon atoms in a chain of carbon atoms. Each double bond in the chain takes the place of two hydrogen atoms. When the carbon chain is saturated with hydrogen atoms, i.e., two hydrogen atoms for each carbon atom, this is called a *saturated fatty acid*. In practical terms, a saturated fat is in the form of a solid, i.e., animal fat, and an *unsaturated fat* is in the form of a liquid, i.e., fish and vegetable oil. Saturated fats are derived primarily from animal sources and unsaturated fats from plant sources.

Fat supplies approximately 40 to 45 percent of the total caloric intake of the American population, and this represents a substantial increase over the percentage of fat consumed in the early 1900s. In addition, fat from animal sources has increased markedly, and that from vegetable sources has decreased. Most nutritionists recommend at least 25 percent of the caloric intake in the form of fat, but this should not exceed 30 to 35 percent. While many agree that the reduction of fat intake should come from saturated fats, there is presently a great deal of controversy on specific recommendations for the intake of saturated fats, particularly in reference to egg and dairy products.

Carbohydrates

Carbohydrates are composed of sugars and starches, and are classified as either monosaccharides, disaccharides, oligosaccharides, or polysaccharides. Monosaccharides are the simple sugars (glucose and fructose are the primary simple sugars) that cannot be hydrolyzed to a simpler form. Disaccharides can be hydrolyzed to two molecules of the same or different monosaccharide (sucrose, lactose, and maltose). Oligosaccharides can be hydrolyzed to yield three to ten monosaccharide units, and polysaccharides can provide more than ten monosaccharide units. The major polysaccharides are starch, dextrin, cellulose, and glycogen, which are composed completely of glucose units. Glucose serves many functions in the body. First, it is a major source of energy, particularly during high-intensity exercise. Glucose also exerts an influence on both protein and fat metabolism, sparing the use of protein as an energy source, and controlling the utilization of fat. Glucose is the sole source of energy for the brain, and is necessary for the functional integrity of nerve tissue.

In the early 1900s, carbohydrates constituted over 55 percent of the total caloric intake. In the 1970s, this figure dropped to approximately 45 percent. In the early 1900s, starches constituted 68 percent of the total carbohydrate intake, but this has dropped to below 50 percent today. Sugar intake, conversely, increased from 32 percent to over 50 percent over the same time period. The major sources of carbohydrates are grains, fruits, vegetables, milk, and concentrated sweets. Refined sugar, syrup, and cornstarch are examples of pure carbohydrates, and many of the concentrated sweets such as candy, honey, jellies, molasses, and soft drinks contain few if any other nutrients. These have been referred to as *empty calories*, for they contribute nothing but calories to the diet.

THE ATHLETE'S DIET

Since athletes place considerable demands on their body every day they train and compete, it is important that the body be as finely tuned as possible. This, by necessity, must include optimal nutrition. Too often, athletes spend considerable time and effort in perfecting skills and attaining top physical condition, only to ignore proper nutrition and sleep. It is not uncommon to trace the deterioration of an athlete's performance back to poor nutrition. What, then, is the best diet for an athlete? Also, will the dietary demands vary with the sport?

While considerable research is presently being conducted, and additional research is needed, the available evidence suggests that the dietary requirements of the athlete are no different than the requirements of the nonathlete, with the exception of the total number of calories consumed. Thus, the optimum diet for athletes, as for nonathletes, must contain adequate quantities of water, calories, proteins, fats, carbohydrates, minerals, and vitamins in the proper proportions, independent of the sport or the event within a sport. In other words, a well-balanced diet appears to be all that is necessary!

What is a well-balanced diet? In the early 1940s, the Food and Nutrition Board of the National Research Council of the National Academy of Sciences was formed to define the nutrient requirements of the American population. At the conclusion of their deliberations, they published a report that became known as the "Recommended Dietary Allowances," or the RDA. The allowances were designed to provide a guideline for planning and evaluating food intake. In 1980, the National Research Council published its most recent of a number of revisions. The allowances for minerals and vitamins have been listed in Tables 10–1 and 10–2, and the protein allowance was discussed in the previous section. With respect to energy intake, males eleven to fifty years of age should consume between 2,700 and 2,900 Kcal, and females between 2,000 and 2,200 Kcal. These figures are calculated on the basis of the average height and weight of the population, for individuals doing light work. Obviously, athletes in intensive training would have considerably higher energy intake demands, as was discussed in Chapter 1.

One of the problems associated with the RDA was the inability of the average individual to understand the specific allowance value, its units of measure, and to translate this information into meaningful terms. This led to a grouping of foods, and the simplified "Basic Seven Food Plan." In 1956, this was simplified even further into the "Four Food Group Plan," which was published in the U.S. Department of Agriculture's publication, "The Essentials of an Adequate Diet." The "Four Food Group Plan" consists of the following four groups: milk and milk products, meat and high-protein foods, fruits and vegetables, and cereal and grain foods. Table 10–3 outlines the basics of the "Four Food Group Plan," including the number of servings per day and the major contributions of each food group. These suggestions are based on the minimal requirements, and will have to be in-creased either by larger servings, or more servings for individuals who are active and expend a considerable amount of additional energy each day. This basic dietary plan is recommended as a base or foundation, as it will assure the athlete of a well-balanced diet, with no deficiencies, providing the energy intake is matching the energy expenditure. With respect to the balance between the basic food groups, protein should constitute 10 to 20 percent of the total caloric intake, fats 30 to 35 percent, and carbohydrates 50 to 55 percent. For athletes who are training to exhaustion on successive days, the carbohydrate fraction could be as high as 70 percent.

Vegetarian Diets

More people appear to be reducing their intake of meat and increasing their intake of vegetables. In some cases, people have made the complete transition to vegetarianism. Vegetarian diets are chosen for a number of reasons, including health, ecological, and economical reasons. Most vegetarians eat any food from plant sources. However, there are several types of vegetarians. Vegans are strict vegetarians and eat only food from plant sources. Lacto-vegetarians eat plant foods plus dairy products. Ovo-vegetarians eat plant foods plus eggs, and lacto-ovovegetarians eat plant foods, dairy products, and eggs. Fruitarians eat fruits, nuts, olive oil, and honey.

Can atheltes survive on a vegetarian diet? The answer is a qualified yes. If the athlete is a strict vegan, he or she must be very careful in the selection of the plant foods eaten to provide a good balance of the essential amino acids, and adequate sources of vitamin A, riboflavin, vitamin B_{12}, vitamin D, calcium, iron, and sufficient calories. More than one professional athlete has noted significant deterioration in athletic performance after switching over to a strict vegetarian diet. The problem was later traced to an unwise selection of plant foods. Inclusion of milk and eggs is highly recommended since their inclusion will lessen the likelihood of nutritional deficiencies. Anyone contemplating a switch from a normal to a vegetarian diet would be well-advised to read authoritative reference material on the subject, written by qualified nutritionists.

Table 10–3 *The Basic Four Food Group Plan*

Food Group	Daily Amounts for Adults	Nutritional Contribution
Milk and milk products	Two or more servings per day either as a milk beverage or a milk product such as cheese and ice cream. A serving would be one cup or its equivalent.	Protein Calcium Riboflavin Vitamin D
Meat and high protein products	Two or more servings of meat, fish, poultry, eggs, or vegetables such as dried beans, lentils, peas, and nuts. A serving of meat, fish, or poultry would be 3.5 ounces of lean and boneless meat.	Protein Thiamin Iron Niacin Riboflavin
Fruit and vegetables	Four or more servings per day of ½ cup or more.	Vitamin A Vitamin C Folic acid
Cereal and grain	Four or more servings per day with one serving equal to one slice of bread, ½ to ¾ cup of cooked cereal, macaroni, spaghetti, etc.	Protein Thiamin Riboflavin Niacin Iron

Dietary Supplements

The food industry makes a considerable amount of money each year in the area of dietary supplements. Is there a need for vitamin and mineral, or protein, supplementation? For the individual who is eating a well-balanced diet with the appropriate number of calories, and who is moderately to highly active, dietary supplementation appears to be totally unnecessary. Supplements may be necessary for the individual or the athlete who is on a restricted caloric diet, where the total energy intake is insufficient to provide the essential requirements. However, for the athlete in training, where the total caloric intake is in excess of 3,000 Kcal, and is as high as 10,000 Kcal, evidence would indicate that there is nothing to be gained by supplementation of any of the dietary constituents. While the requirements for the various nutrients increase in direct proportion to the increase in energy expenditure, the increase in nutrient intake increases correspondingly. This will be discussed in more detail in the following section on ergogenic properties of basic nutrients.

Pre-Contest Meal

For years, the athlete has been given the traditional steak dinner several hours prior to competition. Possibly, this practice originated from the early belief that the muscle consumed itself as fuel for muscular activity and that steak provided the necessary protein to counteract this loss. It is now recognized that this is probably the worst possible meal that the athlete could eat prior to competition. Steak contains a high percentage of fat which takes many hours to be fully digested. The digestive process competes for the available blood with the muscles that are used in the contest. Because of this, the pre-contest meal, no matter what its content, should be given no later than three hours prior to the contest. Another factor to consider is the emotional climate at the time of this meal. Extreme nervousness is frequently present, and even the choicest steak is not enjoyed. The steak would be psychologically more satisfying to the athlete either the night before or the night following the contest.

Nathan J. Smith, in his book, *Food for Sport*, lists

five goals that should be considered in planning the pre-contest diet. These are as follows:

1. Energy intake should be adequate to ward off any feeling of hunger weakness during the entire period of the competition. Although pre-contest food intakes make only a minor contribution to the immediate energy expenditure, they are essential for the support of an adequate level of blood sugar, and for avoiding the sensations of hunger and weakness.
2. The diet plan should ensure that the stomach and upper bowel are empty at the time of competition.
3. Food and fluid intakes prior to and during prolonged competition should guarantee an optimal state of hydration.
4. The pre-competition diet should offer foods that will minimize upset in the gastrointestinal tract.
5. The diet should include food that the athlete is familiar with, and is convinced will "make him win."

It is also important that the athlete not eat anything with a high sugar content two hours or less before competition. Some athletes will ingest two or three candy bars thirty minutes to one hour prior to competition. With such a heavy sugar load, the body reacts by substantially increasing the insulin levels in the blood. In fact, the body overreacts and produces more insulin than is needed. This results in a very sharp decrease in the blood sugar level and the athlete becomes hypoglycemic (Costill, 1979). This condition will definitely reduce the performance potential of the athlete. Foster et al. (1979) found that glucose feedings thirty to forty-five minutes before endurance exercise increased the rate of carbohydrate oxidation and impeded the mobilization of free fatty acids, thereby reducing the exercise time to exhaustion by 19 percent.

Many athletes are starting to use a liquid pre-game meal, since it is palatable, digests relatively easily, and is less likely to result in nervous indigestion, nausea, vomiting, and abdominal cramps. Those who have experimented with liquid pre-contest meals have found them to be highly satisfactory. At the present time, this would appear to be the best available choice as a pre-game meal.

ERGOGENIC PROPERTIES OF BASIC NUTRIENTS

Erogogenic aids are substances or phenomena that elevate or improve the performance of the individual above that expected. The subject of ergogenic aids will be discussed in detail in Chapter 12. In this chapter, however, we will look at the ergogenic properties of various nutrients. Is it possible to manipulate the diet to achieve improvement in performance? The answer is a qualified yes, although improvement is limited to manipulation in only one or two nutritional areas, and the degree of improvement is still debatable. Unfortunately, much of the research that has been conducted in this area has lacked adequate controls. Despite this rather major limitation, however, a great deal of information has accumulated that provides valuable insights for the coach and athlete.

Protein

Is it necessary for the athlete who is in training for the purpose of increasing strength and muscle bulk to supplement his or her normal dietary intake of protein? Protein is essential for the growth and development of the various tissues of the body, since amino acids are the body's "building blocks." It was thought for many years that protein had to be supplemented in rather large quantities. In fact, at one time it was thought that the muscle consumed itself as fuel for its own contractions, and the protein supplementation was essential to prevent the muscles from wasting away. It is now recognized that little protein is consumed as fuel for muscular work. If fats or carbohydrates are available, they are selected in preference to proteins as sources of energy.

Studies have shown that work performance is neither enhanced nor inhibited, by protein supplementation or deprivation. Horstman (1972) summarizes the situation well when he states that the average diet on our Western culture provides adequately for our protein needs. With heavy physical training or work, the caloric intake may exceed 5,000 Kcal, which should provide adequate total protein if the proportion of protein from the total calories is maintained. One possible exception to this is the finding that substantial increases in muscle mass and strength, when under the influence of anabolic steroids, appear to be dependent on protein supplementation.

Consolazio et al. (1975) observed two groups of men who consumed two levels of protein (1.4 and 2.8 g/kg body weight per day) during a forty-day experimental period. Physical activity and sweat rates were relatively high during the entire experimental phase. Body protein stores, and muscle mass was increased with the high-protein diet. However, the additional body protein did not enhance physiological work performance.

Marable et al. (1979) conducted a study using four groups of college men who consumed two levels of protein (0.8g or 2.4g/kg body weight per day) for twenty-eight days, while serving either as controls or as subjects in a progressive resistance exercise program. Independent of the level of protein intake, the exercising subjects experienced a 3.2-kg weight gain, while the weight of the two control groups changed by less than 1.0 kg. The mean urinary nitrogen values expressed as a percentage of the total nitrogen intake were decreased in both exercise groups, but were more pronounced in the group receiving 0.8g/kg of body weight per day. The authors concluded that the magnitude of the decrease for the 0.8g/kg group suggests that their protein intake was marginal during muscle-building exercise.

Fat and Carbohydrate

At one time, carbohydrate was regarded as the chief fuel for muscular contraction. It is now realized that fat is a major, if not the most important, source of fuel for light-to-moderate levels of exercise. This does not imply that athletes should attempt to store more body fat, since they probably are already storing more than needed. Less than a pound of fat is sufficient to provide the total energy needed for a grueling 26.2 mile, three-hour marathon run. A theory has been proposed that the higher levels of fat found in women, coupled with a better ability to utilize fat, provide them with an advantage in long-distance races, but recent work by Costill et al. (1979) has proven this theory to be in error. Thus, fat is not considered to have any special ergogenic properties.

The biggest breakthrough in athletic nutrition came in the 1960s when a group of Scandinavian researchers started experimental observations of carbohydrate storage and utilization with prolonged, endurance-type exercise. Earlier work had suggested that carbohydrate supplementation would facilitate endurance performance. This was confirmed by the finding that exhaustion was always accompanied by hypoglycemia or low blood sugar. Studies in the early 1960s confirmed the importance of carbohydrates when they demonstrated a depletion of the muscle glycogen stores concomitant with hypoglycemia and the attainment of the exhausted state. The use of the muscle biopsy, introduced in the 1960s, enabled scientists to discover these facts. Typically, studies have shown that as the work is prolonged, the glycogen stores in the muscles become progressively depleted. As the individual reaches the state of exhaustion, the glycogen stores are nearly or totally depleted. These studies all suggest that the initial glycogen content of the active muscle is important with respect to defining the endurance potential of the individual, i.e., the greater the glycogen content, the higher the endurance capacity.

From these findings, it is evident that the endurance athlete could improve performance considerably if he or she could increase the glycogen content of his or her muscles. Bergström et al. (1967) investigated this problem. Each of the subjects was given three different diets, each for a prescribed period of time. One diet was high in carbohydrate, one high in fat and protein, and one was a mixed diet; each contained the same number of calories. Prior to starting the diet, the subject depleted his muscle glycogen stores by riding a bicycle ergometer to exhaustion at approximately 75 percent of his maximal oxygen uptake. This was followed by three days on the prescribed diet and then a second ride to exhaustion. Prior to the second ride, a muscle biopsy was obtained to determine glycogen content. The total length of time the subject could ride before reaching exhaustion and the initial glycogen content are shown on the following page. These results support the conclusion that endurance performance can be significantly altered by manipulating the diet, in this case by loading up on carbohydrates prior to competition to enhance the glycogen stores.

A similar example of this phenomenon was

Diet	Glycogen Content, gm/100 gm of wet tissue	Riding Time to Exhaustion, min
Mixed	1.93	125.8
High fat and protein	0.69	58.8
High carbohydrate	3.70	189.3

shown in an experiment by Karlsson and Saltin (1971). Their subjects each participated in two thirty-kilometer races, one preceded by a high carbohydrate diet following muscle glycogen depletion, and the other preceded by a normal, mixed diet. The average muscle glycogen content was elevated on the high carbohydrate diet to nearly double the level attained on the mixed diet. In addition, the times in the thirty-kilometer race were substantially faster following the high carbohydrate diet; the improvement coming primarily in the last half of the race!

With this information available, how does the athlete proceed to enhance muscle glycogen stores? Londeree (1974) has summarized the steps necessary to optimize the glycogen loading phenomenon. First, he points to the fact that carbohydrates are normally stored in limited quantities and that only a limited quantity of carbohydrate can be absorbed from the intestine during the actual competition; thus, it is necessary to enlarge the glycogen stores. To increase glycogen storage, the individual must, first, totally deplete his or her glycogen stores. This can be accomplished by an exhaustive exercise bout of an extended duration, i.e., greater than sixty to ninety minutes. This should be done approximately seven days prior to the competition. The greater the depletion, the greater the additional storage of glycogen. Once depleted, the glycogen stores are maintained in this depleted state by continued training and a low carbohydrate diet. A certain amount of carbohydrate is essential, so the diet should not be totally void of carbohydrate. Approximately three to four days prior to competition, the diet is changed to one that is predominantly carbohydrate. Additional fluids must also be ingested since three to four grams of water are stored with each gram of glycogen. While on the high-carbohydrate diet, activity should be tapered to low

levels to maximize the additional storage of glycogen. Costill (1979) feels the phase of low carbohydrate intake following the depletion phase is unnecessary.

A warning must be given to those who advocate this type of dietary manipulation. Several physicians have become concerned about the possibility of medical risks associated with this kind of dietary practice. Angina-like symptoms (chest pain) have been noted in several athletes who have used this diet. In one case, this was associated with an abnormal electrocardiogram. It is not possible, at the present time, to establish a cause-effect relationship. It seems unlikely that carbohydrate loading would be dangerous to the young, healthy athlete. It might be wise for the older athlete to proceed with caution, however, until this phenomenon is better understood. Most endurance athletes are unknowingly practicing carbohydrate loading to a great extent just by the nature of their rigorous training programs. While they might not go through a three- to four-day extensive reduction in carbohydrate intake following an exhaustive, glycogen-depleting workout, they do periodically deplete their glycogen stores and consume considerable quantities of carbohydrates.

Carbohydrate loading increases the total quantity of glycogen available in the muscle. How does this, in itself, improve performance? During prolonged endurance competition when the body depletes its carbohydrate stores, can't the body perform equally well by using fat as the main source of fuel? A number of studies have shown conclusively that while fat is a major source of fuel for low-intensity exercise—up to 70 percent—that, as the intensity of the exercise increases, the reliance on carbohydrates increases. Once the anaerobic threshold is reached and the oxygen supply is unable to meet the oxygen demands, the body shifts to a dependence on carbohydrate utilization. Horstman (1972), in his review of athletic nutrition, has provided an insight into why this shift occurs. In calculating the actual energy production from a given fuel, it is possible to calculate the efficiency of utilization. This is defined simply as the kilocalories of energy produced per minute from a specific fuel per liter of oxygen consumed, or the energy derived per liter of oxygen. Glucose yields 5.01 Kcal/liter of oxygen, and fat yields only 4.65 Kcal/liter of oxygen. This provides a distinct advantage for carbohydrate utilization when the exercise intensity reaches the upper levels, since there is a greater energy yield for the same amount of oxygen that is consumed.

Vitamins and Minerals

Historically, massive doses of various vitamins and minerals have been taken by certain athletes with the hope of improving their athletic performance. The many problems and diseases associated with various vitamin deficiencies are well known, but do athletes generally have vitamin or mineral deficiencies? Even if deficiencies do not exist, will supplementation of any one vitamin or mineral above the recommended daily dose result in better performance by an athlete? While these questions have been researched extensively, debate still continues over the conflicting results.

B-complex vitamins are among those vitamins known to influence physical performance. They are involved in co-enzyme activity with the metabolism of fats and carbohydrates. Deficiencies have been shown to decrease athletic performance. On the other hand, supplementation with B-complex vitamins, primarily thiamine (B_1), has been shown to both improve performance, as well as to have no influence on performance. Additional research is needed to provide a conclusive answer to the question of whether B-complex supplementation is of any value for the athlete.

Vitamin C also plays an important role in energy metabolism. Similar to a deficiency in the B vitamins, a deficiency in vitamin C will result in a decrease in physical performance. With regard to the question of supplementation, the research literature is equivocal. Early studies of vitamin C supplementation and physical performance showed no distinct advantage in levels of vitamin C in excess of the recommended daily dosage. More recent studies, however, have reopened interest in this area. A number of studies conducted since 1960 have shown vitamin C supplementation to result in prolonged endurance capacity. These more recent findings point to the need for additional studies to clarify the role of vitamin C in endurance performance relative to its mechanism of operation and to the optimal dosage.

Vitamin E must be considered the wonder vitamin of this century since it has been touted as the cure for almost every one of our ills. As with the vitamins discussed previously, research literature relative to the influence of vitamin E on athletic performance conflicts. Using wheat germ oil, a rich source of alpha tocopherol and a most potent source of vitamin E, several studies have shown improvements in endurance performance, while several have shown little or no effect from the vitamin. Again, the evidence must be considered inconclusive at this time, indicating the need for further study of a highly controlled nature.

From these studies, it would appear that the B-complex vitamins and vitamins C and E have ergogenic properties, but this conclusion is certainly open to debate. Additional studies are essential, since vitamin supplementation is expensive and can even be toxic as in the case of the fat-soluble vitamins, i.e., A, D, E, and K, which are stored in the body. The water-soluble vitamins are rapidly excreted in the urine; thus, supplementation with these vitamins, even if they have no measurable effect on performance, leaves the athlete with nothing more than expensive urine.

With minerals, it is well known that deficiencies can reduce the efficiency of the athlete, particularly when exercising in the heat. Sweating reduces the body's sodium and chloride stores. In addition, exercise can substantially alter the body's balance for potassium, calcium, magnesium, and phosphorus. Again, as in the case of vitamins, it is essential to replace those minerals that have been lost, but is supplementation above normal levels an aid to performance?

The use of salt tablets has been advocated for years to supplement the normal salt ingested in food when the athlete is exercising under conditions where there is excessive water and mineral loss through sweating. While replacement of sodium chloride lost in sweat is desirable, care must be taken not to ingest more salt than necessary. Excessive salt intake can lead to undesirable potassium loss and increased water retention. Generally, according to most review articles, a liberal salting of food or the ingestion of an electrolyte solution, such as Gatorade, Sportade, ERG, or other similar, readily available commercial beverages, is sufficient to maintain sodium and chloride levels, without having to ingest salt tablets.

Aspartates have been used as ergogenic aids for a number of years. Aspartates are potassium and magnesium salts of aspartic acid, which supposedly work in an intermediate position in the Krebs cycle to reduce the accumulation of blood ammonia. Increased levels of blood ammonia are thought to be one possible cause of fatigue; thus, aspartates are considered to have possible ergogenic effects by delaying the onset of fatigue. In Golding's review of aspartates (1972), it is again clear that the existing literature is not in agreement. Several studies of a well-designed and controlled nature demonstrated rather remarkable gains in endurance from aspartate administration, but several have shown aspartates to have no influence at all. Again, additional research is needed to clarify the actual role of aspartates in prolonging activities of an endurance nature.

Water

Seldom is water regarded as an ergogenic aid. It is consumed by everyone, has no caloric or nutritional benefits, but is essential to life. From the discussion of dehydration in Chapter 11 and from Costill's (1972) extensive review, it appears that water is an ergogenic aid. Ingesting fluids prior to endurance competition is an effective way to maintain the body temperature at a reduced level and limit the extent of dehydration. For a more detailed discussion of this, refer to the section on dehydration in Chapter 11, Environmental Factors and Athletic Performance.

Caffeine

While at one time carbohydrate was considered the primary, if not the only fuel for muscular exercise, it is now recognized that the role of fat as a primary energy source during exercise is considerable. Fat is essentially an inexhaustible source of fuel, while carbohydrate stores are greatly limited, providing for not more than 60 to 120 minutes of moderately heavy exercise. Since the supply of carbohydrate is limited, it would facilitate performance if either or both carbohydrate stores could be increased, or if fat could be utilized in place of carbohydrate, sparing carbohydrate stores, and theoretically prolonging endurance exercise. The potential for increasing carbohydrate stores was discussed earlier in this section. The discussion will now focus on the use of fat as an alternative energy source, sparing carbohydrate.

In 1977, three studies were published observing the influence of increasing free fatty acid levels in the blood on the subsequent substrate utilization during exercise. Ahlborg and Hagenfeldt (1977) examined leg and splanchnic exchange of free fatty acids and glucose during a ninety-minute bicycle exercise both before and after heparin administration. Heparin increases plasma lipoprotein lipase activity, which in turn increases the availability of free fatty acids. They found the free fatty acid uptake in the exercising legs was augmented following heparin administration, but they concluded that the inhibitation of glucose uptake by the enhanced free fatty acid uptake was of minor importance in the regulation of muscle substrate utilization during exercise. Costill et al. (1977) used a similar design. Seven men were studied during thirty minutes of treadmill exercise at approximately 70 percent of their $\dot{V}O_2$ max, to determine the effects of increased availability of free fatty acids and elevated plasma insulin on the utilization of muscle glycogen. Using heparin to increase the plasma-free fatty acids, they found that the rate of muscle glycogen depletion was decreased by 40 percent. Thus, increasing the availability of free fatty acids in the blood slows the rate of carbohydrate utilization, i.e., a muscle glycogen sparing effect. Hickson et al. (1977) conducted a similar experiment on rats and found that the increased availability of fatty acids delayed the development of exhaustion from prolonged running. They concluded that it appeared likely that the carbohydrate-sparing effect of fatty acids was largely responsible for the increase in endurance.

This series of three experiments led to a second series of experiments investigating the role of caffeine on endurance performance. Caffeine is known to stimulate the mobilization of free fatty acids, and to increase the oxidation of fats. Thus, caffeine was suspected of having carbohydrate-sparing qualities, which could have substantial implications for endurance activities. Costill et al. (1978) had nine competitive cyclists exercise until exhaustion on a bicycle ergometer at 80 percent of $\dot{V}O_2$ max after ingesting either decaffeinated coffee or regular coffee containing 330 mg of caffeine. Endurance time on the bicycle ergometer was increased by 19 percent, which was largely the result of an increased rate of fat oxidation. Ivy et al. (1979) conducted a similar study, and found that the ingestion of 250 mg of caffeine significantly increased work production by 7.4 percent. In an earlier study, Perkins and Williams (1975) were unable to demonstrate increased endurance with the ingestion of caffeine.

These results must be treated with caution. It does appear that caffeine is an ergogenic agent for endurance activity. However, many individuals have tried this with negative results. Caffeine appears to have a variable effect, depending on one's tolerance. For the individual who never drinks coffee or other drinks that have a high caffeine content, the sudden use of caffeine can have undesirable side effects. For the coffee addict, however, the tolerance level may be too high to demonstrate an ergogenic effect.

GENERAL SUMMARY

For hundreds of years, it has been assumed that nutrition can influence the quality of one's athletic performance. The present chapter reviewed the six classes of nutrients, i.e., water, minerals, vitamins, proteins, fats, and carbohydrates, discussing the importance of each relative to general nutrition. This provided the background for a discussion of the athlete's diet. It was concluded that the optimum diet for athletes, as for nonathletes, must contain adequate quantities of water, calories, proteins, fats, carbohydrates, minerals, and vitamins in the proper proportions. In addition, diet is generally independent of the sport, or the event within a sport. A well-balanced diet, as exemplified by the "Four Food Group Plan" appears to provide the base or foundation for the athlete, assuring him or her that there will be no deficiencies, providing the total caloric intake is sufficient. Athletes can do very well on vegetarian diets providing they make a careful selection of their plant food sources, to provide a good balance of the essential amino acids, and adequate sources of vitamin A, riboflavin, vitamin B_{12}, vitamin D, calcium, iron, and sufficient calories. Finally, the pre-contest meal should be light, taken at least three hours prior to the contest, and should be easily digestible. A liquid pre-contest meal appears to have many advantages over solid food.

Does food have ergogenic qualities, or can you alter what you eat to improve performance? While it appears that the average athlete consumes a sufficient quantity of protein and that supplementation has little additional effect, there is evidence to indicate that carbohydrate loading is an effective nutritional manipulative technique, which can increase general cardiovascular endurance by increasing the storage of muscle glycogen. The technique of carbohydrate loading is discussed in detail. Various vitamins and minerals have been proposed as ergogenic aids. From the available research, it appears that the B-complex vitamins, and vitamins C and E, may have ergogenic properties, but the evidence is not conclusive and additional research is needed. Aspartates have been proposed as ergogenic aids, but, again, the research literature is equivocal about their effectiveness. Finally, water is definitely an ergogenic aid, and caffeine appears to have ergogenic properties for endurance activities.

STUDY QUESTIONS

1. What are the six categories of nutrients?
2. What role does water play in body function? Why is it classified as a nutrient?
3. What are the major macrominerals of importance to sport and activity?
4. What are the major functions of the primary macrominerals?
5. What are the major roles of vitamins in the body?
6. Which vitamins are fat soluble? Why is this important?
7. What are the major food sources for the individual vitamins?
8. What are essential amino acids, and why are they important relative to food intake?
9. What is an appropriate protein allowance for the adult male? Female?
10. What is the difference between saturated and unsaturated fats?
11. What is the difference between glucose and glycogen?

12. Describe an ideal athlete's diet for football, and for swimming.
13. Can an athlete survive on a vegetarian diet? Explain.
14. Describe the ideal pre-contest meal.
15. Discuss the ergogenic properties of the various nutrients. Which nutrients have definite ergogenic properties?

REFERENCES

Ahlborg, G., and Hagenfeldt, L. "Effect of Heparin on the Substrate Utilization during Prolonged Exercise." *Scand. J. Clin. Lab. Invest.* 37 (1977):619–624.

Åstrand, P.-O. "Nutrition and Physical Performance." In *Nutrition and the World Food Problem,* edited by M. Rechcigl. Switzerland: S. Karger, Basel, 1979.

Bergström, J.; Hermansen, L.; Hultman, E.; and Saltin, B. "Diet, Muscle Glycogen, and Physical Performance." *Acta Physiol. Scand.* 71 (1967):140–150.

Consolazio, C. F.; Johnson, H. L.; Nelson, R. A.; Dramise, J. G.; and Skala, J. H. "Protein Metabolism during Intensive Physical Training in the Young Adult." *Amer. J. Clin. Nutr.* 28 (1975):29–35.

Costill, D. L. "Water and Electrolytes." In *Ergogenic Aids and Muscular Performance,* edited by W. P. Morgan. New York: Academic Press, 1972.

Costill, D. L. *A Scientific Approach to Distance Running.* Los Altos, Calif.: Track and Field News, 1979.

Costill, D. L.; Bennett, A.; Branam, G; and Eddy, D. "Glucose Ingestion at Rest and during Prolonged Exercise." *J. Appl. Physiol.* 34 (1973):764–769.

Costill, D. L.; Coyle, E.; Dalsky, G.; Evans, W.; Fink, W.; and Hoopes, D. "Effects of Elevated Plasma FFA and Insulin on Muscle Glycogen Usage during Exercise." *J. Appl. Physiol.* 43 (1977):695–699.

Costill, D. L.; Dalsky, G. P.; and Fink, W. J. "Effects of Caffeine Ingestion on Metabolism and Exercise Performance." *Med. Sci. Sports.* 10 (1978):155–158.

Costill, D. L.; Fink, W. J.; Getchell, L. H.; Ivy, J. L.; and Witzmann, F. A. "Lipid Metabolism in Skeletal Muscle of Endurance-Trained Males and Females." *J. Appl. Physiol.* 47 (1979):787–791.

Dairy Council Digest. "Nutrition and Athletic Performance." 46 (1975):7–10.

Dairy Council Digest. "Nutrition and Human Performance." 51 (1980):13–17.

Farrell, P. M., and Bieri, J. G. "Megavitamin E Supplementation in Man." *Amer. J. Clin. Nutr.* 28 (1975):1381–1385.

Foster, C.; Costill, D. L.; and Fink, W. J. "Effects of Preexercise Feedings on Endurance Performance." *Med. Sci. Sports* 11 (1979):1–5.

Golding, L. A. Drugs and Hormones. In *Ergogenic Aids and Muscular Performance,* edited by W. P. Morgan. New York: Academic Press, 1973.

Hickson, R. C.; Rennie, M. J.; Conlee, R. K.; Winder, W. W.; and Holloszy, J. O. "Effects of Increased Plasma Fatty Acids on Glycogen Utilization and Endurance." *J. Appl. Physiol.* 43 (1977):829–833.

Helgheim, I.; Hetland, Ø.; Nilsson, S.; Ingjer, F.; and Strømme, S. B. "The Effects of Vitamin E on serum Enzyme Levels following Heavy exercise." *Eur. J. Appl. Physiol.* 40 (1979):283–289.

Horstman, D. H. "Nutrition." In *Ergogenic Aids and Muscular Performance,* edited by W. P. Morgan. New York: Academic Press, 1972.

Howald, H., and Segesser, B. "Ascorbic Acid and Athletic Performance." *Annals NY Acad. Sci.* 258 (1975):458 464.

Ivy, J. L.; Costill, D. L.; Fink, W. J.; and Lower, R. W. "Influence of Caffeine and Carbohydrate Feedings on Endurance Performance." *Med. Sci. Sports* 11 (1979):6–11.

Karlsson, J., and Saltin, B. "Diet, Muscle Glycogen and Endurance Performance." *J. Appl. Physiol.* 31 (1971):203–206.

Krause, M. V., and Hunscher, M. A. *Food, Nutrition and Diet Therapy.* 5th ed. Philadelphia, W. B. Saunders Co., 1972.

Lawrence, J. D.; Bower, R. C.; Riehl, W. P.; and Smith, J. L. "Effects of Alpha-Tocopherol Acetate on the Swimming Endurance of Trained Swimmers." *Amer. J. Clin. Nutr.* 28 (1975):205–208.

Londeree, B. "Pre-Event Diet Routine." *Runner's World* 9 (1974):26–29.

Marable, N. L.; Hickson, J. F.; Korslund, M. K.; Herbert, W. G.; Desjardins, R. F.; and Thye, F. W. "Urinary Nitrogen Excretion as Influenced by a Muscle-Building Exercise Program and Protein Intake Variation." *Nutr. Reports Int.* 19 (1979): 795-805.

Perkins, R., and Williams, M. H. "Effect of Caffeine upon Maximal Muscular Endurance of Females." *Med. Sci. Sports* 7 (1975): 221–224.

Smith, N. J. *Food for Sport.* Palo Alto, Calif: Bull Publishing Company, 1976.

Williams, M. H. *Nutritional Aspects of Human Physical and Athletic Performance.* Springfield, Ill.: Charles C. Thomas, 1976.

Young, D. R. *Physical Performance Fitness and Diet.* Springfield, Ill.: Charles C. Thomas, 1977.

11

Environmental Factors and Athletic Performance

INTRODUCTION

Frequently, the athlete is expected to perform under less than optimal environmental conditions. The athlete who trains at sea level is forced to make rather extensive physiological adjustments to compete successfully at higher altitudes. Training in cool climates does little to prepare the athlete to compete under conditions of extreme heat and humidity. Similarly, sudden exposure to cold can have a dramatic influence on athletes' performances if they have not had an opportunity to acclimatize to the colder environment.

The environment dictates to a large extent the quality of an athlete's performance. There are many things the athlete can do or adaptations he or she can make to better prepare for variations in the environment, either expected or unexpected. The purpose of this chapter is to inform the athlete and coach as to how they can make these necessary preparations. This chapter will be of limited value for those sports that are performed in a controlled indoor environment, such as basketball, wrestling, and swimming, with the exception of competition at altitudes. However, for sports such as cross country, football, and soccer, the importance of preparing for radical changes in environmental conditions must be recognized. Football provides an excellent example. The football season usually starts in July or August, depending on the level, i.e., high school, college, or professional, and the region. In most regions of the United States, this is the hottest season of the year. When the heat is combined with the high humidity in certain sections of the country, there is a potentially lethal situation. The padding and clothing worn by football players add another stress, since they create a closed microenvironment in which it is difficult to lose body heat. Even under normal conditions of temperature and humidity, this clothing creates potential problems of heat stress. During one three-year period, seven high school and five college football players died as a result of heat stress.* At the other extreme, while of considerably less consequence, football players are exposed to subfreezing temperatures in certain regions of the United States as the season draws to a close. This, too, can create many problems, such as frost bite and an increased potential for serious injury.

VARIATIONS IN TEMPERATURE AND HUMIDITY

The topic of body temperature regulation reviewed in Chapter 2, Responses to Acute Exercise, is considerably important to an understanding of the problem of exercising in extremes in temperature. Since the body is substantially less than 100 percent efficient, it will produce a considerable amount

*From D. K. Mathews and E. L. Fox, *The Physiological Basis of Physical Education and Athletics* 2nd ed. (Philadelphia: W. B. Saunders Co., 1979) p. 104.

of heat as it generates energy to perform various physical tasks. In cold environments, this metabolic heat production is necessary to assist in maintaining the body temperature. In hot environments, however, it is a liability, since it adds to the body's heat load. Chapter 2 describes how the body's temperature is regulated very precisely by the hypothalamus through four major processes: convection, radiation, conduction, and evaporation. At rest, temperature is closely regulated at approximately 98.6° F, but during exercise a much higher level is attained, sometimes exceeding 105° F (Costill, 1979). The body appears to select a new thermostatic "set-point" as the athlete goes from rest to strenuous exercise. This allows him or her to function more efficiently, since chemical reaction rates and oxygen availability are increased. When these regulatory mechanisms fail or when the environmental conditions are such that these four processes are inadequate to cope with the environmental stress, heat or cold, the athlete is placed in a potentially lethal situation. Therefore, a basic knowledge of how the body performs under various environmental temperatures and how to cope with environmental extremes is essential for both the coach and the athlete.

Exercise in the Heat

The ability of the athlete to successfully perform in the heat depends on the degree of heat, the humidity, the air movement, intensity and duration of effort, and the extent of previous exposure to similar environmental conditions. The latter factor is referred to as *acclimatization*. Also of major importance is the athlete's fluid and mineral intake schedule both prior to, as well as during, competition. Each of these factors must be considered when preparing the athlete for competition in the heat.

Degree of heat. The higher the ambient, or existing, temperature, the greater the stress placed on the athlete. At rest, with a "neutral" temperature of 70–80° F, the average individual gives off an excess of 80 Kcal of heat per hour as the by-product of producing metabolic energy. Of this, approximately 25 percent or 20 Kcal/hour are dissipated or removed from the body by evaporation; the remainder is lost by radiation, convection, and conduction. As the athlete exercises at different levels of intensity

up to exhaustion, the metabolic needs of the body increase in a linear manner and up to 900 Kcal/hr or more can be produced as a by-product of metabolism. This presents the body with a considerably greater challenge in dissipating, or ridding itself of, this excess heat. When exercising in a cold environment, this heat load is actually beneficial, assisting in the maintenance of a normal body temperature. However, even when the exercise is conducted in a thermally neutral environment, i.e., 70–80° F, the metabolic heat load places a considerable burden on the cardiovascular system, since the heat must be transported from the central core of the body out to the periphery.

As the temperature of the surrounding environment increases, the gradient between the athlete and the environment decreases, i.e., the temperature of the environment approaches, and can even exceed, the skin and core, or deep body, temperature. This results in an even greater reliance on evaporation as the major avenue of heat loss, since radiation, convection, and conduction lose effectiveness as the environmental temperature increases. Evaporation requires sweating, therefore, an increased dependency on evaporation means an increased demand for sweating. Since a high percentage of the fluid lost in sweat comes from the blood plasma, an even greater demand is imposed on the cardiovascular system. As the environmental temperature increases, more blood is needed to transport heat to the periphery, and an increasing sweat rate reduces the existing blood volume causing the total volume of blood that is available to supply the exercising muscles to be reduced in direct proportion to the intensity of the heat. This results in a reduction in overall performance potential, particularly for activities of an endurance nature. In long-distance runners, sweat losses may approach 6 to 10 percent of the runner's body weight. Such severe dehydration limits subsequent sweating and makes the athlete susceptible to heat cramps, heat stroke, or heat exhaustion.

Radiation, conduction, and convection, while working to cool the athlete on cool days when there is a breeze and partial or total cloud cover, can actually contribute to the heat load of the body if the climatic conditions are right. The athlete exercising at 75° F on a crystal-clear day with no measurable wind will notice considerably more heat stress than when exercising at the same temperature but with a cloud cover and slight breeze. At temperatures above 88–92° F, radiation, convection, and conduction will substantially add to the heat load rather than acting as an avenue of heat loss.

Clothing is an important consideration for the problem of heat stress. Obviously, the more clothing worn, the smaller the available area for evaporation to take place. The foolish practice of exercising in a rubberized suit to promote weight loss is an excellent illustration of how a microenvironment (environment inside the suit) can be created in which the temperature and humidity can reach a sufficiently high level to cause heat stroke or exhaustion if exercise is continued. A football uniform provides a similar microenvironment that is inherently dangerous in hot weather. It is strongly advocated by exercise scientists and sports physicians that the athlete wear as little clothing as possible when heat stress is a potential problem. Where clothing is necessary or required, it should be of loose weave to allow the skin beneath to breathe.

Humidity. An additional factor that is of considerable importance with regard to exercise in the heat is the relative humidity, or the degree of moisture in the surrounding air. Sweating contributes to the loss of body heat *only* if the sweat evaporates from the skin. It is the process of evaporation that results in a heat loss, since the evaporation of one milliliter of water requires 0.58 Kcal; thus the evaporation of a liter (approximately a quart) of water would yield a heat loss of 580 Kcal. The human is capable of sweating up to two liters or more per hour. If the surrounding air is totally saturated with water vapor, i.e., 100 percent humidity, it is impossible for sweat to evaporate, since there is no dry or unsaturated air available to pick up the resulting water vapor. A perfect example of this is the contrast between the bodily sensations in the middle of the desert at a temperature of 100° F, and 10 percent relative humidity compared to those in Houston, Texas, at 80° F, and 95 percent relative humidity. In the former, the body sweats profusely, but evaporation occurs so rapidly that the individual is not conscious of the fact that he or she is sweating. In the latter situation, only a limited amount of sweat can evaporate, since 95 percent of the surrounding air is filled with water vapor. The result is a continuous bath of sweat, which never seems to stop.

This example points to the importance of humidity in athletic performance in the heat. In the previous section, it was stated that evaporation is the major method of regulating body temperature in the heat. If the air is saturated with water vapor, no evaporation can occur even at the lower environmental temperatures, and at the higher temperatures, the body has no way of losing heat, so the body temperature will rise until death results.

It is clear that temperature by itself is not an accurate index of the total physiological stress imposed on the athlete. Humidity, air velocity, and the degree of cloud cover (radiation), as well as temperature, all directly influence the degree of stress felt by the athlete. The proportional contribution to the total stress from each of these factors is not clearly understood, and it probably varies with changing environmental conditions. Efforts have been made to quantify these four factors into a single index. In the 1920s, the effective temperature index was developed, which was later altered to account for the effect of radiation. The latter index was called the corrected effective temperature. In the 1970s, a wet globe thermometer was devised to simultaneously account for conduction, convection, evaporation, and radiation, providing a single temperature reading to estimate the potential cooling capacity of the surrounding environment. Unfortunately, this instrument has not been widely used to monitor the environmental conditions for various athletic events.

Dehydration. One of the greatest problems associated with exercise in the heat, particularly under conditions of high humidity, is dehydration. Since sweating is the major avenue of heat loss when exercising in the heat, the total amount of fluid lost becomes very important as the duration of the activity is extended over time. Humans are able to sweat at the rate of two liters per hour for short periods of time and are able to sustain sweating at the rate of one liter per hour, or more, for periods of three hours or longer. Marathon runners commonly lose five to seven pounds as a result of the 26.2-mile race, even though they are drinking freely during the race. Along with water, salts and other critical electrolytes are also lost at a substantial rate.

Dehydration presents a serious threat to the athlete. It is estimated that the deep body temperature will rise from 0.3 to 0.5° F for every 1 percent loss in body weight. This rise is the result of several factors, one of which is the loss in blood volume, i.e., a large percentage of the water lost in sweating comes from the blood volume. This reduces not only the blood available to transport heat from the core to the periphery but also the effective blood volume available to supply the exercising muscles. The result is a decrease in performance capacity.

The problem of dehydration is not unique to those athletes competing under conditions of thermal stress. In 1967, a county medical society in Iowa recommended that high school wrestling be abolished as a sport. This group of physicians was concerned with the hazardous health practices used by high school wrestlers to "make weight" for a specific weight class. This recommendation created a major wave of hysteria that quickly spread to other states. In the athletic world, Iowa and wrestling are considered inseparable. To ban wrestling in Iowa would be comparable to banning skiing in Colorado, swimming in California, or football in Texas.

Why were these physicians concerned? A group of researchers from the University of Iowa (Tipton, Zambraski, and Tcheng, 1974) set out to define the problem and recommend a solution. They found that the high school wrestlers were losing a considerable amount of body weight over a period of seventeen days, some losing nearly thirty pounds, or almost two pounds per day! In addition, they found that most of the weight loss occurred in the last few days prior to certification and that the greatest weight loss occurred in the youngest boys and lightest weight classes. Simple calculations indicated that most of the weight that was lost came from dehydration, not from a loss of body fat. Analysis of the wrestlers' urine samples confirmed the fact that substantial dehydration had occurred. It is a well-known fact that physical performance is impaired when fluid and electrolyte balances are upset by dehydration, and, as described above, it is apparent that the temperature regulatory mechanisms would also be compromised. In addition, possible signs of kidney damage were identified.

From this, it appears that voluntary dehydration, exemplified by the wrestler, is an undesirable practice and should be discouraged. This would apply to any athlete trying to make weight through a rapid loss of body fluids, e.g., football players, boxers, and even jockeys. The advantages gained are far outweighed by the disadvantages and the primary danger is the potential for serious medical complications. The athlete should focus on weight loss as a long-term process, losing no more than one to two pounds per week. A ten- to fifteen-pound weight loss over a seven-to fourteen day period is essentially a loss of body fluids, not fat. A fat loss should be the desired goal, since excess fat reduces the athlete's performance potential, while the body fluids are essential for optimal performance.

Fluid and Mineral Replacement. For many years, it was considered dangerous for athletes to stop and drink water or other fluids either during practice or competition. It was feared that the intake of fluids would cause cramping of the stomach and intestine; therefore, all fluids were generally withheld until after the practice or competition. Then, coaches started to realize that with copious sweating, large quantities of salt were being lost, and salt losses were associated with muscle cramps. This led to the practice of requiring athletes to take salt tablets by the handfuls, yet fluids were still withheld!

From our present knowledge of dehydration and fluid ingestion during exercise, we now know how dangerous and foolish such practices were. Ingestion of fluids during exercise is essential whenever dehydration is a potential problem. Fluid ingestion both before and during exercise in the heat has been shown to reduce the increase in rectal temperature, as exercise is prolonged up to two hours. For the same level of work and thermal stress, exercise with fluid ingestion results in a deep body temperature that is approximately 1.5° F lower compared to the same situation with no fluid ingestion. Most teams with sound medical leadership are now periodically stopping during practice for a fluid break. Either water or some other fluid fortified with minerals and electrolytes is distributed freely. The frequency of such breaks is dictated by the climatic conditons; the more severe the heat stress and subsequent dehydration, the more frequent the breaks. In the game situation, fluid should be made available at all times that the athlete is not in competition, and he or she should be encouraged to drink as much as possible. Since research shows that one does not drink as much as he or she should to replace the fluid that is lost, athletes should be told to drink even more than their thirst tells them they need.

Fluid intake prior to competition or practice should be encouraged.

Little is known about the most appropriate time and proportions of mineral and electrolyte intake. Under no circumstances should salt tablets be given and fluid withheld. This creates a situation where sweating is impaired and the body temperature will continue to rise. It is also known that fluids containing sugar reduce the speed by which the fluid is removed from the stomach.

Gisolfi (1975) has made several recommendations with regard to fluid replacement. In addition to ingesting fluid prior to exercise, he suggests drinking 200–300 ml (approximately one half of a pint) of a glucose-electrolyte solution every fifteen to twenty minutes. Since it is essential to replace as much fluid as possible, the glucose content should be less than 2.5 gm/100 ml. The solution should be cool, slightly hypotonic, and palatable to the individual. Lastly, he states that the loss of salt in sweat is usually insignificant compared to the water lost and that a liberal salting of foods at meal time is the most effective method of replacing the lost salt.

Acclimatization. Do repeated exposures to hot environments help the athlete adapt better to thermal stress, thus improving his or her athletic performance? Many studies have investigated this problem and have concluded that repeated exposure to heat causes a gradual adjustment that enables the athlete to tolerate the associated stress better. Apparently, almost total acclimatization can occur within a five- to fourteen-day period.

What changes take place as a result of acclimatization? First, the body has an increased ability to produce sweat, although at lower levels of heat stress less sweat is produced. The sweat that is produced is a more dilute sweat, thus conserving the body's mineral stores. There is a lowered skin and body temperature for the same level of work, and the heart rate response to a standardized, submaximal level of exercise is reduced. This latter response is the result of either or both an increased blood volume and a reduction in skin blood flow, both of which would increase the stroke volume. In addition, more work can be accomplished prior to reaching the point of fatigue or exhuastion.

The acclimatization process seems to require more than just exposure to a hot environment.

While the research literature is not in total agreement on this point, it does appear that exercise in a hot environment is required in order to attain acclimatization that will carry over to exercise in the heat. For individuals or teams that are training in environments cooler than those in which they will be competing, it is important to achieve thermal acclimatization prior to the contest or event. This would improve the individual's performance, in addition to reducing the associated physiological stress. Normal workouts in the heat for five to seven days should provide nearly total acclimatization, although the intensity of the workout should be reduced to 70–80 percent during the first few days to prevent heat stress.

Heat Disorders and Their Prevention. When the body is unable to successfully adapt to thermal stress, three forms of failure exist. *Heat cramps*, the least serious of the three heat disorders, is the result of dehydration and the salt loss accompanying high rates of sweating. It is characterized by severe cramping of the skeletal muscles, primarily those muscles used in the exercise. *Heat exhaustion* is the second type of heat disorder and is characterized by a body temperature of 101–104° F, extreme tiredness, breathlessness, dizziness, and tachycardia or rapid pulse. These symptoms appear to be the result of a reduced sweat production, thus limiting the body's major avenue of heat loss. *Heat stroke* is the most serious of the three disorders and is characterized by a body temperature of 105–106° F or higher, cessation of sweating, and total confusion or unconsciousness. If left untreated, the victim of heat stroke is likely to die. While a few people under normal, nonexercising conditions in the heat experience either heat stroke or exhaustion, many athletes push themselves to the point where they are extremely vulnerable to a serious heat disorder. The football player who is wearing a full uniform and protective equipment is particularly vulnerable in a hot environment. The uniform restricts evaporative cooling. The layer of air between the skin and the uniform becomes saturated with water vapor, thus sweat pours off, but little evaporative cooling takes place. The obese player, or the player with a thick layer of subcutaneous fat, has the added problem of the fat providing a thermal barrier to heat dissipation which makes a substantial contribution to his or her total heat stress.

To prevent heat disorders, several simple precautions should be taken. Competition and practice outdoors should not be held when the wet bulb temperature is over 78° F. Wet bulb temperature reflects the humidity as well as the absolute temperature, therefore, it is a more sensitive indication of the physiological stress. Scheduling practices and contests either in the early morning or at night is one way of overcoming the severe heat stress of midday. Fluids should be made readily available and the athlete required to drink as much as he or she can, stopping every ten to twenty minutes in the higher temperatures for a "fluid break." Clothing should be as brief as possible, loose-weaved, and of a light color, since dark colors absorb heat while light colors reflect. The athlete should always "underdress" because the metabolic heat load will soon make extra clothing an unnecessary burden. The athletes should be closely watched for the clinical signs mentioned—sure warnings of impending danger.

The American College of Sports Medicine issued a position statement in 1975 which dealt specifically with heat injuries during distance running. The following statement, in part, applies to all sports where heat injuries might be a problem.

Prevention of Heat Injuries
During Distance Running*

Based on research findings and current rules governing distance running competition, it is the position of the American College of Sports Medicine that:

1. Distance races (> 16 km or 10 miles) should not be conducted when the wet bulb temperature − globe temperature** exceeds 28° C (82.4° F).
2. During periods of the year, when the daylight dry bulb temperature often exceeds 27° C (80° F), distance races should be conducted before 9:00 A.M. or after 4:00 P.M.
3. It is the responsibility of the race sponsors to provide fluids which contain small amounts of

sugar (less than 2.5 g glucose per 100 ml of water) and electrolytes (less than 10 mEq sodium and 5 mEq potassium per liter of solution.)
4. Runners should be encouraged to frequently ingest fluids during competition and to consume 400–500 ml (13–17 oz.) of fluid 10–15 minutes before competition.
5. Rules prohibiting the administration of fluids during the first ten kilometers (6.2 miles) of a marathon race should be amended to permit fluid ingestion at frequent intervals along the race course. In light of the high sweat rates and body temperatures during distance running in the heat, race sponsors should provide "water stations" at 3–4 kilometer (2–2.5 mile) intervals for all races of 16 kilometers (10 miles) or more.
6. Runners should be instructed in how to recognize the early warning symptoms that precede heat injury. Recognition of symptoms, cessation of running, and proper treatment can prevent heat injury. Early warning symptoms include the following: piloerection on chest and upper arms, chilling, throbbing pressure in the head, unsteadiness, nausea, and dry skin.
7. Race sponsors should make prior arrangements with medical personnel for the care of cases of heat injury. Responsible and informed personnel should supervise each "feeding station." Organizational personnel should reserve the right to stop runners who exhibit clear signs of heat stroke or heat exhaustion.

It is the position of the American College of Sports Medicine that policies established by local, national, and international sponsors of distance running events should adhere to these guidelines. Failure to adhere to these guidelines may jeopardize the health of competitors through heat injury.

Exercise in the Cold

Exercise in the cold presents far fewer problems of a severe medical nature. Additional clothing can always be worn during the athletic contest to maintain the athlete in a warm and comfortable environment. The extremities, particularly the hands and feet, are most subject to discomfort and injury from exposure to cold.

*Position statement of the American College of Sports Medicine which appeared in *Medicine and Science in Sports*, vol. 7, no. 1, 1975.

**Adapted from D. Minard, "Prevention of Heat Casualties in Marine Corps Recruits." *Milit. Med.* 126:261 (1961). WB-GT = 0.7 (WBT + 0.2 (GT) + 0.1 (DBT).

As with heat, the temperature alone is not a valid index of the degree of stress felt by the individual. The wind creates a chill factor, and the more moist the surrounding air, the greater the physiological stress. A dry, still day at 10° F in the direct sun can be quite comfortable, yet on a moist, windy day with complete cloud cover at 40° F, the cold can be quite penetrating. Table 11–1 lists equivalent temperatures for various absolute, dry bulb temperatures and wind velocities.

The ability to acclimatize to cold is open to question. If acclimatization does occur as a result of repeated exposures, it is of relatively little value with regard to athletic performance. Of much greater significance are the protective measures taken by physicians, trainers, and coaches to assure the most favorable circumstances for the athlete. Proper protective clothing is important. Tightly woven garments will help maintain a small heat pocket between the skin and clothing. Gloves, hats or caps, and double pairs of stockings are also helpful. Thermal underwear is recommended for the arms, legs, and torso in extreme cold, but as the temperature rises and metabolic heat builds, a serious heat problem could develop. Once the athlete starts to warm up and starts to sweat, he or she should remove excess clothing. Sweat-soaked, wet clothing can create problems in a dry environment where evaporation occurs naturally with its resultant cooling effect.

ALTITUDE

With the awarding of the 1968 Olympic Games to Mexico City came a number of questions and a great deal of confusion as to what influence competition at 7,340 feet would have on athletic performance. Physiologists had been interested in altitude as a physiological stressor for a number of years prior to this time, but with the reality of Olympic competition only a few years away, physiologists, athletes, and coaches alike began to realize that little was known about athletic competition at moderate and high altitudes. Would performance in all activities suffer, or would altitude influence only the endur-

Table 11–1 *Wind-Chill-Factor Chart* *

Estimated wind speed (mph)	Actual Thermometer Reading (°F)											
	50	40	30	20	10	0	−10	−20	−30	−40	−50	−60
	Equivalent Temperature (°F)											
calm	50	40	30	20	10	0	−10	−20	−30	−40	−50	−60
5	48	37	27	16	6	−5	−15	−26	−36	−47	−57	−68
10	40	28	16	4	−9	−24	−33	−46	−58	−70	−83	−95
15	36	22	9	−5	−18	−32	−45	−58	−72	−85	−99	−112
20	32	18	4	−10	−25	−39	−53	−67	−82	−96	−110	−124
25	30	16	0	−15	−29	−44	−59	−74	−88	−104	−118	−133
30	28	13	−2	−18	−33	−48	−63	−79	−94	−109	−125	−140
35	27	11	−4	−20	−35	−51	−67	−82	−98	−113	−129	−145
40	26	10	−6	−21	−37	−53	−69	−85	−100	−116	−132	−148
	Green			Yellow			Red					

(Wind speeds greater than 40 mph have little additional effect.)	LITTLE DANGER (for properly clothed person). Maximum danger of false sense of security.	INCREASING DANGER Danger from freezing of exposed flesh.	GREAT DANGER

Trenchfoot and immersion foot may occur at any point on this chart.

Adapted from Runner's World *8 (1973): 28. Reproduced by permission of the publisher.*

ance activities? Would performance in the long jump, high jump, pole vault, shot put, javelin, discus, and hammer be improved due to the lower density of the surrounding air? Would those who live at altitude have an advantage when competing at altitudes, and if so, could the sea level resident move to altitude for several weeks or a month and achieve acclimatization? These and many other questions stimulated a great deal of research between 1963 and 1968, research which has continued to the present time.

Oxygen Transport

The major problem associated with competition at altitude is the reduced availability of oxygen at the tissue level. The surrounding air has the same percentage of oxygen as that found at sea level (20.93 percent), but due to the lower total pressure, the partial pressure of oxygen is reduced in inverse proportion to the increase in altitude. At sea level, the partial pressure of oxygen is 159 mmHg (760 × 0.2093), while at 8,000 feet the total pressure drops from 760 to 564 mmHg, and the partial pressure of oxygen drops to 118 mmHg. This only reduces the saturation of hemoglobin from 97 percent at sea level to approximately 92 percent at 8,000 feet. It was once thought that it was this small drop in saturation that reduced $\dot{V}O_2$ max approximately 15 percent at this altitude. However, it is also important to remember that the partial pressure of oxygen in the arterial blood drops from about 94 mmHg at sea level to 60 mmHg at 8,000 feet. Assuming a tissue partial pressure of 20 mmHg, the pressure differential drops from 74 to 40 mmHg, or nearly a 50-percent reduction in the diffusion gradient. If the tissue partial pressure were to drop to 0 mmHg, which may be possible for small localized areas of tissue under conditions of exhaustive exercise, the respective gradients would be 94 and 60, or a 36-percent reduction in the diffusion gradient. Since the diffusion gradient is responsible for driving the oxygen from the blood into the tissue, this is an even greater consideration than the small 5-percent reduction in hemoglobin saturation.

From the data, it appears that the oxygen delivery system is restricted in direct proportion to the decrease in total pressure or in inverse proportion to the altitude. Are similar decrements noted in performance and in the various physiological parameters assessed during exercise?

Physical Performance at Altitude. Sprint-type or anaerobic activities are generally not influenced to a great extent by altitude (Åstrand and Rodahl, 1977). These are activities that require only a matter of seconds for completion. Consequently, the demands on the oxygen transport system are minimal, which explains why performance is generally unaffected. It has been postulated that at the higher altitudes, 8,000 feet and above, sprint-type or throwing performances may even be enhanced due to the decreased air density which reduces the frictional resistance of air to running or to the objects being thrown. Limited experience tends to support this theory.

Activities requiring a longer duration, i.e., those with a higher aerobic component, are influenced by increases in altitude (Åstrand and Rodahl, 1977). It appears that the greater the aerobic component, the more the activity will be influenced by altitude, and the higher the altitude, the greater the decrement in performance. The decrement in performance is approximately proportional to the decrease in maximal oxygen uptake.

Physiological Function at Altitude. As was mentioned, there is a reduction in maximal oxygen uptake in inverse proportion to the increase in altitude. This is illustrated in Figure 11–1. Consequently, at submaximal levels of work, the individual will be working at a higher percentage of his or her capacity. It also appears that the individual calls on his or her anaerobic metabolism, i.e., reaches anaerobic threshold, at a much lower absolute level of work but probably at approximately the same relative level.

The pulmonary ventilation is increased at higher altitudes, both at rest and during exercise (Lenfant and Sullivan, 1971). Since the air at higher altitudes is less dense, the increase in ventilation is a compensatory mechanism to bring the same number of molecules of oxygen into the lung as the individual would take in at sea level. Since the number of molecules of oxygen for a given volume of air is less at higher altitudes, an additional volume of air is necessary to supply the same total number of molecules of oxygen. This increased ventilation

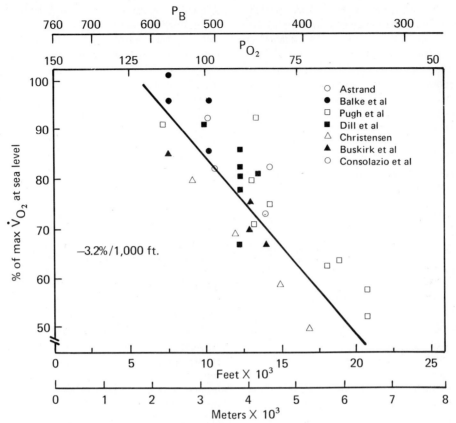

Figure 11–1   Reduction in maximal oxygen uptake in relation to increases in altitude, and a decrease in the barometric pressure (PB) and partial pressure of oxygen in the ambient air (pO₂). The symbols represent data of various authors. (From E. R. Buskirk et al., "The Effects of Altitude on Physical Performance, pp. 65–71, edited by R. F. Goddard. Chicago: Athletic Institute, 1967.)

acts much the same as hyperventilation at sea level, in that the CO_2 in the alveoli is reduced, causing more CO_2 to diffuse from the blood, which results in an increase in pH of the blood. This is referred to as a *respiratory alkalosis* and is compensated for by the kidneys where the excess bicarbonate is removed to normalize the blood pH.

The cardiovascular system also undergoes substantial changes to compensate for the increase in altitude and decrease in partial pressure of oxygen (Lenfant and Sullivan, 1971). The heart rate at standardized submaximal levels of work is elevated in direct proportion to the decrease in oxygen partial pressure. The stroke volume appears to be uninfluenced by altitude, since studies have shown

no change in stroke volume for the same absolute level of work when sea-level values are compared with values at different altitudes. However, this point is unresolved at the present time, since studies have also shown slight increases, as well as decreases, in stroke volume for the same level of work at higher altitudes compared to sea level. This apparent conflict is probably the result of the methodological problems of obtaining accurate estimates of stroke volume from determinations of cardiac output. However, since the change in stroke volume, if real, is small at best, the elevated heart rate at submaximal levels of work results in an increase in cardiac output, Thus, since the amount of oxygen available to the tissues from a certain volume of blood is limited due to the reduced partial pressure of oxygen and the subsequent drop in diffusion gradient, a greater volume of blood is delivered to the exercising tissues.

This discussion of cardiovascular alterations refers only to submaximal levels of work. At maximal or exhaustive levels, the maximal stroke volume does not appear to be influenced, but the peak or maximal heart rate is reduced at higher altitudes. This results in a decrease in the maximal cardiac output (Lenfant and Sullivan, 1971). With a decrease in the diffusion gradient to push oxygen across the membrane from the blood into the tissues along with this reduction in maximal cardiac output, it is not difficult to understand why both maximal oxygen uptake and performance in aerobic activities are affected by increases in altitude. The reason for the decrease in maximal heart rate is not known at the present time.

Acclimatization

As one extends his or her exposure to altitude for days and weeks, the body gradually acclimatizes. The body is able to partially adapt to the decreased partial pressure of oxygen found with increasing elevations. However, the athlete is never able to completely compensate for the increased elevation. While performance will improve with continued exposure, it will never reach the level that the athlete could attain at sea level, providing his or her general level of conditioning has not changed (Åstrand and Rodahl, 1977).

One of the first adaptations made at altitude is an increase in the number of circulating red blood cells (Lenfant and Sullivan, 1971). The actual amount of increase is not well understood, however, as there is also a substantial loss in plasma volume due to a generalized dehydration (Åstrand and Rodahl, 1977). This causes a concentration of the existing red cells, i.e., hemoconcentration. Further research using isotopically tagged, or labeled, red cells will enable a more accurate quantification of this response. Along with the increase in red cells there is an increase in hemoglobin. The net effect of both the red cell and hemoglobin increase is to increase the oxygen-carrying capacity of a fixed volume of blood.

The loss in plasma volume that occurs immediately upon arriving at a higher altitude is a transient response (Åstrand and Rodahl, 1977).

After a week or more at this altitude, the plasma volume will start to increase back to sea-level values. Whether it fully returns to sea-level values is not clear on the basis of the existing research. Several studies have shown a complete recovery, others have shown only a partial recovery, while still others have shown an increase above sea-level values.

Maximal oxygen uptake is decreased upon first reaching higher altitudes, but the adaptive changes in blood volume, red cell mass, and hemoglobin will gradually increase the maximal oxygen uptake, but not to the prealtitude, sea-level values (Åstrand and Rodahl, 1977). Performance in activities of a predominantly aerobic nature will show a similar improvement as the athlete becomes acclimatized, but the ultimate performance will still be below that observed at sea level.

Altitude Training

Researchers in several early studies on the influence of altitude on athletic performance, trained athletes at higher altitudes and found, on returning to sea level, that their performances had improved over their prealtitude sea-level performances. Athletes themselves have noted similar improvements following altitude training. Frederick (1974) states that altitude training has become a basic ingredient of success for many world-class distance runners. He further states that every gold medal winner in the 1972 Munich Olympic Games from the 1,500 meters through the marathon were altitude trained.

While these practical examples are impressive, they are not totally supported by controlled research studies. Several studies have shown no improvement in sea-level performance following altitude training. In several studies where altitude training was found to have an influence on post-altitude, sea-level performance, the subjects were not well trained prior to going to altitude, so it is difficult to discern how much of their post-altitude improvement was due solely to training, independent of altitude.

While the research literature is in apparent conflict on this matter, it is possible to construct a strong theoretical argument for altitude training. First, altitude training evokes a substantial tissue hypoxia (reduced oxygen supply), which is felt to be essential for initiating the conditioning response. Second, the major adaptations of increased red blood cell mass and hemoglobin levels will provide a major advantage with regard to oxygen delivery on return to sea level. While evidence suggests these latter changes are transient, lasting only several days, this would still provide an advantage for the athlete. Maximum ventilation volume appears to be enhanced, as does maximum cardiac output, although the latter is not well documented. Putting all of these adaptations together would give the endurance athlete a distinct advantage upon returning to sea level.

What about the athlete who normally trains at sea level and must compete at altitude? What can he or she do to prepare most effectively for competition? While the research is not clear on all aspects of this question, it appears that the athlete should either compete within twenty-four hours of arrival at higher altitudes, or train at higher altitudes for at least two weeks prior to competition. Even two weeks, however, is not sufficient for total acclimatization. That would require a minimum of four to six weeks. Competing within the initial twenty-four hours does not provide much in the way of acclimatization, but the exposure is brief enough that the classic systems of altitude sickness have not become totally manifest.

When training at higher altitudes, the coach or athlete should select an altitude between 5,000 and 10,000 feet, since the former is considered the lowest level at which an effect will be noticed, and the latter is the highest level for efficient conditioning. When first reaching higher altitudes, the magnitude of the workout should be reduced to approximately 60–70 percent of the intensity of the sea-level workout schedule, gradually working up to a full workout within ten to fourteen days. Symptoms of altitude sickness may persist for a few days, e.g., shortness of breath, headache, dizziness, nausea, and disturbed sleep, but they will gradually disappear.

AIR POLLUTION

During the past ten years, there has been increasing concern relative to the possible problems associated with exercising in polluted air. Ambient air in many cities is contaminated with small quantities of gases and particulates that are not among its normal constituents. When air becomes stagnant or when a temperature inversion occurs, some of these air pollutants reach levels of concentration that produce significant detrimental effects on athletic performance. Carbon monoxide, photochemical oxidants, and sulfur oxides are the major contaminants of concern.

Carbon monoxide is essentially an odorless gas that is rapidly absorbed from inspired air due to the high affinity of hemoglobin for carbon monoxide. The affinity of hemoglobin for carbon monoxide is approximately 240 times greater than its affinity for oxygen. Several studies have reported an inverse, linear decrease in $\dot{V}O_2$ max with increases in blood levels of carbon monoxide, and the blood levels of carbon monoxide are a direct function of the levels of carbon monoxide in the inspired air. Raven (1979) has recently reviewed the literature in this area and indicates that the reduction in $\dot{V}O_2$ max is not statistically significant until blood carbon monoxide levels exceeded 4.3 percent, although performance time on the treadmill has been found reduced at levels as low as 2.7 percent. Submaximal performance does not appear to be greatly affected until the blood levels exceed 15 percent. This would correspond to oxygen uptake values between 35 and 60 percent of maximum.

Ozone is the primary photochemical oxidant that produces many subjective complaints when breathed at high ambient levels of concentration. Eye irritation, chest tightness, a feeling of breathlessness, coughing, and a feeling of nausea are the primary complaints. Ozone has its primary influence on the lungs and respiratory tract. Decrements in lung function occur with increasing concentrations of ozone, as well as with increases in time of exposure and level of ventilation. $\dot{V}O_2$ max has been found to be significantly decreased following two hours of intermittent exercise exposure to 0.75 ppm ozone. This decrease in $\dot{V}O_2$ max is thought to be associated with a reduced oxygen transfer at the lung resulting from a reduced alveolar air exchange (Raven, 1979).

Sulfur dioxide is the major sulfur oxide contaminant of concern during exercise. While the research on sulfur dioxide and exercise is limited, it is certain that ambient levels above 1.0 ppm will cause significant discomfort and will prove detrimental to performance (Raven, 1979). Sulfur dioxide is primarily an upper-airway and bronchial irritant.

Certain cities have initiated air pollution or smog alerts. These are usually color-coded with the colors indicating the degree of severity of pollution. Standards need to be established nationally, and the air monitored accordingly. Increasing evidence is pointing to the wisdom of canceling all games and practices when pollution levels reach a certain point. Considerable research is presently in progress that will hopefully allow a better definition of this area.

DIVING

As one takes to water, an entirely different physical and physiological environment is encountered, which requires a full understanding on the part of the diver. As he or she dives below the surface of water, the diver is subjected to an increasing pressure; while at higher altitudes, the problem was one of a decreasing pressure. Fresh water weighs 62.4 pounds per cubic foot while salt water, due to the salt content, weighs 64.0 pounds per cubic foot. Descending to a level of thirty-three feet produces 14.7 pounds *per square inch* (psi) pressure on the diver from the water alone. Since the atmosphere provides an additional 14.7 psi, the total pressure on the diver would be 29.4 psi (water pressure + air pressure). As the diver descends to sixty-six feet, the water pressure doubles from 14.7 to 29.4 psi which, when added to the air pressure of 14.7 psi, makes a total pressure of 44.1 psi.

The data in the previous discussion is critical to the diver for several important reasons. First, the air he or she breathes on the surface will be compressed to one-half of its original volume in the lung at thirty-three feet below the water's surface. Conversely, the volume of air in his or her lung at a thirty-three-foot depth will expand to twice its original volume by the time he or she reaches the surface. If breathing from a self-contained underwater breathing apparatus (SCUBA), it would be extremely dangerous for the diver to take in a deep breath at a depth of thirty-three feet and to hold this breath as he or she ascended to the surface. Overdistension of the lung would result, with rupturing of the alveoli and pulmonary hemorrhage. If air bubbles end up in the circulatory system as a result

of this extensive damage, emboli develop and can block major vessels, leading to extensive tissue damage, if not death. Thus, it is important for the diver to always blow out or exhale as he or she ascends to the surface.

An additional factor that must be considered relative to the increased pressure with dives is the increased partial pressure of the individual gases. Breathing air at a depth of thirty-three feet doubles the partial pressure of each of the gases. At depths approaching one hundred feet, the partial pressures are four times greater than on the surface. It is at one hundred feet, when breathing air, that problems of *nitrogen narcosis* develop. Nitrogen narcosis is known as the "rapture of the deep." The diver develops symptoms similar to those of alcohol intoxication in which the effect is primarily on the central nervous system. Judgment is distorted, and foolish decisions frequently result in serious injury or death.

Another problem caused by the high partial pressures at the lower depths is oxygen poisoning. Breathing high concentrations of oxygen for long periods of time during deep dives drives a great deal of oxygen into solution. The oxygen in solution is used preferentially over that carried in combination with hemoglobin in the red blood cell. Consequently, oxygen is not released from the red cell and a carrier is not available to remove the CO_2 produced. An excess of both O_2 and CO_2 develops in the tissues, causing visual distortion, confusion, rapid and shallow breathing, and convulsions. The use of oxygen in diving is to be avoided whenever possible.

The high partial pressures of nitrogen in diving will force nitrogen into the blood and tissues. If the diver attempts to ascend too rapidly, this additional nitrogen cannot be delivered to and released through the lungs quickly enough, and it becomes trapped as bubbles in the circulatory system and tissues, causing discomfort and pain. While the joints and ligaments are most often involved, occasionally emboli can form in the circulatory system. causing more serious complications. This is referred to as *decompression sickness*, or *the bends*. Treatment involves placing the diver into a recompression chamber, where the pressure of nitrogen is increased again and then gradually returned to the ambient pressure. This period of recompression forces the nitrogen back into solution and the gradual decrease in pressure then allows the nitrogen to escape through the respiratory system. To prevent this condition, charts have been created that provide the necessary information relative to the time sequence for ascending from various depths. Strict adherence to the respective time table for the depth submerged will allow a safe ascent without the problem of decompression sickness.

One last word of caution: Annually, a number of deaths result from underwater swimming. Typically, the diver forcefully hyperventilates and then attempts to swim as far as possible on a single breath of air. Unfortunately, the individual may become unconscious and drown before realizing he or she is in trouble and needs to come to the surface for a breath of air. In hyperventilating, the CO_2 levels are greatly reduced. Since CO_2 is a potent stimulus for breathing, its reduction in the blood decreases the stimulus for breathing and the oxygen concentration drops below critical levels, resulting in a loss of consciousness. While hyperventilation will allow new records to be set in underwater swimming, it is a practice that must be strongly discouraged due to this inherent danger.

GENERAL SUMMARY

Frequently, athletic competition is conducted under environmental conditions that are less than optimal. Heat, cold, humidity, and altitude each present unique problems for the athlete, which need not seriously handicap performance if he or she understands the situation and plans in advance the proper preventive and precautionary procedures.

This chapter attempts to briefly summarize the nature of these various environmental stresses and to provide the coach and athlete with suggestions for coping with them more successfully. In hot environments, performance is compromised in proportion to the severity of the heat stress. Evaporation becomes the most important avenue of heat loss, but this presents potential problems of dehydration if the fluid loss is not rapidly replaced. As the humidity increases, the problem becomes considerably more serious. Practicing in the heat for a week or two will almost fully acclimatize the athlete to the heat stress. In addition, ingestion of fluids before practice and frequently during practice and competiton will reduce the degree of heat stress and aid performance. In cold environments, acclimatization

does not significantly contribute to the athlete's performance, but proper clothing can play a major role. It is important to dress warmly but not to overdress, for this can cause heat stress.

Altitude directly influences the oxygen transport system. As the altitude increases, the total atmospheric pressure decreases, and this results in a proportional decrease in the partial pressure of the respiratory gases. The partial pressure of oxygen decrease reduces slightly the degree of saturation of the arterial blood with oxygen, but more importantly, it decreases the partial pressure of oxygen in the arterial blood, thus substantially lowering the diffusion gradient. The result is a decreased maximal oxygen uptake and a decrement in performances of an aerobic nature. Acclimitization will reduce the magnitude of these performance decreases but will not totally overcome the influences of altitude, i.e., performance will not equal that at sea level.

Air pollution is another area of concern relative to athletic performance. Carbon monoxide, ozone, and sulfur dioxide are the primary contaminants that can have a detrimental effect on athletic performance when their concentrations reach critical threshold levels. Activities of an endurance nature are those primarily affected.

Lastly, diving involves another unique environment for performance in which the major consideration is the increased pressure under the surface of the water. This increased pressure will have a substantial influence on the breathing pattern of the diver and will also affect the amounts of nitrogen and oxygen that are driven into solution in the tissues and blood. If these are too great, they can lead to problems of nitrogen narcosis, decompression sickness, and oxygen poisoning.

STUDY QUESTIONS

1. What are the four major pathways available for loss of body heat?
2. Which of the above four pathways is most important for controlling body temperature during exercise?
3. What happens to the body temperature during exercise, and why?
4. Why is humidity an important factor when performing in the heat?

5. What is the purpose of a wet globe thermometer? What does it measure?

6. What is the relationship between dehydration and increasing body temperature during exercise?

7. How important is fluid ingestion during practice or competition in the heat?

8. What physiological adaptations occur allowing one to acclimate to exercise in the heat?

9. Differentiate between heat cramps, heat exhaustion, and heat stroke.

10. What factors should be considered to provide maximum protection when exercising in the cold?

11. How does altitude influence athletic performance? Does it influence all sports or events to the same degree?

12. Physiologically, how does altitude affect endurance performance?

13. Would an endurance athlete profit by training at altitude? Why or why not?

14. With underwater diving, what specific problems must one be aware of to avoid serious injury or death?

15. How is endurance exercise performance affected by high concentrations of air pollutants?

REFERENCES

Astrand, P.-O., and Rodahl, K. *Textbook of Work Physiology*, 2nd ed. New York: McGraw-Hill Book Co., 1977.

Balke, B. "Variation in Altitude and its Effect on Exercise Performance." In *Exercise Physiology*, edited by H. B. Falls. New York: Academic Press, 1968.

Buskirk, E. R.; Kollias, J.; Piconreatique, E.; Akers, R.; Prokop, E.; and Baker, P. In *The Effects of Altitude on Physical Performance*, pp. 65–71, edited by R. F. Goddard. Chicago: Athletic Institute, 1967.

Costill, D. L. "Hazards of the Heat." In *The Complete Runner*. Mountain View, Calif.: World Publications, 1974.

Costill, D. L. *A Scientific Approach to Distance Running*. Los Altos, Calif.: Track and Field News, 1979.

deVries, H. A. *Physiology of Exercise for Physical Education and Athletics*. 2nd ed. Dubuque, Iowa: William C. Brown Co., 1974.

Folinsbee, L. J.; Wagner, J. A.; Borgia, J. F.; Drinkwater, B. L.; Gliner, J. A.; and Bedi, J. F., eds. *Environmental Stress: Individual Human Adaptations*. New York: Academic Press, 1978.

Fox, E. L. *Sport Physiology*. Philadelphia: W. B. Saunders Co., 1979.

Frederick, E. C. "Training at Altitude." In *The Complete Runner*. Mountain View, Calif.: World Publications, 1974.

Gisolfi, C. V. "Exercise, Heat, and Dehydration Don't Mix." *Rx Sports and Travel* (May–June 1975): 23–25.

Karpovich, P. V., and Sinning, W. E. *Physiology of Muscular Activity*, 7th ed. Philadelphia: W. B. Saunders Co., 1971.

Lenfant, C., and Sullivan, K. "Adaptation to High Altitude." *N.E.J. Med.* 284 (1971): 1298–1309.

Margaria, R., ed. *Exercise at Altitude*. Amsterdam: Excerpta Medica Foundation, 1967.

Mathews, D. K., and Fox, E. *The Physiological Basis of Physical Education and Athletics*. Philadelphia: W. B. Saunders Co., 1971.

Nadel, E. R., ed. *Problems with Temperature Regulation during Exercise*. New York: Academic Press, 1977.

Raven, P. B. "Heat and Air Pollution: The Cardiac Patient." In *Heart Disease and Rehabilitation*, edited by M. L. Pollock and D. H. Schmidt. Boston: Houghton Mifflin, 1979.

Robertshaw, D. *Environmental Physiology II*. Baltimore: University Park Press, 1977.

Sharkey, B. J. *Physiology of Fitness*. Champaign, Ill.: Human Kinetics Publishers, 1979.

Tipton, C. M.; Zambraski, D. J.; and Tcheng, T. K. "Iowa Wrestling Study: Lessons for Physicians." *Rx Sports and Travel* (January–February 1974): 19–22.

Van Handel, P. "Drinks for the Road." *Runner's World* 9 (July 1974): 29–31.

12

Ergogenic Aids*

INTRODUCTION

As the skill level of athletes in various sports improves from year to year and as athletic records reach new heights, the margin between success and failure in the world of sport becomes smaller. Consequently, coaches and athletes alike look for that slight edge that might assure victory and delay defeat. For some athletes, a special diet may be the deciding factor, others may rely on altering psychological states, while still others may try various hormones or pharmacological agents. Substances or phenomena that elevate or improve the performance of the individual above the expected level are referred to as *ergogenic aids* (Morgan, 1972a). Weight lifters have taken anabolic steroids in an attempt to increase muscle mass and strength. Distance runners have loaded up on carbohydrates two to three days prior to competiton in an attempt to pack extra glycogen into the active muscles. Hypnosis has been tried on a number of athletes in various sports in an attempt to get them over specific "hang-ups." Even the cheers of the crowd supporting the home team may place the visiting team at a distinct disadvantage.

While a number of substances and phenomena have been labeled as ergogenic aids, it must be proven that they actually facilitate the athlete's performance before they can be legitimately classified as ergogenic. The purpose of this chapter is to investigate the various substances and phenomena that have been used by athletes in order to determine their ergogenic potential. Simply because a professional all-star athlete consumes large quantities of a particular substance several hours prior to game time and attributes his success to this practice does not prove that this substance has mystical, power-inducing qualities that will assure other athletes of similar success. While science, with carefully controlled investigations, does not have all of the answers, this is an area where scientific studies are essential to differentiate between a truely ergogenic response and a pseudo-ergogenic response in which the performance is improved simply because the athlete expects it to improve.

DRUGS AND HORMONES

Numerous drugs and hormones have been suggested as having ergogenic properties. Golding (1972) has listed a number of these including:

Adrenaline	Coramine
Alcohol	Lecithin
Alkalies	Metrazol
Amphetamines	Noradrenaline
Caffeine	Steroids
Cocaine	Sulfa drugs

*Sections of this chapter were adapted from William P. Morgan, ed., *Ergogenic Aids and Muscular Performance*. (New York: Academic Press, 1972.)

This section will be confined to a study of alcohol, amphetamines, and anabolic steroids—the three major drugs or hormones that have received the most widespread use and national attention.

Alcohol

Cooper (1972a) states that alcohol is the number one drug problem in the United States. While others classify alcohol as a food, Cooper feels that alcohol is correctly classified as a drug, due to its influence on the central nervous system. Unfortunately, little is known about the influence of varying amounts of alcohol on athletic performance. Obviously, alcohol intake to the point of intoxication would result in an erratic, unpredictable performance. The influence of small amounts of alcohol just prior to or during a contest is not clearly understood.

Several studies have been conducted in the laboratory to observe the effects of small and moderate doses of alcohol on strength, muscular endurance, and cardiovascular endurance. The results from these studies conflict somewhat since several found improved performance and several found decreased performance, but the majority found no difference in performance. It would appear safe to conclude that alcohol has little, if any, ergogenic properties, but that it could be detrimental to optimal performance if taken in sufficient quantity. Recently, there has been considerable concern over increasing numbers of athletes who are becoming alcoholics as a result of indiscriminate use of alcohol.

Amphetamines

Amphetamines are prescription drugs that stimulate the central nervous system. They have been used as appetite suppressants for individuals on weight-loss programs under close medical supervision. Unfortunately, they have found their way into the athletic arena as a stimulant with possible ergogenic properties. Amphetamines have been referred to as "pep pills," "uppers," "bennies," "greenies," and "dexies," just to name a few of the many words or terms popularly used to identify this particular drug. Athletes have found amphetamines readily available, even though they are a prescription drug. Supposedly, amphetamine usage

by an athlete will help him or her run faster, throw farther, jump higher, and prolong the time it takes to reach total fatigue, or exhaustion. Do controlled scientific research studies support these claims?

Physiologically, amphetamines are known to increase alertness; reduce sense of fatigue; increase vasoconstriction, blood pressure, and heart rate; elevate blood sugar; and increase muscle tension. It is generally regarded as a potent, central nervous system stimulant. Does this insure that the drug will aid physical performance?

A number of studies have been conducted to answer this question, but, unfortunately, as in other areas, the results are in direct conflict with one another.

Two of the most widely read and quoted studies were supported by the American Medical Association and published in 1959. Smith and Beecher (1959) observed the influence of 14–21 mg of amphetamine sulfate per 70 kg of body weight on running, swimming, and weight throwing performance. They found that 75 percent of the tests resulted in an improved performance of 1 to 4 percent with amphetamine administration. This was a double-blind study in which neither the experimenter nor the athlete knew which capsules were being administered, the amphetamine or a placebo, i.e., a capsule of identical size, shape, and color containing sugar, gelatin, or some similar ingredient that has no direct specific effect. Karpovich (1959) conducted a similar study, using 10–20 mg of amphetamine sulfate prior to track running, swimming, and treadmill running. Of the fifty-four subjects, the performance of three improved, the performance of one was poorer, and the remaining fifty showed no difference in performance as a result of the amphetamine administration.

Possibly the best designed and controlled study conducted in this area was reported by Golding and Barnard in 1963. They used a double-blind procedure in which either 15 mg of d-amphetamine sulfate or a placebo were administered, three times each. Approximately two to three hours after either the drug or the placebo was administered, the subject was given two treadmill tests to exhaustion, the second following the first by twelve minutes. The purpose of having two treadmill tests to exhaustion was to determine whether amphetamines would "pick up" the subject after one exhaustive bout and make him better able to tolerate the second bout.

Amphetamines supposedly abolish or delay the onset of fatigue. Two groups of subjects were used, one that was considered to be conditioned and a second that was considered to be unconditioned. No differences were found between the placebo and amphetamine treatments for either the first or second treadmill runs for either the conditioned or the unconditioned groups.

Chandler and Blair (1980) conducted a double-blind, placebo-controlled study on the effects of amphetamines on strength, muscular power, running speed, acceleration, aerobic power and anaerobic capacity. The subjects received either a placebo or 15 mg of Dexedrine per 70 kg of body weight two hours prior to testing. When testing following amphetamine administration, improved performance was found in knee extension strength, acceleration, anaerobic capacity, time to exhaustion, and pre-exercise and maximum heart rates. Even though the time to exhaustion on the treadmill was increased, there were no differences in aerobic power. In studies dealing with fatigue, or with the sensation or feeling of fatigue, administration of amphetamines may have a small, but significant effect.

From these results, it is difficult to draw conclusions about amphetamines as an ergogenic agent. While most studies suggest that amphetamines do little to facilitate performance, those few studies that have reported significant improvements in performance point to the need for additional studies of a highly controlled and more comprehensive nature. It is quite possible that the laboratory tests used in some studies do not accurately duplicate the conditions in the playing situation. Treadmill-running time, reaction time, and oxygen debt may be far removed from the actual stress encountered in the sport or event. Future studies must be sensitive to this point. Also, it is quite possible that athletes may be consuming far greater doses of amphetamines than allowed in controlled research studies. If future studies show amphetamines to be potent ergogenic aids, the moral and ethical issue of whether they should be allowed in sport must be considered, in addition to the critical problem of the potential medical risks associated with acute and extended usage of amphetamines.

The use of amphetamines in athletics has become widespread over the past twenty years. During the mid-1970s, many law suits were filed against team trainers and team physicians for administering amphetamines to injured athletes in an effort to get them back into action sooner. While these occurred primarily at the professional level, evidence is also plentiful indicating extensive use of amphetamines by athletes even at the high school level. Since these are prescription drugs, the amphetamines that are being used at each level of competition have to be prescribed by a physician. In no other way can they be legally obtained! The prevalent practice of having amphetamines readily available for individual athletes or athletic teams would suggest that a number of physicians have disregard for the standards of their profession.

Are amphetamines potentially harmful? Experience would tend to suggest that they are inherently dangerous. Deaths have been attributed to excessive amphetamine usage where the athlete pushed beyond his or her normal state of exhaustion. One of the claims made for amphetamines is that they delay the onset of fatigue. It is possible that, rather than delaying the onset, they delay the sensation of fatigue, enabling the individual to push dangerously beyond normal limits to the point of circulatory failure. Amphetamines can be highly toxic, and they also can be physically addictive if taken regularly. Extreme nervousness, acute anxiety, aggressive behavior, and insomnia are also frequently mentioned side effects of regular usage (Golding, 1972).

When used in athletic contests, do amphetamines improve actual performance? Many physicians and scientists have observed that the player on amphetamines frequently feels he or she is having an outstanding performance, when in actuality the performance may be well below normal. The player's self-image appears to be grossly distorted. Jim Bouton, a former major league pitcher, told in his book, *Ball Four*, of the pitcher who was visited on the mound by his manager. He told the manager that he was throwing as well as anyone and that he never felt better. It must have been quite a shock to that pitcher when the manager sent him to the showers for giving up three home runs on three consecutive pitches. Cooper (1972b) cites several examples of bicycle races where all of the participants were given a detailed urine analysis to determine amphetamine usage at the conclusion of the race. Interestingly, traces of amphetamines were found only in those who finished the race at the back of the pack. Thus, it should be concluded that the possible benefits of taking amphetamines, if any, are far outweighed by the potential risks.

Anabolic Steroids

It has been estimated that over 70 percent of world-class weight lifters, shot putters, discus throwers, and javelin throwers either have used anabolic steroids in the past or are presently using them. Androgenic-anabolic steroids are nearly identical to the male sex hormones. The androgenic properties of these hormones accentuate secondary, sexual characteristic development. The anabolic properties are responsible for acceleration of growth through accelerated bone maturation and increased development of muscle mass. The synthetic steroids have been altered to reduce the androgenic properties and increase the anabolic effects. Anabolic steroids have been given for years to youngsters with delayed growth patterns to normalize their growth curves. Theoretically, steroid administration will result in both increased weight, as well as increased strength. Consequently, the athlete who is dependent on size and strength would naturally be interested in steroids. Are anabolic steroids ergogenic in nature? Can they facilitate the actual performance of the athlete? Second, and of greater importance, are there inherent medical risks in taking steroids?

A number of studies have attempted to investigate these questions in an organized and systematic fashion. Fowler, Gardner, and Egstrom (1965) conducted a controlled study of anabolic steroid usage relative to physical performance in healthy young men. Ten of the subjects were athletes, five received the steroid (20 mg of androstenolene per day) and five received a placebo. An additional thirty-seven untrained subjects were randomly assigned to one of four groups: placebo; steroid; placebo + exercise; steroid + exercise. No differences were noted between the placebo and steroid groups following sixteen weeks of training, although the exercising subjects exhibited improved performances. Steroid usage did not result in either a strength or weight gain.

Johnson and O'Shea (1969) created quite a stir in athletic circles when they reported that a group that lifted weights and took anabolic steroids for a three-week period of time had substantially greater increases in weight, strength, muscle girth, and maximal oxygen uptake than a matched group that only lifted weights. Protein powder was given to all of the subjects to supplement their diets during the training period. Weight gain in the steroid group averaged 2.5 kg, or 5.5 lb, while the nonsteroid group gained only 0.3 kg. The most amazing finding from this study was the increase of more than 15 percent in $\dot{V}O_2$ max with essentially no aerobic training. These changes also occurred over a period of only three weeks. Unfortunately, both investigators and subjects knew what supplements each subject was receiving. Subsequent studies have not found changes in $\dot{V}O_2$ max.

Recent studies have been evenly balanced between those that have found no statistically significant change in body size and physical performance attributable to taking steroids, and those who have found steroids to have a considerable influence on weight and strength. How can this basic inconsistency be explained? It may be due to lack of proper controls; an inadequate number of subjects in the study; failure to use a protein supplement; different drugs, dosages, or methods of drug administration; or any one or a combination of these causes; or it may be due to any of a number of other possiblities. The basic problem, however, is not the inconsistency of the findings in these studies but the inability to scientifically observe the effects of the drug dosages that are actually being used in the athletic world. It is estimated that some athletes are taking five to ten times the recommended daily dosage. For obvious reasons, it would be unethical to design a study that used a dosage that exceeded the recommended dosage.

Golding (1972) reported interviews by Dr. Fritz Hagerman with athletes competing in the World Pentathlon Games in 1966 and in the 1968 Olympic Games in Mexico City. Using just two examples, one shot-putter's weight increased from 225 to 280 pounds over a two-year period with anabolic steroids, and the athlete achieved his lifetime best performance during this time. In the second example, a discus thrower's weight went from 220 to 268 pounds in less than six months while taking steroids and his throws increased from the low 180s to 207 feet. In both examples, the dosage was from two to eight times the recommended dosage. This response does appear to be typical of the athlete who takes exceptionally high doses. Thus, if the dosage is high enough, the drug does appear to have a substantial effect on weight gains. Controlled research has failed to identify the source of these weight gains. Is it muscle, water, or fat? Likewise, it is not clear as to whether these weight gains translate into improved athletic performance. An additional twenty pounds of fat or water would be detrimental for most athletes, and even if the twenty-pound gain were muscle, there is no evidence that this would aid performance. Unfortunately, because of the inability to study these higher doses in a controlled study, most of these questions will never be properly answered.

Even if anabolic steroids are eventually shown to be beneficial for athletic performance, two questions must be resolved. First, is it morally and ethically right for the athlete to artificially induce changes in his or her performance potential? Most athletes feel it is wrong for their competitors to do anything that might artificially improve performance, yet many of these same athletes are "forced" into taking steroids in an effort to "keep up" with the other athletes in their sport or event who are chronic steroid users. Cooper (1972b) has quoted an estimate that 80 percent of all weight lifters, shot putters, discus throwers, and javelin throwers of national caliber are using anabolic steroids! It is difficult to be the only athlete in an event at a particular meet who has not been using steroids. It has also been reported that certain female athletes are now taking anabolic steroids in an attempt to increase both size and performance. Although the pressures on the athlete are great, are the potential gains worth the possible risks associated with steroid use?

This leads to the second question: What are the potential risks associated with the recommended doses of anabolic steroids? First, there is evidence that demonstrates that the use of steroids by individuals who are not fully mature will lead to an early closure of the epiphysis of the long bones. Since steroid use is also associated with an increase in the rate of growth of the long bones, it is difficult to determine whether the individual's final height will be less than, greater than, or the same as the height that would have been achieved without steroids. At least the potential for reducing height exists. Large doses of anabolic steroids suppress the natural secretion of gonadotropin and may cause atrophy of the tubules and interstitial tissue of the

testes and possible atrophy of the testicles themselves. Enlargement or hypertrophy of the prostate is another possible side effect. Liver damage from a form of chemical hepatitis has also been identified. Lastly, and possibly of greatest concern, neither scientists nor physicians know the potential long-term effects of chronic steroid usage. The American College of Sports Medicine issued a position statement on the use of steroids in 1977 which contained a comprehensive review of the existing research literature.

One alternative to steroids that has recently been proposed is cyproheptadine. Cyproheptadine is a prescription drug, i.e., a histamine and serotonin antagonist, which has been shown to induce weight gains in underweight adults, probably through appetite stimulation. This drug is being used with athletes, but no controlled studies have been conducted to determine the results of its use. Even with the underweight adults, the composition of the weight gain was not analyzed. Since cyproheptadine is basically an appetite stimulant, it is probable that the weight gain is largely the result of fat accumulation and fluid retention and not due to an increase in muscle mass. Such a weight gain would have little value in athletics.

NUTRITION

The possible influence of nutrition on athletic performance was discussed in great detail in Chapter 10, Nutrition and Athletic Performance. Considerable evidence was provided in that chapter to indicate that certain nutritional manipulations can substantially alter athletic performance.

OXYGEN

During the professional football game of the week on television, it is not uncommon to see the premier running back break loose for a thirty-five-yard touchdown run, struggle back to the bench, grab a face mask, and start breathing 100 percent oxygen. How much does he gain over a normal recovery breathing the surrounding air?

Initial attempts to scientifically investigate the ergogenic properties of oxygen began in the early 1900s, but it was not until the 1932 Olympic Games that oxygen was considered to be a potential ergogenic aid for athletic performance. At that time, the Japanese swimmers won great victories, and many attributed their success to the fact that they breathed pure oxygen prior to competition. Was this success due partly to their use of oxygen, or was it solely due to the fact that they were better athletes at the time of competition?

Oxygen can be supplemented in one of three ways: increasing the partial pressure of oxygen in the inspired gas mixture, using the normal concentration of oxygen in air under compression, or using an increased partial pressure of oxygen in the inspired gas mixture that is under compression. Also, oxygen can be supplemented prior to competition, during competition, during recovery from competition, or during any combination of these three.

Oxygen breathing prior to exercise has a limited effect on that exercise (Wilmore, 1972). If the bout is of a short duration, the total amount of work performed or the rate of work can be increased by breathing oxygen, and submaximal work can be performed at a lower pulse rate. For exercise bouts in excess of two minutes, or when the interval between the oxygen breathing and actual performance exceeds two minutes, the influence of breathing oxygen is greatly diminished. This simply reflects the limits of the oxygen storage potential of the body.

When oxygen is administered during the exercise, definite improvements in performance are noted (Wilmore, 1972). The amount of work performed and the rate of work are substantially increased. Likewise, submaximal work is performed more economically, at a lower physiological cost to the individual. The ergogenic properties of oxygen are not as clearly defined during the recovery period (Wilmore, 1972). The few studies that have been conducted have shown little, if any, effect. However, the studies that have been conducted have not used maximal, exhaustive exercise, which may account for their inability to demonstrate a substantial effect.

From a practical standpoint, oxygen administration prior to exercise would have little value because of the time limitations in athletics previously mentioned. Likewise, administration during exercise would have limited value, for obvious reasons. Oxygen breathing during the recovery period could have some limited value, although this needs to be confirmed by a well-controlled research study. The recovery period would appear to be the only practical time to administer oxygen, but only if it speeded up the recovery process, allowing the athlete to re-enter the contest or game in a more fully recovered state. Wilmore (1972) provides an extensive review of this entire area.

BLOOD DOPING

Ekblom, Goldbarg, and Gullbring (1972) created quite a stir in the sports world in the early 1970s. Their research indicated that by withdrawing between 800 and 1,200 ml of blood from a subject and then reinfusing the red cells back into that subject some four weeks later, a considerable improvement in $\dot{V}O_2$ max and treadmill performance time could be demonstrated. The subjects in this study were divided into two groups: Group I had 800 ml of blood withdrawn in a single day, and Group II had 1,200 ml of blood withdrawn over an eight-day period. Immediately following the blood withdrawal, hemoglobin concentration dropped 13 and 18 percent and $\dot{V}O_2$ max decreased by 13 and 18 percent in groups I and II respectively, while both groups decreased 30 percent in treadmill performance. At the end of four weeks, the red cells were reinfused. Treadmill performance time increased 23 percent and $\dot{V}O_2$ max increased 9 percent over those values prior to the initial blood withdrawal.

Williams (1975), in a review of all research on blood doping through 1975, concluded that while there were several studies that supported the enhancement of athletic performance with blood doping, the bulk of evidence does not substantiate that contention. Shortly after Williams's review article, Ekblom, Wilson, and Åstrand (1976), in a second study of blood doping, reported results that were in agreement with their initial study in 1972, i.e., an increase of 8.0 percent in $\dot{V}O_2$ max following reinfusion of the red blood cells. In 1978, Williams, Lindhjem, and Schuster found no significant differences in ratings of perceived exertion or in treadmill time to exhaustion following reinfusion of red blood cells. In this study, two groups of subjects were used, both having 460 ml of blood withdrawn following the initial testing sessions. However, only one of the two groups had their red blood cells reinfused. The other group received 460 ml of normal saline (placebo).

The most recent study by Buick, et al. (1980) used a well-conceived, double-blind design, in which eleven highly trained distance runners were studied before the blood withdrawal, following the normal restoration of the red blood cells, following a sham reinfusion of 50 ml of saline, and following the actual reinfusion of 900 ml of blood which had been originally withdrawn and freeze-preserved. They also conducted one more observation on these subjects, once their elevated red blood cell levels had returned to normal. They found a substantial increase in VO_2 max following the reinfusion of the red blood cells, and no change following the sham reinfusion.

While the results of these studies are in conflict, the balance of the evidence appears to point to a substantial ergogenic effect from infusing or reinfusing red blood cells. However, it must be pointed out that all testing has been of a laboratory nature, and there is absolutely no evidence that athletic performance is improved by this procedure. While this procedure is relatively safe in the hands of competent physicians, it nevertheless has inherent dangers associated with it. The potential risks of such a procedure seem to outweigh any potential benefits, above and beyond the ethical issue involved.

WARM-UP AND TEMPERATURE VARIATIONS

Most athletes warm-up prior to competition. For some this may consist of simple stretching, while for others it may be a time for an intensive bout of work. Does this precompetition activity facilitate the athlete's performance during the competition, or is this merely a traditional formality that has been carried down through the years? Before this question can be answered, it is important to recognize the different forms of warm-up. Warm-up activities can be identical to those used in competition, or they can be directly related (free-throw shooting drill without the stress of actual competition) or indirectly related (calisthenics for some muscle groups) activities. Lastly, warm-up can be passive, e.g., hot showers or a massage.

Attempting to determine the specific effects of warm-up is extremely difficult, since the effect appears to differ with the activity, as well as with the form of the warm-up. Franks (1972) has provided an outstanding summary of the research through the early 1970s. There is evidence to support both the beneficial and detrimental effects of the warm-up. Warm-up facilitates accuracy, movement time, range of motion, and strength in movements of selected parts of the body, but it does not appear to affect reaction time. Sprints and distance runs are improved with warm-up, but agility runs are not. Baseball throwing speed and softball distance throw are improved with warm-up, but not the accuracy of the throw. Franks (1972) concludes that some forms of warm-up can be detrimental to jumping, agility, running, sprinting, baseball throw for accuracy, and cycle endurance and speed tasks.

While many coaches and athletes feel that the warm-up is essential to prevent injuries, there is little direct research evidence to support this contention. This lack of supporting evidence is true for burst-type activities, as well. However, until this critical aspect of warm-up can be explored more fully, it would seem wise to continue using the warm-up as a precautionary, preventive procedure.

It appears that the efficacy of the warm-up depends on the type of warm-up as well as on the sport. The coach or athlete who has questions about a particular sport should refer directly to the specific research studies dealing with that sport. Unfortunately, no general conclusions can be drawn at this time.

Passive hot and cold applications have also been proposed as potential ergogenic aids. Falls (1972) concludes that cold applications are more likely to provide an ergogenic effect than hot applications. The benefit of a cold application, e.g., a shower, lies in its effect on circulatory function. Cold causes a peripheral vasoconstriction and possibly a reflex vasodilation within the muscle, which makes more blood available for the active tissues. In addition, the cold application cools the body surface which enhances its ability to dissipate body heat. Heat applications have the opposite effect and tend to reduce efficiency in performances of an endurance nature. Heat applications that are used for warming and loosening a joint, e.g., shoulder of the pitcher in baseball, may have a substantial effect, but this depends largely on the individual.

SOCIAL AND PSYCHOLOGICAL FACTORS

What advantage does the home team have when two teams, which are evenly matched, struggle to the last second to determine who wins? Does the cheering crowd give the home team a distinct advantage in this situation and put the visiting team at a disadvantage? Does hypnosis and post-hypnotic suggestion influence the athlete's performance? These and other related questions will be discussed in this section. The social and psychological factors associated with athletic performance are difficult to assess with any degree of validity and reproducibility. This is unfortunate, since these factors may be much more significant in determining the final outcome of competition than the physiological factors discussed previously.

Social Facilitation

While the field of social facilitation encompasses a broad range of specific areas, this section will focus on the area of audience effect, i.e., how performance is influenced by the presence of others. Singer (1972) presents an extensive review of the entire field of social facilitation as an ergogenic aid for those who desire additional information.

When observing the effect of an audience on performance, the nature of the audience must be defined. How large is the audience? Are they hostile (visiting team) or supportive? Are they of the opposite sex compared to the performers? Is the audience active or passive? Singer (1972) noted the problems of conducting a controlled research study with an active audience. The principal problem in a controlled research setting is motivating the audience to be consistent in their active encouragement of the athlete or team. Thus, most studies have involved a passive audience that simply observes and gives no verbal encouragement.

Most of the available research supports the theory that a passive audience facilitates physical performance, although some experiments show the audience to have an inhibiting and disturbing effect on the individual. Where the audience has been shown to have a disturbing effect, it is not clear whether this is a function of the situation or the subject. Competition in front of a passive audience might be a stimulus to the skilled athlete but may threaten the unskilled, nonathlete. Some evidence

exists that suggests that the more highly skilled the performer, the more positive the influence exerted by the audience.

Singer (1972) points out that task difficulty and anxiety level, as well as skill level, influence the effect of the audience on the subsequent performance. In an attempt to integrate these factors, he concludes that simple tasks demanding physical energy, repetition, power, strength, or endurance are probably enhanced by an audience. Motor skills requiring complex coordination, finely executed movements, and intense concentration may be impaired by the presence of observers until the skills are well learned. The more highly skilled athlete in any activity should be favorably influenced by an audience. Singer feels that the most highly skilled athletes are, in most instances, unaffected by the crowd's behavior, whether they are encouraged or "booed." Some athletes become too "psyched" playing in front of an audience and never attain the potential they exhibit in practice. Also, there is some evidence suggesting that performance can be impaired by a hostile audience.

Hypnosis

Morgan (1972b) conducted an extensive review of the existing research literature relative to hypnosis as an aid to athletic performance. Unfortunately, as mentioned in previous sections of this chapter, the literature is in conflict. While some investigators have reported absolutely no improvement in muscular strength and endurance with hypnosis, others have reported that simply being in a trance can either decrease or increase performance. Most people assume that superhuman feats of strength can be performed under the influence of hypnosis on the basis of the many popular accounts in the media. A critical look at the existing literature, however, does not totally support this assumption. In fact, the research studies are nearly evenly balanced between those that show improvement and those that show no difference between the hypnotic and the waking state. Controlled research in this particular area is extremely difficult to design and execute, due to various methodological problems and the variability of the subjects' response to hypnosis. Morgan (1972b) concludes by stating that while hypnotic suggestions of enhanced muscular strength and endurance are sometimes effective, they cannot be counted upon to consistently facilitate performance.

It appears that hypnosis is most effective when used to correct psychomotor problems, reduce pain, resolve aggression conflicts, and control anxiety states in the competitive athlete (Morgan, 1972b). Certainly, considerable additional research will be necessary before the coach and athlete, as well as the scientist, understand fully the potential of hypnosis in sport.

Mental Practice

When the athlete mentally rehearses an event or sport using the image of a perfectly executed, skilled performance, this is referred to as *mental practice*. How effective is this imaginary practice? Will it facilitate the performance of the skilled athlete?

It appears from a recent review by Corbin (1972) that mental practice does facilitate the performance of a skilled performer. While some studies showed little or no improvement with mental practice, most of the studies reviewed showed a substantial influence. The degree of improvement, however, depends on several factors. The individual must have had some previous experience with the task, although it is not fully understood whether the skill level of the performer is a factor or not. The ability to conceptualize also appears to influence the athlete's success. Possibly one of the most important results of the athlete's use of mental practice is the improvement in the ability to concentrate on that specific task. Constant mental rehearsals in practice may allow the athlete to focus more fully on the task during the actual competition.

GENERAL SUMMARY

In his or her never-ending search for excellence and improved performance, the athlete has tried numerous drugs, hormones, and diets, as well as many other physical substances and phenomena such as hypnosis and mental practice. Often, the athlete has used these aids indiscriminately with complete disregard for health and safety. Furthermore, if an athlete becomes successful after using one of these substances or phenomena, the word spreads quickly, and, soon, athletes in all parts of the world are using the substance or phenomena without waiting for evidence of its effectiveness or information about its side effects. Just as important are the moral and ethical considerations.

This chapter has reviewed the more widely used substances and phenomena thought to have ergogenic properties, and has raised more questions than it has answered. With regard to drugs and hormones, it was concluded that alcohol had no apparent effect on athletic performance when consumed in small doses, but that it can have a substantial detrimental effect when given in large doses. Amphetamines have been shown to improve, as well as have no influence on, athletic performance, which suggests a need for further study of a more highly controlled nature. Anabolic steroids have been shown to cause great increases in weight and strength in individual athletes who have taken extremely high doses. However, controlled research studies using only the recommended daily dosage have shown both increases, as well as no change, in weight and strength. With both amphetamines and steroids, the potential medical risks must be given serious consideration.

One of the areas that receives great attention and interest from athletes who are concerned with improved performance is nutrition. This was discussed in detail in Chapter 10, Nutrition and Athletic Performance.

Oxygen is an ergogenic aid when given immediately before a short duration contest, i.e., less than two minutes in length, or when given during the contest or work bout. These ergogenic properties are not as certain when oxygen is administered during the period of recovery. The issue of blood doping has yet to be resolved, although the evidence would suggest that it is an ergogenic aid.

Warm-up and hot and cold applications were also discussed as potential ergogenic aids. While warm-up appears to be beneficial for certain activities or contests, for others, it either has no effect or it can actually be detrimental. Cold applications, such as cold showers, do appear to improve the cardiovascular function of the individual during controlled bouts of exercise.

Lastly, the area of social and psychological factors was investigated. It appears that the influence of social facilitation and hypnosis are unpredictable and may depend entirely on the subject, the task, and the surrounding environment. Mental practice, however, does appear to facilitate the performance of even highly skilled athletes, possibly through improving their ability to concentrate.

STUDY QUESTIONS

1. What is the meaning of the term *ergogenic aid*?
2. What is presently known about the use of amphetamines in athletic competition? Is there an enhancement of performance? What are the potential risks of using amphetamines?
3. Does the use of alcohol in moderate or large doses improve athletic performance?
4. What are anabolic steroids? What are the differences between the androgenic and anabolic characteristics of steroids?
5. Does the use of anabolic steroids result in improved athletic performance?
6. What are some of the medical risks of steroid use?
7. How beneficial is the breathing of oxygen prior to the start of competition, during competition, and during the recovery from competition?
8. What is blood doping? Does blood doping improve athletic performance?
9. How important is warm-up in improving athletic performance? Is it essential for injury prevention?
10. How is social facilitation likely to influence athletic performance? Is there a differential response depending on the skill level of the athlete?
11. Does hypnosis improve athletic performance? Mental practice?

REFERENCES

American College of Sports Medicine Position Statement. "The Use and Abuse of Anabolic-Androgenic Steroids in Sports." *Med. Sci. Sports* 9 (1977): xi–xiii.

Bergström, J.; Hermansen, L.; Hultman, E.; and Saltin, B. "Diet, Muscle Glycogen, and Physical Performance." *Acta Physiol. Scand.* 71 (1967): 140–150.

Buick, F. J.; Gledhill, N.; Froese, A. B.; Spriet, L.; and Meyers, E. C. "Effect of Induced Erythrocythemia on Aerobic Work Capacity." *J. Appl. Physiol.* 48 (1980): 636–642.

Chandler, J. V. and Blair, S. N. "The Effect of Amphetamines on Selected Physiological Components Related to Athletic Success." *Med. Sci. Sports Exercise* 12 (1980): 65–69.

Cooper, D. L. "Understanding the Drug Menace." *Bulletin Nat. Assoc. Secondary School Principles.* 56 (1972a): 53–60.

Cooper, D. L. "Drugs and the Athlete." *J. Amer. Med. Assoc.* 221 (1972b): 1007–1011.

Corbin, C. B. "Mental Practice." In *Ergogenic Aids and Muscular Performance*, edited by W. P. Morgan. New York: Academic Press, 1972.

Costill, D. L. "Water and Electrolytes." In *Ergogenic Aids and Muscular Performance*, edited by W. P. Morgan. New York: Academic Press, 1972.

Ekblom, B.; Goldbarg, A. N.; and Gullbring, B. "Response to Exercise after Blood Loss and Reinfusion." *J. Appl. Physiol.* 33 (1972): 175–180.

Ekblom, B.; Wilson, G.; and Åstrand, P.-O. "Central Circulation during Exercise after Venesection and Reinfusion of Red Blood Cells." *J. Appl. Physiol.* 40 (1976): 379–383.

Falls, H. B. "Heat and Cold Applications." In *Ergogenic Aids and Muscular Performance*, edited by W. P. Morgan. New York: Academic Press, 1972.

Fowler, W. H.; Gardner, G. W.; and Egstrom, G. H. "Effect of Anabolic Steroid on Physical Performance in Young Men." *J. Appl. Physiol.* 20 (1965): 1038–1040.

Franks, B. D. "Physical Warm-up." In *Ergogenic Aids and Muscular Performance*, edited by W. P. Morgan. New York: Academic Press, 1972.

Golding, L. A. "Drugs and Hormones." In *Ergogenic Aids and Muscular Performance*, edited by W. P. Morgan. New York: Academic Press, 1972.

Golding, L. A., and Barnard, R. J. "The Effect of d-amphetamine Sulfate on Physical Performance." *J. Sports Med. Phys. Fit.* 3 (1963): 221–224.

Horstman, D. H. "Nutrition." In *Ergogenic Aids and Muscular Performance*, edited by W. P. Morgan. New York: Academic Press, 1972.

Johnson, L. C., and O'Shea, J. P. "Anabolic Steroid: Effects on Strength Development." *Science* 164 (1969): 957–959.

Karlsson, J., and Saltin, B. "Diet, Muscle Glycogen, and Endurance Performance." *J. Appl. Physiol.* 31 (1971): 203–206

Karpovich, P. V. "Effect of Amphetamine Sulfate on Athletic Performance." *J. Amer. Med. Assoc.* 170 (1959): 558–561.

Londeree, B. "Pre-event Diet Routine." *Runner's World.* 9 (1974): 26–29.

Morgan, W. P. (ed.) *Ergogenic Aids and Muscular Performance.* New York: Academic Press, 1972a.

Morgan, W. P. "Hypnosis and Muscular Performance." In *Ergogenic Aids and Muscular Performance*, edited by W. P. Morgan. New York: Academic Press, 1972b.

Singer, R. N. "Social Facilitation." In *Ergogenic Aids and Muscular Performance*, edited by W. P. Morgan. New York: Academic Press, 1972.

Smith, G. M. and Beecher, H. K. "Amphetamine Sulfate and Athletic Performance." *J. Amer. Med. Assoc.* 170 (1959): 542–557.

Williams, M. H. "Blood Doping—Does it Really Help Athletes?" *Physician Sportsmed.* 3 (1975): 52–56.

Williams, M. H.; Lindhjem, M.; and Schuster, R. "The Effect of Blood Infusion upon Endurance Capacity and Ratings of Perceived Exertion." *Med. Sci. Sports* 10 (1978): 113–118.

Wilmore, J. H. "Oxygen." In *Ergogenic Aids and Muscular Performance*, edited by W. P. Morgan. New York: Academic Press, 1972.

13

The Female Athlete

INTRODUCTION

While females have competed successfully in athletics for many years, the athletic arena has traditionally been the domain of the male. During the early 1970s, female athletics underwent a dramatic revolution. Demands were made for equality in budget, facilities, equipment, coaching, and competitive opportunities for a position in the world of athletics comparable to that enjoyed by the male. While the demand for equality of opportunity was generally met, with moderate to major reluctance, the demand by some females that traditionally all male sports be sexually integrated was met with heated discussion and debate. In this controversy the question arose, repeatedly, whether female athletes were genetically inferior to male athletes in physical and physiological characteristics. Were the sexes created equal in their potential athletic ability? These questions and their answers have important implications, not only for the athletic world, but also for many areas of employment in which physical performance characteristics are critical. Can females perform the duties of firefighting, police work, flying commercial airplanes, working on telephone lines, or similar positions that require unusual physical demands?

This chapter will focus on similarities and differences between males and females in those areas that directly influence athletic performance. Of primary concern will be the areas of body build and composition, strength, cardiovascular endurance capacity, and motor skill development and athletic ability. By looking at the record books, it is apparent that the female athlete performs at a substantially lower level than her male counterpart in almost all athletic events or contests. On the basis of world records in the year 1978, the male was 9.3 percent faster in the 100-meter dash, jumped 16.9 percent higher in the high jump, ran 11.2 percent faster in the 1,500-meter run, and swam 7.3 percent faster in the 400-meter freestyle swim. Do these differences result from biological differences between the sexes, or do they reflect the social and cultural restrictions that have been placed on the female during her preadolescent and adolescent development?

BODY BUILD AND COMPOSITION

The statement that the mature male and female differ in body build and composition does not require scientific validation. However, even in the mature adult, the differences that presently exist between the male and female are considerably greater than they need to be. At the time when full maturity is reached, the average female is five inches shorter than the average male, thirty to forty pounds lighter in total weight, forty to fifty pounds lighter in lean body weight, and considerably fatter, i.e., 25 versus 15 percent relative body fat (Behnke and Wilmore, 1974). Up to the age of thirteen to fourteen years, however, the average female is either equal to, or greater than, the average male in both height and weight. This is undoubtedly due to the earlier maturation of the female. Once full maturity is reached, the male will have broader shoulders, narrower hips, and a greater chest girth relative to his total body size. In terms of absolute values, the male has a greater amount of subcutaneous fat in the abdominal and upper regions of the body, while the female carries substantially more fat in the hip and lower regions of the body. The female's hips are equal in width to the males even though the width of the other bones and areas are, on the average, 10 percent, or more, greater in the male. The two sexes are equal in girth measurements at the abdomen, hips, and thigh. Additionally, the average female, on the basis of somatotype, tends more toward endomorphy, or fatness, while the average male tends to be more linear (ectomorphy) and muscular (mesomorphy).

In terms of body composition, the eighteen- to twenty-two-year-old female will average between 22 and 26 percent relative body fat, while the male of similar age will average between 12 and 16 percent. These differences are due to both a lower absolute lean weight and a higher absolute fat weight in the female. Whether these differences are primarily biological or genetic in nature, or whether environmental and cultural factors are of major importance is not clearly understood at the present time. However, evidence is now available that shows that each of these factors is important and that each of them makes a significant contribution to the total differences observed.

The higher levels of the androgen hormones in the male are undoubtedly responsible for his greater lean body weight. Similarly, the higher levels of the estrogen hormones in the female are at least partially responsible for her greater amount of fat weight. The mature female has higher amounts of essential fat due to the fat in breast and in other sex-specific tissues. The significant question that needs to be answered is how much additional fat the female should possess? At what point does this additional fat become nonessential and limit athletic performance?

It is difficult to design a research experiment to answer these questions. However, insight into the problem is gained by observing the relative body fats of national and world-class athletes whose sport, event, or activity require speed, endurance, and mobility. Figure 9–1 illustrates the relative body fat values for a large number of track and field athletes. While the values are highly variable for the group as a whole, close inspection of the data reveals that the runners are considerably leaner than those competing in the field events. Of the seventy-eight runners evaluated, twelve had relative fat values under 10 percent and many had values under those of the college-age male (approximately 15 percent). Costill, Bowers, and Kammer (1970) reported an average value of 7.5 percent fat for 114 male competitors at the 1968 United States Olympic marathon trial. Two of the women in Figure 9–1 had values of approximately 6 percent fat (determined by underwater weighing). One of these women had started running because she was considered obese and wanted to use exercise in addition to diet to reduce her weight to a more normal level. She became enthusiastic with her running program, expanded it, and became a world-record-holding, long-distance runner. While the low relative body fats for these runners may be largely the result of their inherited constitutions, this illustration suggests that the high intensity, endurance type of exercise engaged in by these female athletes is also a most significant factor. Training at distances of up to one hundred miles, or more, per week requires extraordinarily high levels of caloric expenditure. Thus, it appears that the female athlete can approach the relative fat values observed in male athletes, although considerably more research will be necessary to confirm this conclusion. In addition, it would seem that the average values of relative fat for the fully mature female are considerably above the level that might be considered ideal. The sedentary life style acquired by the average female once she reaches puberty undoubtedly accounts for these comparatively high values. Likewise, it is difficult to justify the extraordinarily high values of the few female shot-putters illustrated in Figure 9–1. These values should not be interpreted as essential for success in this event. Refer to Chapter 7, Body Build and Composition, and to Chapter 9, Profiles of Elite Athletes, for further discussion of this topic.

STRENGTH

It is well recognized that the average male is considerably stronger than the average female. Composite strength scores from several different studies suggest that men are approximately 30 to 40 percent stronger than women. Even at ages of seven through seventeen years, while the values are relatively close, the female is not able to exhibit the same level of strength. These results are somewhat misleading, however, for when individual values are considered for specific areas of the body, it is found that leg strength is nearly identical in the two sexes. When expressed relative to body size, leg strength is identical, and when leg strength is expressed relative to lean body weight, to more accurately reflect muscle mass, the females are slightly stronger! With reference to upper-body strength, however, females are only 30 to 50 percent as strong as males.

Can females benefit from strength-training exercises? Several studies have confirmed that weight training in adolescent girls and college-age women can produce significant gains in strength in each of the areas trained. Brown and Wilmore (1974) reported bench-press strengths of 115 to 187 pounds and leg-press strengths of 125 to 175 pounds in seven, nationally ranked, female, track-and-field throwing-event athletes, five of whom had just completed a six-month, intensive weight-training program. These values are considerably greater than those reported for normal, untrained males of similar ages, but well below values reported for male weight lifters. Another study (Wilmore, 1974) has demonstrated that the mean strength of young, nonathletic women can be improved by as much as 30 percent consequent to a ten-week weight-training program. Some of the women in this study doubled their strength in selected areas during this relatively short training period. In comparison with a group of nonathletic young men on an identical program, these women exhibited greater gains in strength, although their initial values were lower.

From these studies, it appears that the female has the potential to develop substantial levels of strength that are considerably higher than those normally identified in the average, typically sedentary, female. Yet, while strength training does produce large increases in the female's total body strength, it does not appear to result in concomitant gains in muscle bulk. This is an important point, since most female athletes would like to increase their basic levels of strength, but many would be quite unwilling to strength train if they suspected that they would develop excessively large, bulky muscles. The inability of the average female to gain substantial amounts of muscle with strength training is undoubtedly due to her relatively low ratio of testosterone to estrogen compared to the average male. Some females will notice an increased bulkiness accompanying their strength training, but it is felt that they probably have naturally high testosterone to estrogen ratios.

Will the female ever be able to attain the same levels of strength as the male for all major regions of the body? From the similarity of the strength of the legs between the two sexes, it appears that the quality of muscle is the same, irrespective of sex. However, because of the higher levels of testosterone in the male, the male will continue to have a larger total muscle mass. If muscle mass is the major determinant of strength, then the male will always have a distinct advantage. If the levels of strength are independent of muscle mass, then the potential for absolute strength may be similar in both the sexes. Since the basic mechanisms allowing the expression of greater levels of strength have yet to be defined, it is impossible to draw any conclusions at the present time.

CARDIOVASCULAR ENDURANCE

In general, the female has a smaller stroke volume than the male for an equivalent, submaximal level of work. She is able to partially compensate for this by increasing her heart rate response to that level of work. This lower stroke volume is at least partially related to her smaller body size. Another factor of importance to the female, when compared to the male, is her lower hemoglobin concentration. Several studies have suggested that females may have values as much as 10 percent lower than males of the same age. Because of a lower maximal stroke volume and a similar maximal heart rate which reduce the maximal cardiac output, in addition to lower hemoglobin levels, the female's oxygen-carrying and oxygen-delivery capacity is apparently considerably less than the male's. This should result in a substantial difference in endurance capacity between the sexes, since the relationship between endurance capacity and $\dot{V}O_2$ max is very high. The values for males and females are quite similar up to ten to fifteen years of age. Beyond this age, however, the female's capacity decreases rather markedly, while the male's continues to improve. For the college-age male and female, this difference is quite large with the female exhibiting a mean $\dot{V}O_2$ max between 30 and 44 ml/kg × min, while the mean value for males ranges between 45 and 53 ml/kg × min (Drinkwater, 1973). These differences would tend to agree with and be partially explained by the physiological observations noted above relative to the female's reduced maximal cardiac output and reduced hemoglobin levels. The lack of an observed difference in $\dot{V}O_2$ max at the younger ages is probably due to similarities in maximal cardiac output and hemoglobin levels up to the age of puberty, at which point the differences start to appear.

While the preceding discussion appears to have resolved this entire area of cardiovascular endurance capacity, recent research indicates that the female's endurance capacity at ages beyond ten years does not necessarily have to be reduced or even substantially below that of the male of similar age. Hermanson and Andersen (1965) investigated the endurance capacity of both sedentary and athletic college-age populations and found the athletic men and women to have $\dot{V}O_2$ max values of 71 and 55 ml/kg × min, respectively, compared with values of 44 and 38 ml/kg × min, respectively, in the sedentary men and women. While the athletic men were noticeably superior, the athletic women had values 25 percent greater than the sedentary men.

Wilmore and Brown (1974) investigated cardiovascular endurance capacity in highly trained, female endurance athletes at various ages up to and including the fourth decade of life. Eleven subjects of national and international caliber were selected from a population of female distance runners. One of these women had won five consecutive United States and International Cross-Country championships. Another held the best time in the world for females in the marathon, and a third held the best time in the world for females in the fifty-mile run. The average $\dot{V}O_2$ max value for this group of women was 59.1 ml/kg × min, which is considerably higher than that for average women and men of similar age. National-caliber, long-distance, men

runners studied by Costill and Winrow (1970) averaged 70.3 ml/kg × min, 15.9 percent higher than these women. However, the three best runners among the eleven women averaged 67.4 ml/kg × min, or only 4.1 percent lower than the average value for the ten, nationally ranked, men marathon runners of almost exactly the same age.

Figure 13–1 demonstrates the range of values for both young and older female distance runners compared to average values for the untrained male and female. It is obvious that females have the potential for levels of endurance that are far greater than they normally possess. When $\dot{V}O_2$ max is expressed relative to the athlete's lean body weight, rather than to total body weight, the female athlete is nearly identical to the male athlete in $\dot{V}O_2$ max. Davies (1971) found that when the $\dot{V}O_2$ max was expressed relative to the actual active muscle mass, the differences between the sexes disappeared entirely. While this may imply that men and women have the same endurance potential, Drinkwater (1973) makes the important observation that women must still carry their entire body weight as part of their total workload, which would undoubtedly hinder their actual performance. However, this would not be a factor in an activity such as bicycling, which provides a more equal opportunity for females to compete against males.

MOTOR SKILLS AND ATHLETIC ABILITY

With the exception of one activity, the softball throw for distance, boys and girls are quite similar in their performance of physical activities up to the age of ten to twelve years. Tests of specific motor skills or general athletic ability show few differences between the sexes during this period of development. Past the age of twelve, however, the male becomes considerably stronger, possesses greater muscular and cardiovascular endurance, and becomes more proficient in almost all motor skills. This phenomenon is illustrated in Figure 13–2 for selected motor skills.

From Figure 13–2 it is obvious that the female lags far behind the male at all ages in the softball throw, the female throwing only half of the distance of the male at any particular age. In an unpublished study, Grimditch and Sockolov investigated why females perform so poorly in the softball throw.

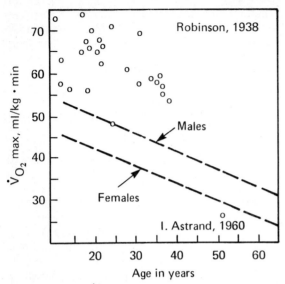

Figure 13–1 $\dot{V}O_2$ max values for female distance runners compared to normal untrained males and females. (Normal male values obtained from S. Robinson, "Experimental Studies of Physical Fitness in Relation to Age," *Arbeitsphysiol.* 10 (1938): 251–323. Normal female values obtained from I. Åstrand, "Aerobic Work Capacity in Men and Women with Special Reference to Age," *Acta Physiol. Scand.* 49, Suppl. 169 (1960).)

Postulating this difference to be the result of insufficient practice and experience, they recruited over 200 males and females from three to twenty years of age to throw the softball for distance with both the dominant and nondominant arms. The results are illustrated in Figure 13–3. As they had theorized, there was absolutely no difference between the males and females for the nondominant arm, up to the age of ten to twelve years, just as with each of the other motor skill tasks shown in Figure 13–2. The results for the dominant arm were in agreement with what had been reported previously (Figure 13–2). Thus the softball throw for distance using the dominant arm appears to be biased by the previous experience and practice of the males. When the influence of experience and practice was removed by using the nondominant arm, this motor skill task was identical to each of the others.

Athletic performance differences were briefly

discussed in the introduction to this chapter. The female is outperformed by the male in almost all sports, events, or activities. This is quite obvious in such activities as the shotput in track and field, where high levels of upper body strength are critical to successful performance. In the 400-meter free style, however, the winning time for the men in the 1924 Olympic games was 16 percent faster than for the women, but this difference decreased to 11.6 percent in the 1948 Olympics and to only 7.5 percent in the 1980 Olympics. The fastest female, 800-meter free style swimmer in 1979 swam faster than the world-record-holding male for the same distance in 1972! Therefore, in this particular event the gap between the sexes is narrowing, and there are indications that this is also true for other events and for other sports. Unfortunately, it is difficult to make valid comparisons, since the degree to which the sport, activity, or event has been emphasized is not constant, and factors such as coaching, facilities, and training techniques have differed considerably between the sexes over the years. While the performance gap appears to be closing, it is far too early to predict whether it will ever close completely for any or all sports.

MENSTRUAL AND GYNECOLOGICAL CONSIDERATIONS

One of the great concerns about female participation in athletics is in the area of gynecological considerations and menstruation. Do females run a high risk of damaging their reproductive organs as a result of vigorous running, jumping, or contact sports? Should females avoid exercise and competition during the flow phase of their menstrual cycle? These and many other questions were the subject of an extensive review article by Ryan in 1975.

First, there appears to be a high degree of variability among females with regard to exercise and competition during the various phases of the menstrual cycle. Many females have few or no menstrual difficulties under any conditions, whether they are active or sedentary. On the other hand, a significant number of females have dysmenorrhea, or other menstrual difficulties, which apparently are neither helped nor aggravated by vigorous

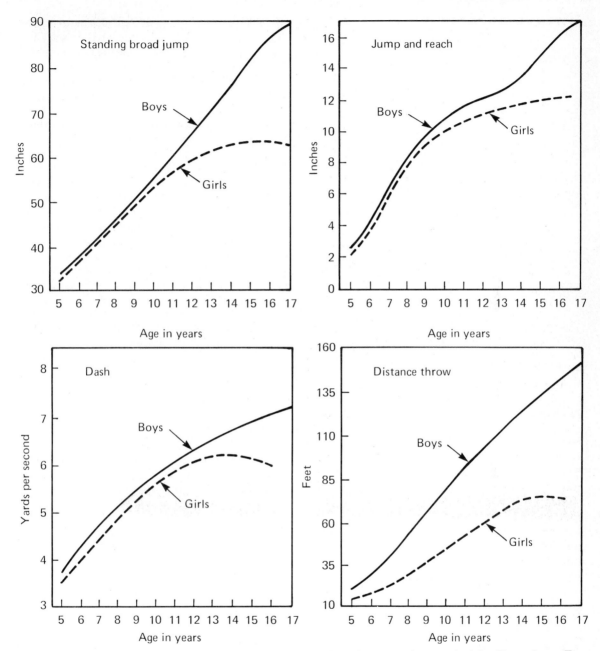

Figure 13–2 Performance of selected motor-skill test items for young boys and girls. (From Anna Espenschade and Helen Eckert, "Motor Development," *Science and Medicine of Exercise and Sport, 2nd ed.,* pp. 326–30. Edited by Warren R. Johnson and E. R. Buskirk. Copyright © 1974 by Warren R. Johnson and Elsworth R. Buskirk. Copyright © 1960 by Warren R. Johnson. Reprinted by permission of Harper and Row, Publishers, Inc.)

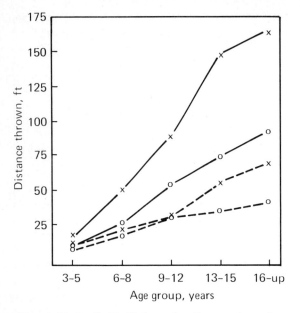

Figure 13–3   Softball throw for distance in males (×) and females (○) using the dominant (———) and nondominant (– – – –) arms. (From G. Grimditch and R. Sockolov, unpublished observations. University of California, Davis, 1974.)

physical activity. Recently, there have been reports of a total absence of menstruation in females who train for long-distance running, gymnastics, ballet, figure skating, and competitive cycling. This may be related to their exceptionally low, total body weight and reduced levels of body fat, since several studies have reported an absence of menstruation in chronically underweight females. Female distance runners frequently train seventy to one hundred miles or more per week, and their relative body fat typically decreases to 10 percent or less. Return of menstruation usually follows a reduction in training intensity. There is considerable interest in this area, and a number of research studies are presently in progress.

Physical performance seems to be best in the immediate post-menstrual period, up to the fifteenth day of the cycle. The number of females who perform poorly during the flow phase of the cycle is about the same as the number who experience no difference. Some have even noted an improved performance during flow, establishing records and winning world class competitions. Again, the individual variability is so great that no general rules of thumb can be given. Full participation in activities of all types should be allowed during the flow phase for those who experience no difficulties, and provisions should be made for those who do experience difficulties, so they are not forced into undesirable activities.

The potential for gynecological injuries has been a major concern in athletics for centuries. Females at one time were discouraged from participating in any activity where there was considerable running, jumping, or bodily contact. The uterus was considered to be highly vulnerable to major injuries, which could have serious consequences later in life. It is now recognized that injuries to the female reproductive organs are rare. Unlike the male, the female's organs are internal and in an extremely well-protected position. The breasts are in a more vulnerable position, but even here, serious injury is extremely rare, even in contact sports. Follow-up studies on former female athletes indicate that they have normal pregnancy and child birth, and, in fact, may have shorter delivery times and a faster return to normal activities.

GENERAL SUMMARY

From the preceding discussion, there appear to be substantial differences between the average female and the average male in almost all aspects of physical performance beyond the age of ten to twelve years. Prior to this time, there are few, if any, differences between the sexes. What happens to the female once she reaches puberty? Is she physically over the hill, reaching her peak at a relatively early age, or are there other factors or circumstances which might account for her reduced physical capabilities? Recent studies on highly trained, female athletes suggest that the female is not appreciably different from her highly trained, male counterpart, at ages beyond puberty. It appears that the average values used for comparative purposes beyond the age of puberty are for relatively active males and relatively sedentary females. Somewhere between the ages of ten to twelve years, the average female substitutes the piano for climbing trees, and sewing for chasing the boys down the street. In Chapter 8 it was pointed out that once one assumes a sedentary life style, the basic physiological components of general fitness deteriorate. Strength, muscular endurance, and cardiovascular endurance are lost, and body fat tends to accumulate. Similar trends can be noted for the male by the time he reaches thirty to thirty-five years of age, an age that corresponds to a reduction in his activity patterns. So, what appear to be dramatic biological differences between the sexes, in fact, may be more related to the cultural and social restrictions placed on the female after puberty. Further research into this intriguing area is certainly needed.

With regard to the female athlete, there appears to be little difference between her and her male counterpart in terms of strength, endurance, and body composition. Strength of the lower extremities, when related to body weight and lean body weight, is similar between the sexes, although the male maintains a distinct superiority in upper-body strength. Strength training, formerly condemned as a mode of training for women because of its supposed masculinizing effects, is now recognized as extremely valuable in developing the strength component, which is usually the weakest link in the physiological profile of the female athlete.

Endurance capacity in the highly trained, female distance runner is approximately equal to the capacity of the highly trained, male distance runner, when the values are expressed relative to lean body weight. For the better female runners, these values are relatively close when expressed relative to total body weight. Although the female is far below the male in lean body weight, the highly trained, female distance runner has a relative body fat similar to the male distance runner.

Because of these similarities, and because their needs are basically the same, there is little reason to advocate different training or conditioning programs on the basis of sex.

STUDY QUESTIONS

1. How do females compare with males relative to fat weight and lean weight?
2. To what levels can females reduce their body fat as a result of training?
3. How do men and women compare relative to upper-body strength? Lower-body strength? Why are there differences between upper- and lower-body strength in men and women?
4. What is the role of testosterone in the development of strength and lean body weight?
5. What differences in $\dot{V}O_2$ max exist between normal males and females? Between highly trained males and females?
6. Why are male and female performances in motor skills similar up to the age of puberty, and yet considerably different once puberty has been attained?
7. How does the menstrual cycle influence athletic performance?
8. What are some of the possible reasons that women athletes in intensive training will, in some cases, stop menstruating for intervals of several years or more?
9. What injuries might female athletes expect to their reproductive organs?

REFERENCES

Astrand, P.-O, and Rodahl, K. *Textbook of Work Physiology*, 2nd ed. New York: McGraw-Hill Book Co., 1977.

Behnke, A. R., and Wilmore, J. H. *Evaluation and Regulation of Body Build and Composition*. Englewood Cliffs, N.J.: Prentice-Hall, 1974.

Brown, C. H., and Wilmore, J. H. "The Effects of Maximal Resistance Training on the Strength and Body Composition of Women Athletes." *Med. Sci. Sport* 6 (1974): 174–177.

Costill, D. L.; Bowers, R.; and Kammer, W. F. "Skinfold Estimates of Body Fat Among Marathon Runners." *Med. Sci. Sports* 2 (1970): 93–95.

Costill, D. L., and Winrow, E. "Maximal Oxygen Intake Among Marathon Runners." *Arch. Phys. Med. Rehab.* 51 (1970): 317–320.

Davies, C. T. M. "Body Composition in Children: A Reference Standard for Maximum Aerobic Power Output on a Stationary Bicycle Ergometer." In *Proceedings of the III International Symposium on Pediatric Work Physiology. Acta Paediatr Scand.* Suppl. 217, 1971.

Drinkwater, B. L. "Physiological Responses of Women to Exercise." In *Exercise and Sport Sciences Reviews*, vol. 1, edited by J. H. Wilmore. New York: Academic Press, 1973.

Hermanson, L., and Andersen, K. L. "Aerobic Work Capacity in Young Norwegian Men and Women." *J. Appl. Physiol.* 20 (1965): 425–431.

Klafs, C. E., and Lyon, M. J. *The Female Athlete: Conditioning, Competition, and Culture*. St. Louis: C. V. Mosby Co., 1973.

Mayhew, J. L. and Gross, P. M. "Body Composition

Changes in Young Women with High Resistance Weight Training." *Res. Quart.* 45 (1974): 433–440.

Plowman, S. "Physiological Characteristics of Female Athletes." *Res. Quart.* 45 (1974): 349–362.

Ryan, A. J. "The Female Athlete: Gynecological Considerations." *J. Health, Phys. Educ. Rec.* 46 (1975): 40–44.

Wilmore, J. H. "Alterations in Strength, Body Composition and Anthropometric Measurements Consequent to a 10-week Weight Training Program." *Med. Sci. Sport* 6 (1974): 133–138.

Wilmore, J. H. "Exploding the Myth of Female Inferiority." *Physician and Sportsmed.* 2 (1974): 54–58.

Wilmore, J. H., and Brown, C. H. "Physiological Profiles of Women Distance Runners." *Med. Sci. Sport* 6 (1974): 178–181.

14

The Growth and Aging Process

INTRODUCTION

Age-group competition has grown considerably over the last decade and is now a major force in the world of sport. Little League baseball and Pop Warner football are examples of this type of sport or activity for boys, as is Bobby Sox softball for girls, and mini-bike racing, swimming, track and field, and long-distance running for many other youngsters of both sexes. Moreover, age-group competition no longer stops with youngsters in their early years but goes on into old age. The man or woman who turns forty can begin a new career in athletics if he or she has an interest and some talent in track and field events. Masters' or seniors' competition in track and field starts at age forty, and competition is broken into age groups by decades, e.g., forty to forty-nine years, fifty to fifty-nine years, sixty to sixty-nine years and above. Men in their eighties have been observed in formal competitions, and many men in their seventies have completed the official, 26-mile, 385-yard marathon! Similar age-group competitive experiences are available in swimming.

With this tremendous interest in age-group competition, many questions have been raised. Is competition physically or psychologically harmful for the preadolescent? Should eight-year-olds be competing in long-distance running? Does pitching a baseball place traumatic stress on the elbow of the youngster's pitching arm? How does a sedentary, forty-five-year-old male prepare himeslf for formal

competition, when, hearing about age-group competition, his urge to be an athlete is rekindled? These and many other questions of a similar nature will be addressed in the following pages as we focus attention on both the growth and aging process.

DEVELOPMENT AND AGING OF THE TISSUES

Bone

The development of bone was discussed in detail in Chapter 1. Briefly, bone is the principal calcified tissue of humans. The bone matrix is formed from collagen fibers in which small cells called osteocytes are embedded. The long bones of the body are preformed of cartilage. Even prior to birth, the cartilage is slowly converted to bone by the process of ossification, which involves the deposition of the bone minerals, calcium and phosphorus, into the bone matrix. Ossification occurs in an orderly process, allowing the bone to grow until ossification is completed. Figure 14–1 illustrates a typical long bone that has not yet reached full growth. The central portion of the bone, or the shaft, is referred to as the diaphysis. The ends of the bone are formed of cartilaginous epiphyseal centers. At birth, the entire shaft, or diaphysis, has been ossified and growth continues at both ends of the long bones. Between the diaphysis and the epiphyseal centers lies the growth plate, or the epiphyseal line. When

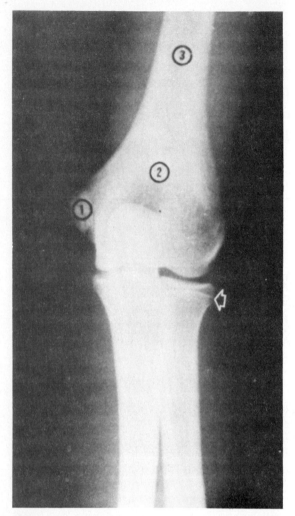

Figure 14–1   Growth of the long bones. (From R. L. Larson, "Physical Activity and the Growth and Development of Bone and Joint Structures." In *Physical Activity: Human Growth, and Development,* edited by G. L. Rarick. New York: Academic Press, 1974. Reproduced by permission of the publisher.) Note: (1) medial epicondylar epiphysis of the humerus, (2) metaphysis of the humerus, (3) diaphysis of the humerus. Arrow refers to the growth plate of the proximal radial epiphysis.

growth is completed, the diaphysis and epiphysis are fused, and the growth plate disappears.

There is a wide variation in the average age at which the different bones reach full growth or maturity, ranging from the preteens to the early twenties. On the average, girls achieve full maturity several years before boys. Exercise, generally, is regarded as being essential for proper bone growth. While exercise does not appear to influence the length of long bone growth, it does increase the width of the bone and gives the bone greater tensile strength.

In this chapter, we are interested in the process of bone growth, primarily, in order to understand the potential for injury. An injury to an immature bone could result in the premature cessation of growth. The greatest concern is with the potential injury of the epiphyses, since a fracture at the epiphyses and growth plate could disturb the blood supply and disrupt the growth process. Fortunately, such injuries are relatively few and seldom occur in sports. In one study of thirty-one epiphyseal injuries, only 23 percent were sports induced, the remainder resulting from falls and vehicular accidents (Larson, 1974).

One type of serious epiphyseal injury that occurs in athletics is called *traumatic epiphysitis.* One form is "Little Leaguer's elbow," a condition resulting from repetitive strains to the medial epicondylar epiphysis of the humerus. According to Larson, studies have shown that twelve-year-old boys can throw a baseball up to seventy miles per hour, causing a sudden pull on the epiphysis, which anchors the tendons of the involved muscles, that may result in its separation (Figure 14–2). The repetitive stress of throwing may produce an inflammatory response, i.e., traumatic epiphysitis. In a well-controlled study published in 1965, Adams found epiphysitis by X-ray examination in *all* 80 pitchers in a group of 162, young boys who were studied, while only a small percentage of the nonpitchers and the control group of nonplayers exhibited similar changes. Subsequent studies have shown a much lower percentage.

Larson and McMahan (1966) reviewed 1,338 consecutive athletic injuries seen by a group of four orthopedists in one practice. They reported that 20 percent of these injuries were in the age range of fourteen years of age and younger. Only 6 percent of all injuries in fifteen-year-olds and younger involved the epiphysis. They also stated that this type of injury does not always result in crippling, or permanent, trauma and that early recognition is important.

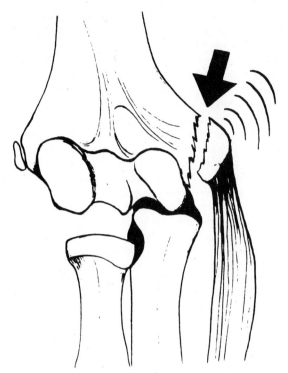

Figure 14–2 An example of a separation of the epiphysis. (From R. L. Larson, "Physical Activity and the Growth and Development of Bone and Joint Structures." In *Physical Activity: Human Growth, and Development,* edited by G. L. Rarick. New York: Academic Press, 1974. Reproduced by permission of the publisher.)

Of all the sports, competitive baseball appears to be the most dangerous on the basis of its potential for serious injuries, which largely result from the pitching motion. Some leagues have replaced the pitcher with a pitching machine. This would seem to be the only sensible approach until the youngster reaches an age at which pitching is not a major source of injuries. Pop Warner football and the other competitive sports and activities have a relatively good record with regard to bone injury. While the potential for injury in football is generally considered high, apparently the small size of the player, the matching of children by size, and good protective equipment provide a relatively safe environment for the young football player.

Older athletes, i.e., those over forty years, have a greater potential for bone injury than the younger athletes who have reached full maturity. While it varies considerably among individuals, the density of bone starts to decrease at about the age of forty. This is due to a decrease in the calcium and phosphorus content of the bone. The result is a more porous bone, which is more likely to break when placed under extreme stress. The more porous bone also takes longer to fully heal when it is broken. Recent evidence suggests that supplementation of calcium intake can reduce the extent of this bone mineral loss. Endurance activities also appear to limit mineral loss.

Muscle

The ultrastructure and growth characteristics of muscle tissue were discussed in detail in Chapter 1. From birth through adolescence there is a steady increase in the muscle mass of the body that parallels the youngster's gain in weight. With puberty, there is a peak acceleration in the development of muscle in boys, which corresponds to the sudden increase in testosterone production. Girls do not experience this period of rapid acceleration, but their muscle mass does continue to increase. Once a girl reaches puberty, her estrogen levels increase, which promotes the deposition of body fat. While muscle is still capable of developing as a girl passes puberty, its rate of development, relative to the increase in body weight, decreases.

When the female reaches sixteen to eighteen years and the male eighteen to twenty-two, the muscle mass is at its peak, unless it is increased further through either diet and exercise, or both. The muscle mass will remain relatively stable from this age through the ages of thirty to forty years, if physical activity levels remain constant and do not decrease. With older age, there is a decrease in the total muscle mass, which may result from both atrophy of selected muscle fibers and a decrease in the number of muscle fibers. The decrease in fibers may be the result of nerve fiber degeneration.

One area of major controversy with regard to muscle development in youngsters is the use of weight training to develop muscular strength and endurance. For many years, young boys and girls were discouraged from using weights for fear that they might injure themselves and prematurely stop their growth processes. Studies on animals suggest that heavy-resistance exercise would lead to a stronger, broader, and more compact bone. However, since it is nearly impossible to load these animals to the same extent as youngsters, it has not been practical to design an experiment that accurately defines the risks associated with heavy-resistance exercise in youngsters. It would appear that the potential for injury and structural damage from heavy-resistance exercise is extremely low, but since the future of the youngster is at stake, it is appropriate to take a conservative approach until additional studies can be conducted. Thus, a program using low weights and high repetitions would be preferred to one using high weights and low repetitions. One of the safest techniques for strength training in youngsters would be to use the isokinetic concept, in which resistance is matched to the force applied, so that the youngster does not have to contend with actual weights, i.e., barbells and dumbbells. Refer to Chapter 4, Strength, Power, and Muscular Endurance, for a more detailed description of this technique.

Changes in strength with age parallel the increases and decreases in muscle mass. Peak strength is usually attained by the age of twenty years in females and between twenty and thirty years in males. Strength remains relatively stable until ages of thirty-five to forty-five years and then decreases gradually with increasing age. deVries (1974) has stated that by sixty years of age, the male has lost not more than 10 to 20 percent of his maximum strength. The loss of strength with aging in the female appears to proceed at a slightly faster rate. This loss of strength with age consists of two components: a decrease in ability to maintain maximum static force, and a decrease in ability to accelerate mass (deVries, 1974).

Fat

Fat cells form and fat starts to deposit in these cells early in the development of the fetus and continues indefinitely. While evidence suggests that the actual number of fat cells becomes constant sometime during the teens, each fat cell has the ability to increase in size at any age. If the number of fat cells is actually fixed early in life, it is important to keep the total fat content of the body low during this period of time. In this way, the total number of fat cells will be minimized, and the chances of extreme obesity as an adult will be greatly reduced. More recent evidence, however, suggests that fat cells can continue to increase in number throughout life (Faust, et al., 1978).

The degree of fat accumulation with growth and aging will depend entirely on the dietary and exercise habits of the individual, in addition to heredity. While heredity is unchangeable, diet and exercise can be manipulated to either increase or decrease the fat stores. At birth, the body weight is 10 to 12 percent fat, and by the time the individual reaches physical maturity, the fat content reaches 15 and 25 percent of the total body weight for males and females, respectively. Figure 14–3 illustrates the relationship between relative, or percent, body fat and age for males and females. Both relative and absolute fat increase with age once physical maturity is reached. This is probably due to an increase in dietary intake, in addition to a decrease in levels of physical activity, although there is a reduced ability to mobilize fat with age. Beyond the age of thirty, there is also a progressive decrease in the lean body weight, which is primarily the result of decreased muscle mass and reduced mineral content of the bones. Both of these decreases are, at least partially, the result of decreased levels of physical activity.

Nervous System

As the child grows, he or she develops better agility and coordination which is a direct function of both the central and peripheral nervous systems. During the early stages of development, myelination of the nerve fibers must be completed before fast reactions and skilled movement can occur. Conduction velocity along a nerve fiber is considerably slower if myelination is absent or incomplete. Late in life, as the aging process progresses, conduction velocity along a nerve fiber may tend to slow. Speed of reaction and movement both slow down with age, and while this may be partially due to a decreased conduction velocity in the peripheral nervous system, both sensory and motor, several investigators feel that the main cause lies in the central nervous system. Some evidence suggests that the more active the individual nerve cells, the more likely they are to retain their optimal function and to resist the aging process. This would be a major benefit of remaining physically active throughout life.

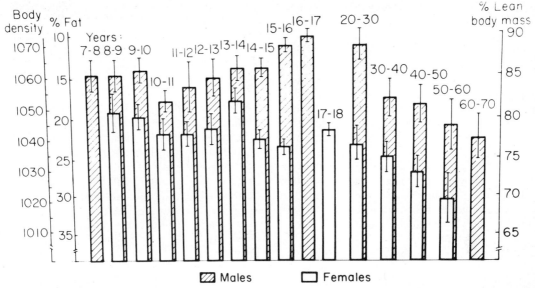

Figure 14–3 Changes in relative body fat with age for males and females. (From J. Parizková, "Body Composition and Exercise During Growth and Development." In *Physical Activity: Human Growth and Development,* edited by G. L. Rarick. New York: Academic Press, 1974. Reproduced by permission of the publisher.)

GENERAL PHYSIOLOGICAL FUNCTION

In almost all of the physiological systems, function appears to improve until maturity, or shortly before, and then plateaus for a period of time, before starting to decline with old age. Unfortunately, it is difficult to define the role of aging apart from the sedentary life style of the average individual. Both lead to a decrease in general physiological function. Recent evidence suggests that the rate of decrease associated with aging can be reduced or slowed by increasing the level of physical activity.

Basal Metabolic Rate (BMR)

The BMR, or lowest metabolic rate that the individual attains during a twenty-four-hour day, decreases at a rate of approximately 3 percent per decade from the age of three through eighty. Longitudinal studies that have followed the same individuals over twenty-year periods, or longer, suggest a more conservative decrease of only 1 to 2 percent per decade. Up to the age of twenty to thirty, this decrease is assumed to reflect a more efficient metabolism. Beyond thirty years of age, this de-

crease could be a result of the decrease in lean body weight referred to earlier in this chapter. It would be interesting to determine if physically active individuals, particularly those performing heavy-resistance exercise on a regular basis, have this same decrease in BMR. Likewise, it would be interesting to determine whether increasing muscle mass through heavy-resistance weight training would increase the BMR in older people. An increased BMR might reduce the degree of fat accumulation that seems to accompany the aging process.

Pulmonary Function

A number of cross-sectional studies have demonstrated that lung function is markedly altered by age. During the period of growth, the static lung volumes, as well as the functional pulmonary tests, increase to the time of physical maturity. Shortly after reaching this peak, however, there is a gradual reduction with age. Vital capacity, $FEV_{1.0}$ (the greatest volume of air that can be exhaled in the first second of a forced vital capacity test) and forced, expiratory flow rate all exhibit a linear decrease with age, starting at twenty to thirty years of age. While these volumes and rates are decreasing, the residual lung volume increases and the total lung capacity remains unchanged; thus, the ratio of the residual volume to the total lung capacity (RV/TLC) increases. In the early twenties, 18 to 22 percent of the total lung capacity is represented by the residual volume, but this increases to 30 percent, and higher, as the individual reaches fifty years of age. Smoking appears to accelerate this process.

The changes in these volumes and flow rates are matched by the changes in maximal ventilatory capacity during exhaustive exercise. Maximal expiratory ventilation ($\dot{V}E$ max) will increase with age to the point of physical maturity, and then it will decrease with the aging process. From cross-sectional data for males, the $\dot{V}E$ max, for four- to six-year-old boys, will average about 40 liters/min, increase to 110–140 liters/min at full maturity, and decrease to 60–80 liters/min for sixty- to seventy-year-olds. Females follow the same general pattern, although their absolute values will be considerably lower for each age level, due, primarily, to their smaller stature.

These changes are probably the result of a combination of factors, but the most important is the loss in elasticity of the lung tissue and chest wall, which increases the work or the effort involved in breathing. The decrease in mobility of the chest wall with age appears to be the major cause of reduction in the function of the lung.

Cardiovascular Function

A number of changes occur in cardiovascular function as the individual ages. Figure 14–4 illustrates the linear decrease in maximal heart rate with age. Children frequently exceed 200 beats/min, while the average sixty-year-old has a maximal heart rate of approximately 160 beats/min. It has been estimated that the maximal heart rate decreases by slightly less than one beat per year as the individual ages. The average maximal heart rate for each age level can be estimated from the following equation:

$$HR_{max} = 220 - age$$

It should be recognized that this represents only an estimate of the mean or average value for the age. Individual values could deviate from this estimated value by ± 20 beats/min, or more.

Peak, or maximum, stroke volume and cardiac output values appear to decline with age, although the number of studies conducted and number of subjects used are quite limited. Peripheral blood flow capacity is reduced with aging, but the density of the capillaries does not appear to change. It is difficult to determine whether the decreases in stroke volume, cardiac output, and peripheral blood flow are directly the result of the aging process or the result of an increasingly sedentary life style, which leads to cardiovascular deconditioning. Recent studies would tend to suggest that both are involved, but the relative contribution by each is not known.

Maximal Aerobic Capacity

The purpose of the basic pulmonary and cardiovascular adaptations that are made with varying levels of exercise is to accommodate the need of the exercising muscles for oxygen. Thus, the decreases in pulmonary and cardiovascular function with age suggest that aerobic capacity, or $\dot{V}O_2$ max, experiences a similar decline with age. Robinson, in 1938, demonstrated this phenomenon in a cross-sectional

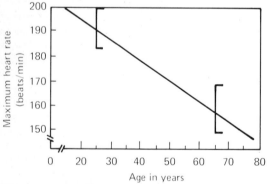

Relation between maximum rate and age*

Figure 14–4 Decrease in maximal heart rate with age. (From K. L. Andersen, R. J. Shephard, H. Denolin, E. Varnauskas, and R. Masironi, *Fundamentals of Exercise Testing*. Geneva: World Health Organization, 1971. Reproduced by permission of the publisher.)

sample of boys and men ranging in age from six to ninety-one years. He found that VO_2 max attained its peak value at seventeen to twenty years of age and then decreased as a linear function of age (see Figures 6–5 and 13–1). Adams, McHenry, and Bernauer (1972) found a similar relationship between $\dot{V}O_2$ max and age (Figure 14–5) in a large population of adult males. Studies of girls and women have shown essentially the same trend, although the female starts her decline at a much younger age (refer to Chapter 13), probably due to an earlier assumption of a sedentary lifestyle.

Again the questions must be asked: How much of the observed decrease is a result of biological aging? How important is the habitual level of physical activity in determining the rate of decline? Andersen and Hermansen (1965) gained insight into these questions when they compared the $\dot{V}O_2$ max values for a group of sixty-three cross-country skiers, fifty to sixty-six years of age, with a group of office workers and a group of industrial workers of

similar ages and with a group of twenty to thirty-year-old students. They found the following:

Group	Age Range (yr)	$\dot{V}O_2$ max (ml/kg × min)
Skiers	50–66	48
Office workers	50–60	36
Industrial workers	50–60	34
Students	20–30	44

These data support the contention that the decline in $\dot{V}O_2$ max with age, demonstrated in several studies, is not strictly a function of age, although the possibility that heredity might be an important factor in the high $\dot{V}O_2$ max values of the older skiers should not be discounted. Figure 6–5, in Chapter 6, illustrates the results of a similar type of study. A group of twenty-five of the best sprint and distance runners over forty years of age in the United States was brought into the laboratory for a comprehensive series of tests. While their $\dot{V}O_2$ max

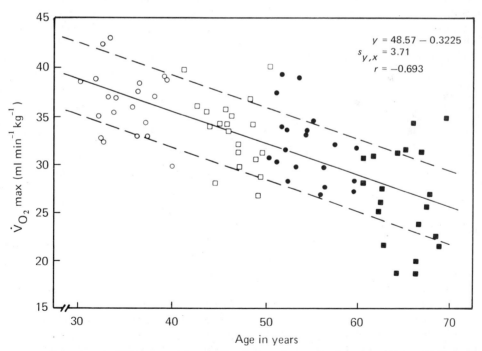

Figure 14–5 Decrease in VO₂ max with age. Symbols refer to the four age groups studied. (From W. C. Adams et al., "Multistage Treadmill Walking Performance and Associated Cardiorespiratory Responses of Middle-aged Men," *Clin. Sci.* 42, 1972. Reproduced by permission of the publisher.)

values were considerably higher than those of average men of the same age, the relative rate of decline with age closely paralleled the rate of decline illustrated by Robinson's (1938) data for normal men. Were these older athletes genetically superior, or can their comparatively high values be attributed to their training programs? The answer to these questions will have to await studies of a longitudinal nature.

It is of considerable interest to look at the extremes in age relative to endurance performance. One five-year-old boy has run a 7:51.1 mile and a 6-hour and 56-minute marathon (26 miles, 385 yards). At the other extreme are individuals in their seventies running full marathon distances, and farther. The human body has a tremendous ability to adapt to physical stress. Is this magnitude of stress harmful in any way to the very young or to the very old athlete? The limited information presently available suggests that no measurable physiological damage results from such training. In most cases, these very young and relatively old endurance runners are some of the best physical specimens for their ages, as determined by routine physical examinations. Still, to be on the cautious side, periodic examination by the family physician is recommended to identify any problems as early as possible. To date, few problems of a significant nature have materialized. Also, whether young or old, the potential athlete should approach his training program in a conservative manner, starting slowly and building up gradually. For the older individual, proper medical clearance, including an exercise electrocardiogram must precede both training and competition. This will be discussed in detail in the following chapter.

PSYCHOLOGICAL ASPECTS

Is formal, organized competition or participation in vigorous physical activity damaging to the emotional health and psychological development of the athlete? For the mature athlete, this presents no major problem, but many parents, educators, physicians, and psychologists have expressed concern over the potential for undesirable, emotional experiences in the developing young athlete. The question has been raised whether children who compete in formal, highly organized activities are likely to develop undesirable behavior patterns or psychological damage as a result of the pressures to win and be successful by adult standards. Does the eleven-year-old boy competing on the all-star Little League team experience pressures and situations that would lead to immediate or future behavior or emotional problems?

Only limited research has been conducted in this area. Skubic (1954, 1955) studied both Little League and Middle League (thirteen to fifteen years of age) baseball athletes in a small community in California. Using parents' opinions and the Galvanic skin-resistance measurement, she found essentially no difference between the athletes in formal competition compared to those who participated informally in physical education softball. There were few athletes who had any serious emotional problems that could be related to the stress of competition. Generally, her results suggested that formal competition at this age level was not detrimental to the child, but actually facilitated social and emotional growth.

On the other hand, Sherif et al. (1961) conducted a fascinating study, which has been referred to as the "Lord of the Flies" or "Robber's Cave" experiment. In this study, a group of boys at a summer camp were divided into two subgroups. During the initial part of the study, the groups were separated during much of the day, but they had periods of interaction. No problems between the groups developed during this part of the study. For the second phase of the study, the groups were put into situations where they were always in competition with each other in camp life, as well as in sports and games, both for recognition and for tangible rewards. During this phase, members of the individual groups developed strong allegiances to their own group and extreme hostility toward the other group. Night raids, cheating, and other forms of aggressive and undesirable behavior began to develop. This phase of the study was discontinued when several members of both groups started developing symptoms of serious psychological disturbances. During the third, and last, phase of the experiment, an attempt was made to bring the two groups back together in cooperative ventures, removing all forms of competition between the groups. It took considerable time to achieve the goal of working in a genuinely cooperative effort.

From these examples, it can only be concluded

that competition can have both positive and negative influences on the emotional development of the youngster. Of major importance is the climate in which the competition takes place. If the climate is

such that winning is the only goal and parents are allowed to say and do whatever they please without giving the child sound guidance in coping with the stress of the situation, the child will be likely to

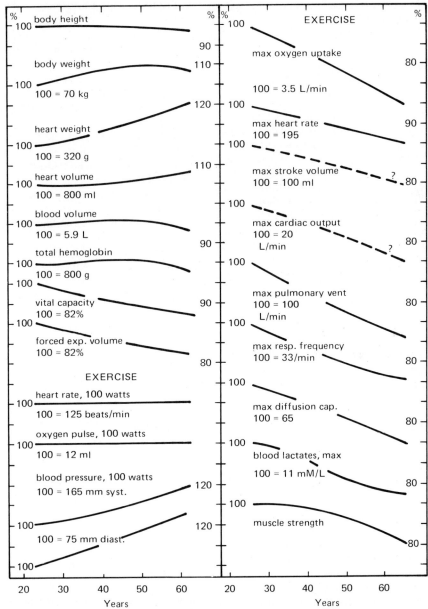

Figure 14–6 Variation in physical dimensions and physiological function with age. (From I. Åstrand, "Aerobic Work Capacity; Its Relation to Age, Sex, and Other Factors." *American Heart Association Monograph,* No. 15, 1967. By permission of the American Heart Association, Inc.)

have a negative experience. In short, the nature of the child's experience will depend almost entirely on the local situation. If competition is organized with this in mind, and the goal is to satisfy the needs of the child and not the adult, the experience should be positive and facilitate sound emotional growth and psychological development.

TRAINING THE YOUNG AND THE OLDER ATHLETE

Must special consideration be given to the young or older athlete when developing individualized programs of training? Generally, both the youngster and the older athlete will adapt well to the same type of training routine designed for the mature athlete. Heavy-resistance exercises with weights should be avoided by the younger athletes and isometric exercises should be avoided by older athletes. The latter suggestion is made because the unusually high increase in blood pressure that is associated with isometric contractions could cause serious complications in the older athlete. Older athletes should progress slowly in the early stages of their training programs to reduce the considerable stiffness and soreness that are likely to occur. Particular attention should be given to stretching exercises to help alleviate the potential joint and muscle problems that seem to be more common in the older athlete.

GENERAL SUMMARY

This chapter has outlined those physiological and body composition alterations that accompany the aging process from birth to old age. Most of these changes are illustrated in Figure 14–6, which summarizes data from a large number of studies and was compiled by Åstrand (1967). In addition, potential physiological and psychological problems associated with competition in the young and older athlete were discussed. It appears that strenuous physical exercise and intense competition can be of considerable value to athletes of all ages providing that the athletes have proper medical clearance and guidance and that the goals of competition are adjusted to serve the needs of the athlete.

STUDY QUESTIONS

1. What is the major concern when a bone breaks that has not reached full growth?
2. What is traumatic epiphysitis?
3. From the aspect of serious injury, which sport, baseball or football, places the youngster at higher risk?
4. At what age does lean body weight reach its peak in both males and females?
5. How dangerous is weight training in young boys and girls? What advice would you give to these youngsters if they wanted to improve their strength?
6. What typical changes occur in fat cells as one ages?
7. As one ages, what happens to the basal metabolic rate?
8. How does pulmonary function change with aging?
9. Why does cardiovascular endurance capacity decrease with age?
10. What does research tell us with respect to the psychological problems associated with competition at early ages?
11. Is it advisable for men and women over forty years of age to begin competition in competitive athletics? What precautions should be taken?

REFERENCES

Adams, J. E. "Injury to the Throwing Arm." *Calif. Med.* 102 (1965): 127–132.

Adams, W. C.; McHenry, M. M.; and Bernauer, E. M. "Multistage Treadmill Walking Performance and Associated Cardiorespiratory Responses of Middle-aged Men." *Clin. Sci.* 42 (1972): 355–370.

Albinson, J. G., and Andrew, G. M. *Child in Sport and Physical Activity.* Baltimore: University Park Press, 1976.

Andersen, K., and Hermansen, L. "Aerobic Work Capacity in Middle-Aged Norwegian Men." *J. Appl. Physiol.* 20 (1965): 432–436.

Åstrand, I. "Aerobic Work Capacity; Its Relation to Age, Sex, and Other Factors." *American Heart Association Monograph* No. 15, New York, 1967.

Corbin, C. B. *A Textbook of Motor Development.* Dubuque, Iowa: W. C. Brown, 1973.

deVries, H. A. *Physiology of Exercise for Physical Education and Athletics.* 2nd ed. Dubuque, Iowa: William C. Brown, 1974.

Espenshade, A. S., and Eckert, H. M. *Motor Development.* Columbus, Ohio: Charles E. Merrill Publishing Co., 1967.

Faust, I. M., Johnson, P. R., Stern, J. S., and Hirsch, J. "Diet-Induced Adipocyte Number Increase in Adult Rats: A New Model of Obesity." *Am. J. Physiol.* 235 (1978): E279–E286.

Goldman, R., and Rockstein, M. eds. *The Physiology and Pathology of Human Aging.* New York: Academic Press, 1975.

Larson, R. L. "Physical Activity and the Growth and Development of Bone and Joint Structures." In *Physical Activity: Human Growth and Development,* edited by G. L. Rarick, New York: Academic Press, 1974.

Larson, R. L., and McMahan, R. O. "The Epiphyses and the Childhood Athlete." *J. Amer. Med. Assoc.* 196 (1966): 607–612.

Rarick, G. L. *Physical Activity Human Growth and Development.* New York: Academic Press, 1973.

Robinson, S. "Experimental Studies of Physical Fitness in Relation to Age." *Arbeitsphysiol.* 10 (1938):251–323.

Rockstein, M., ed. *Theoretical Aspects of Aging.* New York: Academic Press, 1974.

Shephard, R. J. *Physical Activity and Aging.* Chicago: Year Book Medical Publishers, 1978.

Sherif, M.; Harvey, O. J.; White, B. J.; Hood, W. R.; Sherif, C. W. *Intergroup Conflict and Cooperation. The Robber's Cave Experiment.* Norman, Oklahoma: University of Oklahoma Book Exchange, 1961.

Skubic, E. "Studies of Little League and Middle League Baseball." *Res. Quart.* 27 (1954): 97–110.

Skubic, E. "Emotional Responses of Boys to Little League and Middle League Competitive Baseball." *Res. Quart.* 26 (1955): 342–352.

Smith, N.; Ogilvie, B.; Haskell, W.; and Gaillard, B. *Handbook for the Young Athlete.* Palo Alto, Calif: Bull Publishing Co., 1978.

Smith, E. L. and Serfass, R. C. ed. *Exercise and Aging: The Scientific Basis.* Hillside, New Jersey: Enslow Publishers, 1981.

15

Physical Activity for Health and Fitness*

INTRODUCTION

Throughout the previous chapters of this book, emphasis has been totally focused on the relationship of physical activity to various aspects of athletic performance. Discussion has centered on the male and the female athlete, the young and the old athlete, the basic elements of athletic performance, the influence of the environment on performance, and the role of selected ergogenic aids. This final chapter will look briefly at the health-related aspects of physical activity, a topic of considerable importance to the athlete and nonathlete alike. How important is physical activity to the health, fitness, and general well-being of the average individual in today's world with its emphasis on sedentary living? Can man, who was designed for strenuous activity, successfully adapt to this newly imposed sedentary lifestyle?

DISEASES OF MODERN LIVING

Chronic and degenerative diseases of the cardiovascular and pulmonary systems are the major causes of serious illness and death in the United States. Cardiovascular disease alone affects more than twenty-seven million Americans each year, resulting in over one million deaths, and costs the individual, government, and private industry over 50 billion dollars annually. While infectious diseases, such as influenza, tuberculosis, and pneumonia, were the major causes of death in the early 1900s, diseases of our modern life style, such as cancer, lung, and heart disease, have now attained the distinction of being the major causes of death. Cardiovascular disease, including heart disease and stroke, now kills more Americans each year than all other causes of death combined, including infant mortality and accidents!

Most individuals consider themselves to be healthy, until they experience some overt sign of illness. However, with chronic degenerative diseases, such as heart disease and cancer, the individual is generally unaware that the disease process is smoldering and slowly progressing from a minor affliction to one of major proportions. As one grows older, the frequency and rate of these undetected disease processes accelerate. Fortunately, early detection and proper treatment of the various chronic diseases can substantially reduce their intensity and the resulting number of deaths. Perhaps even more important, alteration of factors associated with an increased risk for a particular disease can either prevent the development of that disease or delay its onset for many years. This would include changing dietary habits, increasing habitual physical activity, abstaining from the use of tobacco, moderating alcohol intake, and improving the ability to handle psychological stress.

*Parts of this chapter were prepared in collaboration with Dr. William L. Haskell, Stanford University School of Medicine, for use by the Preventive Medicine Center, Palo Alto, California.

A discussion of each of the various chronic diseases would require considerably more space than is available. Consequently, discussion has been limited to those two areas where physical activity is known to play a predominant role—heart disease and obesity. Both are now considered to be of childhood origin; thus, the preventive aspects are very important.

Heart Disease

As humans age, their coronary arteries, i.e., those arteries that supply the heart muscle itself, become progressively narrower as a result of fat being deposited along the inner wall of the artery. This process of progressive narrowing is referred to as atherosclerosis. Kannel and Dawber (1972) have stated that atherosclerosis is not only a disease of the aged but that it is primarily a pediatric problem, since the pathologic changes that lead to atherosclerosis begin in infancy and progress during childhood. Fatty streaks, or lipid deposits, which are thought to be the probable precursors to atherosclerosis, are common in children by the age of three to five years. Enos, Holmes, and Beyer (1953) demonstrated that over 70 percent of autopsied Korean War combat casualties, with an average age of 22.1 years, already had at least moderately advanced coronary atherosclerosis. McNamera et al. (1971) found evidence of coronary atherosclerosis in 45 percent of Vietnam war casualties, with 5 percent exhibiting severe manifestations of the disease.

Between the years 1900 and 1970, heart disease tripled as a major cause of death. This three-fold increase is a relative increase, expressed in deaths per 100,000 population. Since the population of the United States has more than doubled over this seventy-year period, the absolute number of deaths from heart disease has risen even more dramatically. It is presently estimated that cardiovascular disease is identifiable in approximately 25 percent of the adult American population. Furthermore, heart disease has become the leading cause of death in men of ages thirty-five to forty-five years. Heart disease has become a national tragedy!

Risk Factors. Over the years, scientists have attempted to determine the basic etiology, or cause, of the atherosclerotic process. Several studies have been conducted that have closely observed selected members of communities for extensive periods of time. When a substantial number of deaths occur over a fifteen- to twenty-year period, it is possible to group those individuals who died from heart attacks to determine what risk factors they possessed in common. While this approach does not specifically define the actual causal mechanisms, it does provide the researcher with a valuable insight into the disease process.

The factors identified in these long-term, longitudinal, population studies are referred to as *risk factors*. The factors associated with an increased risk for the premature development of heart disease can be grouped into those over which the individual has no control and those that can be altered through basic changes in life style. Those that are beyond the individual's control include heredity, sex, age, and race. Those factors that can be altered include elevated blood fats (cholesterol and triglycerides), elevated blood pressure (hypertension), cigarette smoking, obesity, diabetes, abnormalities of the electrocardiogram, anxiety and tension (stress), and physical inactivity. Evidence is now available suggesting that these risk factors can be identified at an early age. Studies of college students indicate that coronary and stroke mortality rate can be predicted at this relatively young age. In a study of ninety-six boys, eight to twelve years of age (Wilmore and McNamara, 1974), 19.8 percent had cholesterol values in excess of the suggested, high-normal value of 200 mg/100 ml, 5.2 percent exhibited abnormal resting electrocardiograms, and 37.5 percent had in excess of 20 percent relative fat. Elevated blood pressure was not observed.

Role of Exercise. A number of research studies have identified inadequate physical activity as a risk factor in heart disease. Naughton and Bruhn (1970) have reported the incidence of heart attack in sedentary populations to be approximately twice that found in men who are physically active, either in their jobs or in their recreational pursuits. They suggest that the clinical manifestations of the disease should be preventable if suitable activity programs are instituted early in life. Fox, Naughton, and Haskell (1971) conclude that the existing evidence suggests, but falls short of actually proving, that an increase in habitual physical activity is beneficial in the prevention of heart disease. There are studies that also suggest that the patient who has survived a first heart attack will be less likely to have a second attack or die from a subsequent attack if he or she has been active in a physical-conditioning, rehabilitation program.

From these data, it is impossible to state, unequivocably, that exercise will provide protection from a premature heart attack. The available evidence suggests that an increase in habitual physical activity is beneficial. Fox (1973) has concluded that the likely benefits of habitual physical activity will be more in the area of an improved quality of life than in life extension. Obviously, the identification of the preventive role of exercise in heart disease must await further study of a longitudinal nature. While this may take fifty years, or more, to resolve beyond a shadow of a doubt, it would be prudent to subscribe to the theory that physical activity is important until it is proven otherwise.

Obesity

Obesity and overweight constitute two of the most serious medical and health problems in the United States today. It is ironic that while millions of people are dying of starvation each year in all parts of the world, many Americans are dying as an indirect result of an overabundance of food. The prevalence of obesity and overweight in this country has increased dramatically over the past fifteen years. Presently, as many as 10 million teenagers are overweight, representing about 20 percent of the total U.S. teenage population. For the adult population over forty years of age, 30 percent of all men and 40 percent of all women are more than 20 percent above their ideal weight. It has also been demonstrated that the average individual in this country will gain approximately one pound of additional weight each year after the age of twenty-five. Such a seemingly small gain, however, results in thirty pounds of excess weight by age fifty-five. Since the bone and muscle mass decreases by approximately one half pound per year, this means a forty-five pound gain in fat over this thirty-year period!

Overweight versus Obesity. What is the distinction between the terms *overweight* and *obesity*? Al-

so, what is meant by the term *ideal weight*? First, overweight is defined as any body weight that exceeds the normal or standard weight for a particular individual, based on his or her age, height, and frame size. These values are established solely on the basis of population averages. It is quite possible to be overweight according to these standards and yet have a body fat content lower than normal. Football players have frequently been found to be overweight, while actually being much leaner than individuals of the same age, height, and frame size who are of normal weight or even underweight. There are also individuals who are not overweight by the standard tables, but who are actually obese.

Obesity refers to the condition in which the total amount of body fat exceeds that considered optimal for a particular individual's body weight. This implies that the amount of body fat must be assessed much more accurately than can be guessed from the standard tables, which are based on height and frame size. The hydrostatic, or underwater, weighing technique is probably the most accurate of the clinical research techniques available for estimating body fat, but it is not practical for the assessment of the general population, due to the length of time and cost for each test. A much simpler technique, which is not as accurate as hydrostatic weighing but is much faster and inexpensive, involves measuring with calipers the thickness of two layers of skin plus the interposed layer of fat at several sites. Theoretically, the skinfold thickness will vary directly with the thickness of the underlying subcutaneous fat, which is related to the total body fat. The quantity of fat is normally expressed as a percentage of the individual's total body weight. Exact standards for allowable fat percentages have not been universally agreed on; however, men with over 25 percent body fat and women with over 35 percent should be considered obese.

The concept of ideal weight is closely related to these upper limits of body fat. It is felt that the average male should possess approximately 15 percent of his weight as fat and the average female approximately 23 percent. This will vary somewhat between individuals, but it does provide a realistic target to aim for. As an example, assume that a 180-pound man had 20 percent of his body weight as fat. He would possess 36 pounds of fat. The remaining weight, 144 pounds, is referred to as the lean body weight, or mass, and consists of bone, muscle, and other nonfat components. In order for this man to reach a level of 15 percent fat, he would have to lose eleven pounds, providing his lean body mass remained the same. (See calculations in Table 15–1). This would give him a target, or ideal, weight of 169 pounds. Ideal weight is determined by dividing the lean body weight by the fraction of the total body weight that is desired to be lean. For 15 percent fat, the fraction would be .85, or 85 percent lean weight.

It should be clear that to identify those people with obesity problems, it is necessary to first determine the actual, or relative, fat content of the body. Simply referring to even the most sophisticated standard weight tables is not sufficient to identify a large percentage of the obese population. It is quite possible to be obese by these criteria and still be within, or even below, the allowable limits established in these tables.

Etiology of Obesity. At one time, obesity was thought to be the result of basic hormonal imbalances in the blood, resulting from a failure of one or more of the endocrine glands. Later, it was believed that only a small fraction of the total obese population could be accounted for in this manner, and that it was gluttony, rather than glandular malfunction, that caused the majority of obesity problems. Fortunately, the results of more recent medical and physiological research show that obesity can be the result of any one, or a combination of many, factors. Its etiology is not as simple or straight-forward as was once believed.

A number of recent experimental studies on animals have linked obesity to hereditary or genetic factors. Indirect studies suggest a similar link for humans. According to several studies (Mayer, 1972), only 8 to 9 percent of children with parents of normal weight were found to be obese, whereas 40 percent and 80 percent were considered to be obese when either or both parents, respectively, were obese.

Obesity has also been experimentally and clinically linked with both physiological and psychological trauma. Hormonal imbalances, emotional trauma, and alterations in basic homeostatic mechanisms have all been shown to be either directly or indirectly related to the onset of obesity. Environmental factors, i.e., cultural habits, inadequate physical activity, and improper diets, have also been shown to contribute to obesity.

Thus, obesity is of complex origin, and the specific causes undoubtedly differ from one person to the next. Recognizing this fact is important both in the treatment of existing obesity and in the application of measures to prevent its onset. To attribute obesity solely to gluttony is most unfair and very damaging psychologically to obese individuals who are concerned and are attempting to correct their problem. Several studies have even shown that obese individuals actually eat less than normal individuals of similar sex and age, although they get far less physical activity.

Health Problems in Obesity. Obesity has been directly related to four different types of health problems: changes in various normal body functions, increased risk of developing certain diseases, detrimental effects on established diseases, and adverse psychological reactions.*

Just as the cause of obesity varies from one individual to another, so do the prevalence and extent of changes in body function. However, there are cer-

*U.S. Department of Health, Education, and Welfare, Public Health Service, *Obesity and Health* (Washington, D.C.: Government Printing Office, 1966).

Table 15–1   *Calculating Ideal or Target Weights*

Weight 180 lb	Relative fat	20%
Total fat = 20% × 180 lb = 36 lb		
Lean body weight = 180 lb − 36 lb = 144 lb		
Ideal weight = 144 ÷ .85 = 169 lb	Ideal relative fat	15%
Target weight loss = 180 lb − 169 lb = 11 lb		

tain trends that are specifically linked to obesity. Respiratory problems are quite common among the obese. They have difficulty in normal breathing, a greater incidence of respiratory infections, and a lower exercise tolerance. Lethargy, associated with increased levels of carbon dioxide in the blood, and polycythemia (increased red blood cell production) due to lowered arterial blood oxygenation, are also common results from obesity. These can lead to blood clotting (thrombosis), enlargement of the heart, and congestive heart failure. Hypertension and atherosclerosis have also been linked to obesity, as have metabolic and endocrine disorders, such as impaired carbohydrate metabolism and diabetes. Obesity has also been associated with an increased risk of gallbladder disease, digestive diseases, and nephritis. More important, the mortality rate of the obese is substantially higher for each of these diseases than for people of normal weight.

The effect of obesity on existing diseases is not clearly understood at the present time. Obesity can contribute to the further development of certain diseases, and weight reduction is usually prescribed as an integral part of the treatment of the disease. Conditions such as angina pectoris, hypertension, congestive heart failure, myocardial infarction, varicose veins, diabetes, and orthopedic problems would benefit from weight reduction.

It is possible that psychological problems actually cause obesity in a substantial percentage of the obese population. Further emotional or psychological problems can arise from the existence of the condition itself. There is definitely a social stigma to obesity in our society, which contributes substantially to the problems of those who are obese. Consequently, obese individuals may also need psychiatric assistance in their efforts to lose weight.

Treatment, Prevention, and Controls. On paper, weight control seems to be a very simple matter. The energy consumed by the body in the form of food must be equal to the energy expended by the body in physical activity. In both cases, the energy is expressed in calories. The body will normally maintain a balance between the caloric intake and the caloric expenditure. However, when this balance is upset, a loss or gain in weight will result. It appears that both weight losses and weight gains are basically dependent on only two factors—dietary and exercise habits.

The sole purpose of a weight-reduction diet is to create a caloric deficiency, i.e., the caloric intake is lowered so that the caloric expenditure exceeds the intake. It has been estimated that the loss of one pound of fat requires a caloric deficit of 3,500 Kcals. To lose one pound a week, the caloric deficit would have to average 500 Kcals/day, which is approximately the equivalent of five scrambled eggs, three and one-half cans of beer (12-ounce can), or a six-ounce sirloin steak. A reasonable or sensible weight loss would be one to two pounds per week. Losses any greater than this should not be attempted, unless under direct medical supervision. By losing just one pound of fat a week, an individual will lose 52 pounds in only one year! Few people become obese that rapidly.

Weight loss should be a long-term project. Research has demonstrated, and experience has proven, that rapid weight losses are usually short-lived and the original weight is quickly regained. Rapid weight losses are generally the result of large losses of body water. Since the body has built-in safety mechanisms to prevent an imbalance in body water levels, the water loss will, eventually, be replaced. Thus, the individual wishing to lose twenty pounds of fat is advised to attempt to attain this goal in a six- to twelve-month period.

Many special diets have been popular in recent years, such as the drinking man's diet, Dr. Stillman's diet, and Dr. Adkin's diet. Each claims to be the ultimate in terms of effectiveness and comfort in weight loss. Likewise, each diet has its loyal following of confirmed believers who make a strong case for the superiority of their particular diet over the others. Is there a superior diet? Research tends to show that almost all of these diets are effective, but *no one single diet has been shown to be any more effective than any other.* Again, the important factor is the development of a caloric deficit, while maintaining a balanced diet that is complete in all respects with regard to vitamin and mineral requirements. The diet that meets these criteria and is best suited to the comfort and personality of each individual is the best diet.

Several agents or aids have been advocated for assisting an individual in reducing his caloric intake. Anorexigenic agents (agents used to decrease or suppress the appetite), such as amphetamines, have been prescribed with varying success, but they produce side effects such as insomnia, irritability, and tenseness. Thyroid hormone has also been used, but its effects are highly questionable and it produces side effects similar to the amphetamines.

Recently, human chorionic gonadotropin, a hormone derived from the urine of pregnant women, has been used to promote rapid weight loss. Daily injections of this hormone, in addition to a 500-Kcal/day diet, supposedly produce a one-pound-per-day weight loss. Recent evidence, however, shows human chorionic gonadotropin to be no more effective than an injection of plain salt water. The weight that is lost appears to be strictly the result of the 500-Kcal/day diet.

Diuretics have been suggested, but the resulting weight loss is almost entirely salt and water. Therefore, these should be used only for those patients who have problems of water retention or hyperhydration. Total fasting has been shown to be helpful in the initial stages of weight loss in highly obese individuals, but hospitalization and close supervision of the patient is required. It must be emphasized that, regardless of their effectiveness, none of these agents or aids should be used except under the prescription and close supervision of a physician.

For many years, it has been a common belief that exercise is of little help in programs of weight reduction and control. The classic examples are the statements that to lose one pound of fat, a person must chop wood for seven hours, walk thirty-five miles, or climb a ten-foot staircase 1,000 times. These examples are intended to show the foolishness of trying to lose weight through exercise. It is also argued that the appetite increases as a result of exercise, and that this increase in caloric intake has the same, or greater, caloric value as the expenditure from the exercise itself.

Both of these concepts have been proven false. In fact, research has proven that exercise is probably the most efficient way to lose weight and that it also results in weight losses of a permanent nature.

Inactivity is a major cause of obesity in the United States. In fact, inactivity may be a far more significant factor in the development of obesity than overeating! Thus, exercise must be recognized as an essential component in any program of weight reduction or control.

When planning an exercise program, it is important to remember that one seldom obtains something for nothing. An effortless exercise program, of course, would be ideal but such a program would be unrealistic. With the popularity of exercise increasing, there are many gimmicks, gadgets, and fads on the market. While some of these are legitimate and effective, many are of no practical value for either exercise or weight loss. To exercise efficiently and make substantial progress requires work and sweat.

The physical activity level of any individual can be increased by concentrating on four basic areas. First, one should have a regular formal exercise schedule, consisting of a warm-up period, the formal exercise or exercises, and a cooling-off period. This formal exercise should be undertaken at least three times a week and can consist of anything from walking to jogging or swimming.

Second, one should have supplementary physical recreation in addition to formal exercise. Gardening, golf, bowling, sailing, and dancing are just a few of the many active recreational pursuits that will result in a far greater expenditure of energy than the more commonly practiced art of television watching. Third, the total daily caloric expenditure can be increased in the course of one's usual daily activities by walking several flights of steps instead of using the elevator, by parking an extra block or more from work or the store, and by performing many of the other routine daily activities in a more active manner. The object is to look for ways of increasing the amount of physical work the body can perform each day, during the daily routine, in spite of mechanization.

Last, the physical activity level associated with one's job can be increased. This can be done in much the same manner as just outlined. Since approximately a fourth to a third of one's life is spent on the job, this time can be used much more efficiently if the basic activity levels on the job are increased.

From this information, it appears that the most efficient and sensible approach to weight loss is through a combination of diet and exercise. Since a caloric deficit is the key to weight loss, the caloric intake would only have to be reduced and physical activity increased half as much as necessary as if either one was used exclusively by itself for weight loss. Thus, routine exercise is effective in weight control and weight reduction. Likewise, sedentary habits tend to lead to problems of overweight and obesity. A word of caution, however. It is quite possible, and even probable, that one's weight on the bathroom scale will change very little, if any, following a month or two of vigorous exercise. While this is discouraging and might lead one to suspect that the exercise program is not helping to reduce body fat, this phenomenon is a natural occurrence. During the initial stages of an exercise program the individual develops muscle as well as loses fat, both of which are highly desirable. For the first month or two, the gains in muscle are nearly the same as the losses in fat. As a result, the bathroom scale does not give an accurate measurement of the actual changes in the body's composition.

THE PRESCRIPTION OF EXERCISE

From the preceding discussion, it is obvious that the sedentary nature of modern man has led to a number of health-related problems. Many of these problems can be either resolved or prevented by prescribing programs of routine physical activity for the young and old, alike. The sport and exercise sciences have now progressed to the point where individualized exercise programs can be prescribed and tailored to the likes, needs, and physical capacity of the individual participant. The era of a single group program to fit people of all ages and capacities has come and gone. The individualized prescription of exercise is now a reality and is being used successfully throughout the United States.

Medical Clearance

Prior to beginning any exercise program, it is important that all individuals over thirty years old have a complete physical examination by their private physicians. This should include a discussion of the proposed exercise program, in the event that there are medical complications that might make a particular activity or sport undesirable. As an example, patients who have elevated blood pressure should be cautioned to avoid activities that use isometric contractions. Isometric contractions tend to cause a considerable rise in blood pressure and usually result in a Valsalva maneuver in which the intra-abdominal and intra-thoracic pressure are increased to the point of restricting the vena cava, thus limiting venous return to the heart. Both responses can lead to serious medical complications.

The physical examination should include a health and family history, a resting electrocardiogram and blood pressure assessment, and an exercise stress electrocardiogram performed on either a bicycle ergometer or treadmill. The stress electrocardiogram is extremely important since between 8 and 14 percent of the normal, asymptomatic adult population with normal resting electrocardiograms will demonstrate abnormalities in their electrocardiograms during or following exercise, which is indicative of coronary atherosclerosis. This does not preclude the participation of these individuals in an exercise program, but it does place them in a special, high-risk category in which exercise should be performed under the supervision of a physician.

Factors in Prescribing Exercise

Once an individual is cleared by the family physician, an exercise program can be prescribed. The exercise prescription involves four basic factors: mode or type of exercise, frequency of participation, duration of each exercise period, and intensity of the exercise bout. Each of these will be discussed individually.

Mode of Exercise. The prescribed exercise program should include, as its focus, a cardiovascular endurance activity. Traditionally, walking, jogging, running, hiking, and swimming have been the activities prescribed most frequently. Unfortunately, these activities do not appeal to everyone, so additional activities need to be identified that will promote similar cardiovascular endurance development. Recently, bicycling and tennis were shown to cause significant improvements in endurance capacity. Strenuous activities, like handball and racketball, probably have a significant endurance component, but this has not, as yet, been substantiated by research. For these types of activities, it is advisable to be preconditioned through one of the standard endurance activities, such as jogging, before undertaking serious competition. This introduces the concept of conditioning activities and maintenance activities. It is felt by some researchers, clinicians, and practitioners that in order to successfully compete in certain sports or activities, a basic preconditioning program is essential.

Rather than using the sport or activity to get in shape, one would get in shape prior to participating in that sport or activity. If the activity required a moderate to high level of cardiovascular endurance, the individual would engage in a jogging, swimming, or bicycling program for several months, until his or her endurance capacity was increased to the necessary level, at which time the person would switch over to the sport. Conditioning activities would be used to bring the individual to the desired fitness level. The sport would then act as a maintenance activity to maintain the individual at that desired level of fitness. This is an important concept that should not be overlooked.

When selecting activities, it is important to match individuals with activities that they will enjoy and be willing to continue throughout life. Exercise must be regarded as a lifetime pursuit, for the benefits are soon lost once participation stops. Motivation is probably the most important factor in a successful exercise program. Thus, selecting an activity that is fun, provides a challenge, and can provide the needed benefits is the most critical task in the exercise prescription process.

Exercise Frequency. The frequency of participation is an important factor to consider, but it is probably less critical than either the exercise duration or intensity. Research studies conducted on this aspect have shown that three to four days per week is an optimal frequency (Pollock, 1973). This does not mean that five, or more, days per week will not give additional benefits, but simply that, for health purposes, you are getting the best return for the amount of time invested. It is important that the individual limit exercise to three to four days per week, initially, and build up to five, or more, days per week, only if the individual enjoys what he or she is doing. All too often, an individual who starts out with great intentions and is highly motivated will exercise every day for the first few weeks, only to stop from utter fatigue. Obviously, additional days per week above the three- to four-day frequency are beneficial for weight loss purposes, but this level should not be encouraged until the exercise habit is firmly established.

Exercise Duration. Several studies have demonstrated improvement in cardiovascular conditioning with endurance-exercise programs as brief as five to ten minutes per day. Recent research (Pollock, 1973) has indicated that twenty to thirty minutes per day is an optimal amount. Again, optimal is used here in the context of greatest return for time invested, and the specified time refers to the time during which the individual is at his or her training heart rate (THR).

Exercise Intensity. The intensity of the exercise bout is undoubtedly the most critical aspect of the three factors, frequency, duration, and intensity. How hard does one have to push himself or herself? Ex-athletes immediately recall the exhaustive workouts they endured to condition themselves for their sport. Unfortunately, this concept gets carried over into the area of exercise for health. Evidence now suggests that a substantial training effect can be accomplished by training at between 60 and 80 percent of an individual's capacity (Pollock, 1973). There appears to be a training threshold above which a training response occurs. Some evidence suggests that training must be at a level that is at least 60 percent of one's capacity, and that training at levels below 60 percent results in little, if any, cardiovascular benefit.

Exercise intensity is quantified by having the individual exercise at his or her own, individualized, training heart rate (THR). The THR is established by determining the individual's exercise capacity on a maximal exercise stress test. He or she is then assigned a heart rate that represents a set percentage of that capacity. A THR set at 75 percent of the individual's HRmax represents a level of only 60 to 65 percent of one's $\dot{V}O_2$ max, but this will be sufficient to initiate a substantial training response. Some clinicians actually measure $\dot{V}O_2$ up to, and including, $\dot{V}O_2$ max. They establish the THR by using the heart rate equivalent to a set fraction of the VO_2 max. As an example, when the individual is tested, heart rate and $\dot{V}O_2$ data for each minute are obtained and plotted against each other. If a training level of 75 percent of $\dot{V}O_2$ max is used, the $\dot{V}O_2$ at 75 percent is determined ($\dot{V}O_2$ max $\times$ 0.75) and the corresponding heart rate is selected as the THR.

The concept of THR is extremely valuable. There is a high correlation between heart rate and the work done by the heart. Heart rate alone is a good index of myocardial oxygen consumption as well as coronary blood flow. If the THR concept is followed, the individual's heart will perform at the same level of work even though the metabolic costs of the work might vary considerably. When exercising at high altitudes or under extremes in temperature, the heart rate will be greatly elevated if the individual attempts to maintain the rate of work, e.g., run at a 6-min/mi pace. With the THR concept, the individual simply does less work under these extreme environmental conditions to maintain the same heart rate (THR). This is a much safer approach to the training program.

The THR concept automatically accounts for improvement. As the individual becomes better conditioned, his or her heart rate decreases for the same level of work, or conversely, the individual must actually perform more work in order to reach his or her THR.

THE EXERCISE PROGRAM

Once medical clearance has been obtained and the exercise prescription determined, it is necessary to integrate all of the previously described information into a total exercise program. That is an integral part of the individual's overall health-improvement plan. The program should be designed, specifically, on the basis of the results of the medical evaluation, as well as on the basis of the individual's exercise capacity, interests, and personal needs. It should be designed to bring one to a reasonable level of fitness for his or her age, health status, occupation, and leisure-time interests. Once an individual has achieved this level, his or her program becomes one of fitness maintenance. At that time, the amount of physical activity required will become less, since the amount of activity needed to stay at the ideal level of fitness is less than it takes to get there. Also, once one reaches the ideal, or optimal, level of fitness, it is possible to safely and enjoyably participate in a much greater variety of exercises and active sports or games.

The exercise program should include the following:

- A conditioning or physical fitness program
- A recreational activities guide
- A daily, living habits guide

The Conditioning Program

Exercise capacity varies widely among individuals, even when they are of similar ages and physical builds. That is why each program is based upon the individual's own, personal test results. The total time to perform the recommended program will vary between thirty and forty-five minutes per session, depending on the individual's present level of fitness and his personal goals.

The recommended conditioning program consists of the following activities listed in the order in which they should be performed:

- A set of warm-up exercises
- A set of flexibility exercises
- An endurance conditioning period
- A set of strength exercises (optional)
- A cooling-down period.

Warm-Up Period. The exercise session should begin with low-intensity, calisthenic and stretching exercises. Such a warm-up period will increase both heart rate and breathing to provide for the efficient and safe functioning of the heart, blood vessels, lungs, and muscles during the more vigorous exercise that follows. A good warm-up will also reduce the amount of muscle and joint soreness that may be experienced during the early stages of the exercise program.

Flexibility-Development Activities. The flexibility exercises, such as those illustrated in Appendix B, are supplementary to those exercises performed during the warm-up period and are intended for those who have poor flexibility, as well as muscle and joint problems, such as low back pain. These exercises are to be performed slowly, as quick stretching movements are potentially dangerous and can lead to muscle pulls or muscle spasms.

Endurance-Development Activities. Physical activities that develop endurance are the "heart" of the exercise program. They are designed to improve both the capacity and efficiency of the cardiovascular and respiratory systems. Also, they are the types of exercises that are most useful in helping to control or reduce body weight.

Activities such as walking, jogging, running, cycling, swimming, and hiking are good endurance activities. Sports such as handball, basketball, tennis, and badminton are also good, providing they are pursued vigorously. Activities such as golf, bowling, and softball are generally of little value from the standpoint of developing cardiorespiratory endurance, but they are fun and have definite recreational value. Tables 15–2 to 15–6 illustrate a progressive walk-jog-run type program.

Strength Exercises. A series of strength-development exercises are illustrated in Appendix A, most of which require strength-training equipment. Access to dumbbells, barbells, weight machines, or other strength-training devices is not essential, however, since one can gain a great deal from exercises that utilize body weight as the resistance.

If one participates in a weight-training program, it is advisable to start with a weight that is exactly one-half of one's maximum strength. The individual should attempt to lift that weight ten consecutive times. If one can just barely do this, he or

Table 15–2 *A Walking Program.*

Step	Peak O_2 Value[a]	Workout Description	Time (min)	Miles
I	8.5	Walk 0.67 mi in 20 min	20	0.67
II	8.5	Walk 1 mi in 30 min	30	1.00
III	10.4	Walk 1.25 mi in 30 min	30	1.25
IV	12.0	Walk 1.50 mi in 30 min	30	1.50
V	14.0	Walk 1.75 mi in 30 min	30	1.75
VI	16.0	Walk 2.0 mi in 30 min	30	2.00

[a]ml/kg · min^{-1}

Table 15–3 *A Walking-Jogging Program.*

Step	Peak O_2 Value[a]	Work Description	Time (min)	Miles
I	17.2	Walk 2.25 mi in 30 min	30	2.25
II	24.5	Walk .25 mi in 3 min 45 sec Jog .25 mi in 3 min Repeat for 31 min	31	2.25
III	24.5	Walk .5 mi in 7 min 30 sec Jog .5 mi in 6 min Repeat for 34 min 30 sec	34.5	2.50
IV	24.5	Walk .25 mi in 3 min 45 sec Jog .75 mi in 9 min Walk .5 mi in 7 min 30 sec Repeat first two steps	33	2.50
V	24.5	Jog 1 mi in 12 min Walk .25 mi in 3 min 45 sec Repeat	31.5	2.50
VI	27.5	Walk .25 mi in 3 min 45 sec Jog 1 mi in 11 min Repeat for 33 min 15 sec	33.25	2.75

[a]ml/kg · min^{-1}

Table 15–4   *A Jogging Program.*

Step	Peak O_2 Value[a]	Workout Description	Time (min)	Miles
I	27.5	Jog 1 mi in 11 min	34	3.00
		Jog .5 mi in 6 min		
		Repeat		
II	27.5	Jog 3 mi in 33 min	33	3.00
III	30.5	Jog 1 mi in 10 min	31	3.00
		Jog 1 mi in 11 min		
		Jog 1 mi in 10 min		
IV	30.5	Jog 3 mi in 30 min	30	3.00
V	33.5	Jog 1 mi in 9 min 15 sec	28.5	3.00
		Jog 1 mi in 10 min		
		Jog 1 mi in 9 min 15 sec		
VI	33.5	Jog 3 mi at 9 min 15 sec/mi	28	3.00

[a] $ml/kg \cdot min^{-1}$

Table 15–5   *A Jogging-Running Program.*

Step	Peak O_2 Value[a]	Workout Description	Time (min)	Miles
I	33.5	Jog 3.25 mi at 9 min 15 sec/mi	30	3.25
II	36.5	Jog 3.375 mi at 8 min 30 sec/mi	29	3.38
III	36.5	Jog 3.5 mi at 8 min 30 sec/mi	30	3.50
IV	39.5	Jog-Run 3.5 mi at 8 min/mi	28	3.50
V	39.5	Jog-Run 3.75 mi at 8 min/mi	30	3.75
VI	39.5	Jog-Run 4.0 mi at 8 min/mi	32	4.00

[a] $ml/kg \cdot min^{-1}$

Table 15–6   *A Running Program.*

Step	Peak O_2 Value[a]	Workout Description	Time (min)	Miles
I	42.5	Run 4 mi at 7 min 30 sec/mi	30	4.00
II	42.5	Run 4.25 mi at 7 min 30 sec/mi	32	4.25
III	42.5	Run 4.38 mi at 7 min 30 sec/mi	33	4.38
IV	45.5	Run 4.5 mi at 7 min/mi	31.5	4.50
V	45.5	Run 4.75 mi at 7 min/mi	33.25	4.75
VI	45.5	Run 5 mi at 7 min/mi	35	5.00

[a] $ml/kg \cdot min^{-1}$

she is starting at the right weight. If one could have done more, he or she should go to the next highest weight for the second set. If the individual did less than eight repetitions on the first set, the weight lifted should be reduced to the next lowest level for the second set. Once a weight gets the person to the point of fatigue by the eighth to tenth repetition, the individual has found his or her starting weight. Two or three sets of each lift should be performed per day, three days per week, in which eight to ten repetitions count as a single set. As the individual increases strength, more repetitions will be able to be done per set. Once he or she hits fifteen repetitions, it is time to increase to the next highest weight. This training technique is referred to as *progressive resistance exercise.* For those lifts where the maximum strength has not been determined, the process of selecting an initial weight is largely one of trial and error.

Cooling-Down Period. Every exercise session should be concluded with a tapering down, or cooling-off, period. This is best accomplished by slowly reducing the intensity of the activity during the last several minutes of the workout. A slow, restful walk for several minutes keeps the blood from pooling in the extremities, and helps reduce the chances of developing muscle soreness. Stopping abruptly following an endurance bout of exercise causes blood to pool in the legs and may actually result in dizziness and fainting.

Recreational Activities

Recreational activities are an important part of any comprehensive, physical activity program. While these activites are primarily engaged in for enjoyment and relaxation, many of them also contribute to fitness development as well. Activities such as hiking, tennis, handball, squash, and certain team sports fall into this category. Guidelines to be used in the selection of these activities include the following: (1) Can they be learned or performed with at least a moderate degree of success? (2) Do they include opportunities for social development? and (3) Are they varied enough to maintain continued interest?

Many excellent opportunities exist for those individuals who have no recreational hobbies or activities but who would like to become involved. Local recreation centers or clubs, YMCAs, YWCAs, public schools, and community colleges offer instructional classes in a wide variety of activities for little or no cost. Often the entire family can participate in these classes, an added bonus to a total health-improvement program.

Several words of caution are necessary. First, one should not be carried away by competitive activities. While the competitive spirit is natural and healthy, it does occasionally tend to overpower one's common sense. Second, contact-type sports or activities should be avoided, except for the exceptional individual who is in a highly trained and conditioned state. Also, it is important to keep in mind that these are primarily recreational activities, which are only one aspect of the total physical activity program. Once the individual has attained a reasonable state of fitness, however, these activities may be adequate to keep him or her there.

Life Pattern Alterations

Man has become a victim of his own technological progress. History has observed the transformation of homo sapiens into homo sedentarius. Fortunately, the trend toward a totally sedentary life style is not irreversible. Simply by consciously altering a few basic habits, one can overcome much of this tendency toward sedentary living. The following suggestions are just a few of many changes that can be made in daily living habits to increase health and fitness levels.

1. Elevators and escalators are convenient but do little for health. Walk those stairways, starting with one or two flights and progressively increase as the body becomes conditioned.
2. Park the car several blocks, or more, from your normal on-the-job parking place and briskly walk this extra distance.
3. Take a brisk walk during coffee or lunch breaks or before dinner.
4. Walk to the corner market or store for those short errands and give the car, the crowded roads, and the polluted air a well-deserved rest.

5. Wash your own car, mow your own lawn, and do your own handiwork. These can become hobbies, and the money saved can be applied toward a new bike.
6. Throw away the remote control for the television set and walk those few extra steps for channel changing or fine tuning. This might be just enough to break many of their TV habit.
7. Do not lie when you can sit, do not sit when you can stand, and do not stand when you can be moving.
8. Be innovative and see how much work you can save the machines.

GENERAL GUIDELINES FOR AN EXERCISE PROGRAM

When an inactive individual begins a physical activity program, there are several very basic and important factors that need to be considered.

Clothing

The choice of clothing will obviously depend upon the weather and the activity in which the individual plans to participate. However, clothing should always be comfortable, reasonably loose, and heavy or light enough to insure protection from heat, cold, and wind. Because of the heat generated with exercise, it is better to underdress rather than overdress. Women should avoid restrictive support garments or clothing that restrict either free movement or blood flow. In conditioning activities, such as jogging, men do not need to wear athletic supporters, since they frequently cause skin irritations.

One should not wear rubberized or plastic clothing while exercising. The increased sweat loss does not result in a permanent loss of body weight, and this practice can be very dangerous. The rubberized or plastic clothing does not allow the body sweat to evaporate, which is the principal mechanism for temperature regulation during exercise. The result can be a dramatic rise in body temperature, excessive dehydration and salt loss, and eventual heat stroke or heat exhaustion.

Shoes

The type and proper fit of shoe is important for any activity program. A good quality of tennis, basketball, or gym shoe is recommended for most types of activities. For programs of running, jogging, or walking, however, special shoes are recommended that have been designed specifically for these activities. These shoes should not fit tightly; the soles should be firm and the tops pliable; and they should have a good supporting heel. Ripple or crepe soles are excellent for use on hard surfaces. It is important to remember that good shoes and socks are the best prevention against blisters and sore and aching feet, ankles, and knees.

Running Surfaces

For those individuals who include walking, running, or jogging in their activity programs, the matter of running surfaces should be given careful consideration. Beginners and individuals who are overweight or who have a history of foot, ankle, or knee problems should avoid hard surfaces, such as running tracks, cement, or asphalt. Grass or dirt paths usually provide good surfaces. Golf courses, parks, or rights-of-way along parkways can provide good variations in scenery and terrain. During bad weather, use the local YMCA, school, or church gymnasium or protected areas around shopping centers and around the home.

When to Exercise

Almost any time of the day is acceptable for exercising, except for an hour or two following a meal and during hot and humid weather. Since man seems to be a creature of habit, a specific time of day should be set aside for the activity program. Early morning before breakfast is often the best time for many people, since they have few conflicting commitments at that time of day.

Illness or Injury

The physical activity program should be modified or temporarily stopped during any illness, injury, or infection that might be aggravated by such a program. Use proper footwear and socks and take it easy at the beginning to avoid potential foot and leg problems. Also, switch to an activity that does not require one to support his or her weight while exercising, such as swimming or bicycling, to help eliminate foot or leg problems, without losing fitness. Any persistent illness or injury should be brought to the attention of the individual's personal physician.

Motivation

Physical activity programs are usually started with the best of intentions, but, all too often, the individual's enthusiasm tends to wane after a short period of time. Since the physical activity program is intended to be a lifetime pursuit, it is important that the indvidual be properly motivated. Several suggestions are listed below to help overcome the motivation problem.

- Either select activities you enjoy or learn to enjoy the activities in which you feel you must participate.
- Exercise at a regular time of the day and make this a part of your daily routine.
- Exercise with a partner or become a member of a formal group. However, do not get talked into competition.
- Take selected physiological and medical measurements and attempt to chart your improvement on each of these.
- Become educated in what you are doing. By reading, attending lectures or seminars, and group discussions, attempt to understand the importance of a physical activity program relative to your total health.

ENERGY EXPENDITURE AND PHYSICAL ACTIVITY

The amount of oxygen consumed is directly proportional to the energy expended in physical activity. At rest, man uses approximately 3.5 ml of oxygen per kilogram (2.2 lb) of body weight per minute (ml/kg × min). When walking slowly at 2 mph, one uses about 9.0 ml, and one uses 24 ml when walking rapidly at 5.0 mph. The amount of oxygen necessary to perform an activity is referred to as that activity's *oxygen requirement*. Thus, all physical activities can be classified according to their intensities as determined by their oxygen requirements.

A simplified system for classifying physical activities has been developed, using the concept of *metabolic equivalents*, or METS. One MET is equal to the resting oxygen uptake, approximately 3.5 ml/kg × min. An activity that is rated as two METS would, therefore, require two times the resting oxygen consumption, or 7 ml/kg × min, and an activity that is rated at 4 METS would require approximately 14 ml/kg × min (4 × 3.5 = 14).

A number of activities and their MET values are presented in Table 15–7. It should be noted that these values are only approximations, due to the variations in metabolic efficiency both within and between individuals. This table can also be used to select activities to supplement the endurance-training program.

Table 15–7 *Selected Activities and Their Respective MET Values.*

Self-Care Activities		*Self-Care Activities*	
Activity	*METS*	*Activity*	*METS*
Rest, supine	1.0	Showering	3.5
Sitting	1.0	Walking downstairs	4.5
Standing, relaxed	1.0	Walking, 3.5 mph	5.5
Eating	1.0	Ambulation, braces and crutches	6.5
Conversation	1.0		
Dressing and undressing	2.0	*Housework Activities*	
Washing hands and face	2.0	*Activity*	*METS*
Propulsion, wheelchair	2.0	Handsewing	1.0
Walking, 2.5 mph	3.0	Sweeping floor	1.5

Table 15–7   *(continued)*

Housework Activities		Physical-Conditioning Activities	
Activity	*METS*	*Activity*	*METS*
Machine sewing	1.5	Swimming, crawl, 1 ft/sec	5.0
Polishing furniture	2.0	Level walking, 3.5 mph (1 mi in 17 min)	5.5
Peeling potatoes	2.5	Level walking, 4.0 mph (1 mi in 15 min)	6.5
Scrubbing, standing	2.5	Level jogging, 5.0 mph (1 mi in 12 min)	7.5
Washing small clothes	2.5	Level cycling, 13 mph	
Kneading dough	2.5	(1 mi in 4 min 37 sec)	9.0
Scrubbing floors	3.0	Level running, 7.5 mph (1 mi in 8 min)	9.0
Cleaning windows	3.0	Swimming, crawl, 2 ft/sec	10.0
Making beds	3.0	Level running, 8.5 mph (1 mi in 7 min)	12.0
Ironing, standing	3.5	Level running, 10.0 mph (1 mi in 6 min)	15.0
Mopping	3.5	Swimming crawl, 2.5 ft/sec	15.0
Wringing wash by hand	3.5	Swimming crawl, 3.0 ft/sec	20.0
Hanging wash	3.5	Level running, 12 mph (1 mi in 5 min)	20.0
Beating carpets	4.0	Level running, 15 mph (¼ mi in 1 min)	30.0
		Swimming crawl, 3.5 ft/sec	30.0

Occupational Activities	
Activity	*METS*
Sitting at desk	1.5
Writing	1.5
Riding in automobile	1.5
Watch repairing	1.5
Typing	2.0
Welding	2.5
Radio assembly	2.5
Playing musical instrument	2.5
Parts assembly	3.0
Bricklaying and plastering	3.5
Heavy assembly work	4.0
Wheeling wheelbarrow 115 lb, 2.5 mph	4.0
Carpentry	5.5
Mowing lawn by handmower	6.5
Chopping wood	6.5
Shoveling	7.0
Digging	7.5

Recreational Activities	
Activity	*METS*
Painting, sitting	1.5
Playing piano	2.0
Driving car	2.0
Canoeing, 2.5 mph	2.5
Horseback riding, walk	2.5
Volleyball, 6-man recreational	3.0
Billiards	3.0
Bowling	3.5
Horseshoes	3.5
Golf	4.0
Cricket	4.0
Archery	4.5
Ballroom dancing	4.5
Table tennis	4.5
Baseball	4.5
Tennis	6.0
Horseback riding, trot	6.5
Folk dancing	6.5
Skiing	8.0
Horseback riding, gallop	8.0
Squash rackets	8.5
Fencing	9.0
Basketball	9.0
Football	9.0
Gymnastics	10.0
Handball and paddleball	10.0

Physical-Conditioning Activities	
Activity	*METS*
Level walking, 2 mph (1 mi in 30 min)	2.5
Level cycling, 5.5 mph	
(1 mi in 10 min 54 sec)	3.0
Level cycling, 6 mph (1 mi in 10 min)	3.5
Level walking, 2.5 mph (1 mi in 24 min)	3.5
Level walking, 3 mph (1 mi in 20 min)	4.5
Calisthenics	4.5
Level cycling, 9.7 mph	
(1 mi in 6 min 18 sec)	5.0

Table 15–8 *Physiological Changes Resulting from Endurance-Type Physical Conditioning.*

Heart
   Reduced resting heart rate
   Reduced heart rate for standardized, submaximal exercise
   Increased rate of heart rate recovery after standardized exercise
   Increased blood volume pumped per heart beat (stroke volume)
   Increased size of heart muscle (myocardial hypertrophy)
   Increased blood supply to heart muscle
   Increased strength of contraction (contractibility)

Blood Vessels and Blood Chemistry
   Reduced resting systolic and diastolic arterial blood pressure
   Reduced risk of hardening of the arteries (arteriosclerosis)
   Reduced serum lipids, i.e., cholesterol, triglycerides
   Increased blood supply to muscles
   Increased blood volume
   More efficient exchange of oxygen and carbon dioxide in muscles

Lungs
   Increased functional capacity during exercise
   Increased blood supply
   Increased diffusion of respiratory gases
   Reduced nonfunctional volume of lung (residual volume)

Neural, Endocrine, and Metabolic Function
   Increased glucose tolerance
   Increased enzymatic function in muscle cells
   Reduced body fat content (adiposity)
   Increased muscle mass (lean body mass)
   Reduced strain resulting from psychological stress
   Increased maximal oxygen uptake

GENERAL SUMMARY

Patterns of modern living have channeled the average American into an increasingly sedentary existence. Man, however, was designed and built for movement, and it appears that, physiologically, he has not adapted well to this reduced level of activity. Regular exercise is necessary to develop and maintain an optimal level of good health, performance, and appearance. It can increase an individual's physical working capacity by increasing muscle strength and endurance, enhancing the function of the lungs, heart, and blood vessels; increasing the flexibility of joints, and improving the efficiency or skill of movement. For many adults with sedentary occupations, physical activity provides an outlet for job-related tensions or mental fatigue. It also aids in weight control or reduction, improves posture, contributes to a youthful appearance, and increases general vitality. Active individuals appear to have fewer heart attacks than their less active counterparts. Furthermore, if an active individual does suffer an attack, it probably will be less severe and his or her chances of survival are greater. Additionally, more than 50 percent of lower back pain or discomfort is due to poor muscle tone and flexibility of the lower back and to inadequate abdominal muscle tone. In many instances, this disability could be prevented or corrected by proper exercise. And finally, much of the degeneration of bodily functions and structure associated with premature aging seems to be reduced by frequent participation in a program of proper exercise.

An individually prescribed exercise program to

supplement the normal daily activities of most adults is essential for good health. There is a sound physiological basis for such a program. The physiological and medical benefits that generally occur as a result of an increased activity program are summarized in Table 15–8. The magnitude of change in each of these measurements is dependent on the types of activities pursued, their frequency and duration, and the degree of effort (intensity) put into the activity.

STUDY QUESTIONS

1. What are the major causes of death in the United States at this time?
2. What is atherosclerosis, and at what age does it begin?
3. What are the basic risk factors for coronary artery disease?
4. What is the role of exercise in the prevention of coronary artery disease?
5. What is the difference between overweight and obesity?
6. What is ideal body weight and how is it determined?
7. What are some of the health-related problems associated with obesity?
8. What is the most effective treatment of obesity?
9. What role does exercise play in the prevention and treatment of obesity?
10. What are the basic steps in prescribing exercise?
11. What four factors must be considered in the exercise prescription?
12. Which of the above four factors is the most important?
13. Describe the components of a good exercise program.
14. How do you effectively motivate individuals to maintain regular exercise habits?

REFERENCES

Amsterdam, E. A.; Wilmore, J. H.; and DeMaria, A. N. *Exercise in Cardiovascular Health and Disease.* New York: Yorke Medical Books, 1977.

Cooper, K. H. *Aerobics.* New York: M. Evans & Co., 1968.

Cooper, K. H. *The New Aerobics.* M. Evans & Co., 1970.

Cooper, M., and Cooper, K. H. *Aerobics for Women.* M. Evans & Co., 1972.

Daniels, J.; Fitts, R., and Sheehan, G. *Conditioning for Distance Running.* New York: John Wiley & Sons, 1978.

Enos, W. F.; Holmes, R. H.; and Beyer, J. "Coronary Disease among United States Soldiers Killed in Action in Korea." *J. Amer. Med. Assoc.* 152 (1953): 1090–1093.

Faria, I. E., and Cavanagh, P. R. *The Physiology and Biomechanics of Cycling.* New York: John Wiley & Sons, 1978.

Fixx, J. F. *The Complete Book of Running.* New York: Random House, 1977.

Fixx, J. F. *Jim Fixx's Second Book of Running.* New York: Random House, 1980.

Foss, M. L., and Garrick, J. G. *Ski Conditioning.* New York: John Wiley & Sons, 1978.

Fox, S. M., III. "Relationship of Activity Habits to Coronary Heart Disease." In *Exercise Testing and Exercise Training in Coronary Heart Disease,* edited by J. P. Naughton, and H. K. Hellerstein. New York: Academic Press, 1973.

Fox, S. M., III; Naughton, J. P.; and Haskell, W. L.

"Physical Activity and the Prevention of Coronary Heart Disease." *Annals Clin. Res.* 3 (1971): 404–432.

Getchell, B. *Physical Fitness: A Way of Life.* 2nd ed. New York: John Wiley & Sons, 1979.

Kannel, W. B., and Dawber, T. R. "Atherosclerosis as a Pediatric Problem." *J. Pediatrics.* 80 (1972): 544–554.

Katch, F. I., and McArdle, W. D. Nutrition, Weight Control, and Exercise. Boston: Houghton Mifflin Company, 1977.

Kuntzleman, C. T. *Activetics.* New York: Peter H. Wyden Publisher, 1975.

Lowenthal, D. T.; Bharadwaja, K.; and Oaks, W. W. *Therapeutics through Exercise.* New York: Grune & Stratton, 1979.

Mayer, J. *Overweight Causes, Cost, and Control.* Englewood Cliffs, N.J.: Prentice-Hall, Inc., 1968.

Mayer, J. *Human Nutrition: Its Physiological, Medical and Social Aspects.* Springfield, Ill.: Charles C. Thomas, 1972, p. 308.

McNamara, J. J.; Molot, M. A.; Stremple, J. F.; and Cutting, R. T. "Coronary Artery Disease in Combat Casualties in Vietnam." *J. Amer. Med. Assoc.* 216 (1971): 1185–1187.

Naughton, J. P., and Bruhn, J. "Emotional Stress, Physical Activity and Ischemic Heart Disease." *Disease-A-Month,* July 1970, pp. 3–34.

Naughton, J. P., and Hellerstein, H. K. eds. *Exercise Testing and Exercise Training in Coronary Heart Disease.* New York: Academic Press, 1973.

Pollock, M. L. "The Quantification of Endurance Training Programs." In *Exercise and Sport Sciences Reviews,* vol. 1, edited by J. H. Wilmore. New York: Academic Press, 1973.

Pollock, M. L., and Schmidt, D. H., eds. *Heart Disease and Rehabilitation.* Boston: Houghton Mifflin, 1979.

Pollock, M. L.; Wilmore, J. H.; and Fox, S. M. *Health and Fitness through Physical Activity.* New York: John Wiley & Sons, 1978.

Sharkey, B. J. *Physiology of Fitness.* Champaign, Ill.: Human Kinetics Publishers, 1979.

Wilmore, J. H., and McNamara, J. J. "Prevalence of Coronary Heart Disease Risk Factors in Boys 8 to 12 Years of Age." *J. Pediatrics* 84 (1974): 527–533.

Appendices

A

Strength Exercises

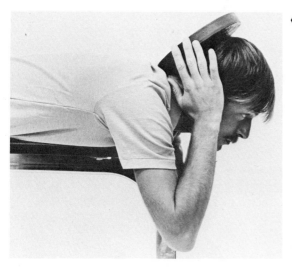

Neck Flexion and Extension. From a sitting position or a supine position on a bench, hold the appropriate weight against the head. Slowly curl or flex the head forward to the chest or extend the head backward as far as it will go.

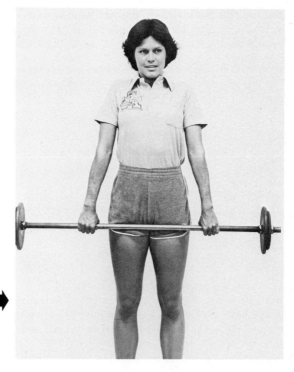

Shoulder Shrug. Holding the weight with an overhand or pronated grip, arms extended downward from a standing position, shrug the shoulders up and back, attempting to increase the range of joint movement with successive repetitions.

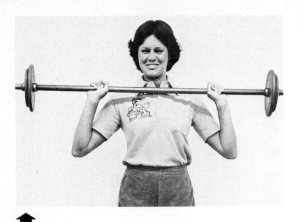

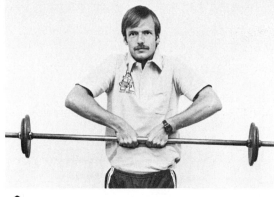

Military or Overhead Press. Standing with the feet shoulder-width apart, bend the knees to a 45-degree angle and reach down and grab the bar with an overhand grip, hands spread shoulder-width apart. Lift the weight to the starting position by straightening the legs. As the bar approaches the hips, bend the knees slightly and snap the elbows under the bar. With the back straight, bar at chest level, lift the weight up and over head, locking the elbows out at full extension. Return the bar to the chest level.

Behind-the-Neck Press. Execute exactly as described for the military press, except return the bar behind the head to the back of the neck with each repetition.

Upright Rowing. Grab the bar with the hands almost touching, using an overhand grip. Starting with the bar at waist or hip level, lift the bar to the height of the chin, elbows extended outward, and return to the starting position.

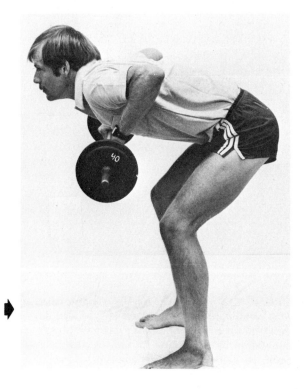

Bent Rowing. With the knees bent to a 45-degree angle, bend over at the waist, back parallel to the ground. Grasp the bar with an overhand grip, hands shoulder-width apart. Using the arms only, lift the bar to the chest, and return to the starting position.

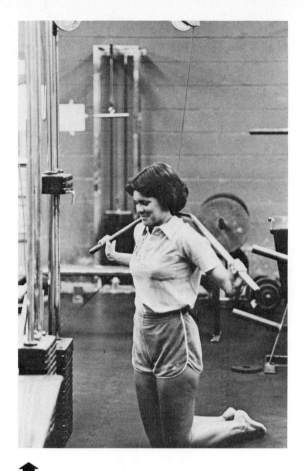

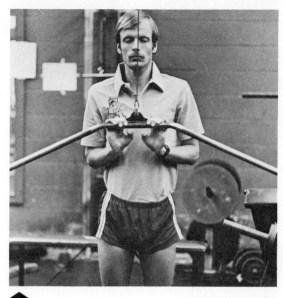

Triceps Extension. From a standing position, hands close together in an overhand grip, bar of the lat machine at eye level, pull or press the bar downward through the full range of motion, and return to the starting position.

Lat Machine or Pull-Down. From a seated or kneeling position, grab the bar of the lat machine with an overhand grip, hands shoulder-width apart. Pull the bar down until it touches the base of the neck and shoulders, and return to the starting position.

Lateral Arm Raise. With one dumbbell in each hand, arms hanging downward to the side of the body, raise both arms out to the side of the body to an overhead position, keeping the elbows locked in extension. Return to the starting position.

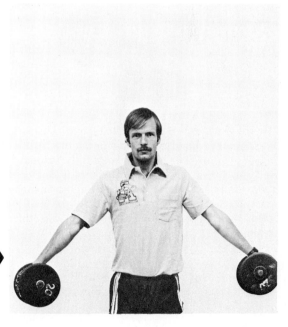

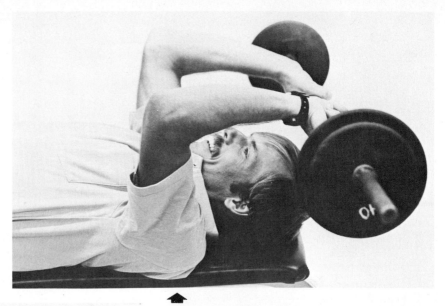

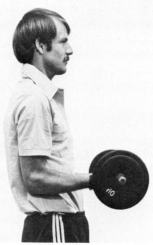

Bent-Arm Pull-Over. Lying supine on the bench, with the barbell in an overhand grasp, hands shoulder-width apart, and with the barbell over head, lower it slowly over and behind the head, as far back as possible, and return to the starting position.

Biceps Curl. Grasp the bar shoulder-width apart, using an underhand grip. Bring the bar to a position of rest against the thighs, elbows fully extended, and feet spread shoulder-width apart. Using only the arms, raise the bar to the chest and return to the starting position. Keep the back straight, and always return to a position with the elbows fully extended.

Dumbbell Curl. Execute in exactly the same manner as the biceps curl, using a dumbbell instead of a barbell.

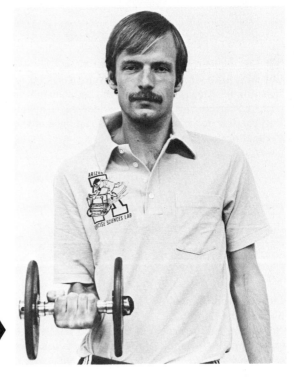

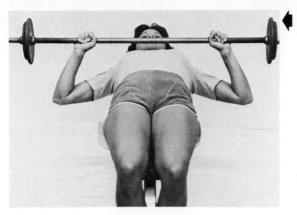

Bench Press. From a supine position on a bench, take the weight with an overhand grip, hands shoulder-width apart, elbows fully extended. Lower the weight to the chest, and return to the starting position.

Incline Press. Execute in exactly the same manner as the bench press, except that the exercise is performed on a bench inclined to approximately a 45-degree angle.

Bar Dip. Starting with the weight supported by both arms extended on two bars, lower the body until the upper and lower arm form a 90-degree angle, and return to the starting position.

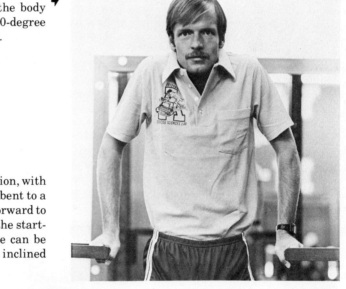

Weighted Sit-Ups. From the supine position, with a weight behind the head and neck, knees bent to a 90-degree angle, curl the head and trunk forward to an upright sitting position, and return to the starting position. A somewhat similar exercise can be performed without a weight by using an inclined board.

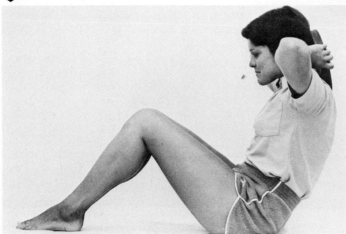

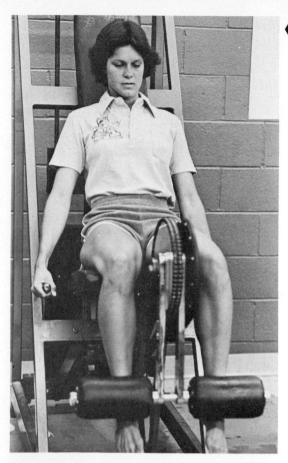

Knee Extension. Sitting on the edge of the leg extension machine with the knee flexed to a 90-degree angle, extend the knee outward, until it locks out in full extension, then return to the starting position.

Knee Flexion. Using a leg machine, assume a prone position, legs extended. Flex at the knee joint through the range of motion, and return to the starting position.

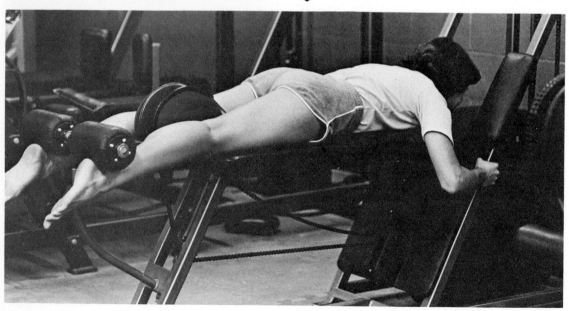

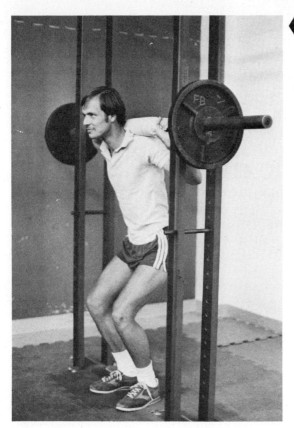

Squat. Standing erect, with the weight balanced comfortably across the top of the shoulders, using an overhand grip, hands spread shoulder-width apart, lower the weight by bending at the knees to a 90-degree angle, and return to the starting position. Keep the back straight.

Hack Squat. Follow the instructions for the squat, except hold the bar behind the legs, and elevate the heels on a block of wood.

Toe Raise. Standing erect, with the balls of the feet on a block of wood, assume the same position described for the squat. Rise up on the toes as far as possible, and return to a position where the heels are slightly lower than the block of wood.

B

Warm-Up and Flexibility Exercises

Head Rotation. Standing up straight, with hands on hips and feet spread shoulder-width apart, slowly rotate the head clockwise in a full circle. Reverse to a counter-clockwise direction.

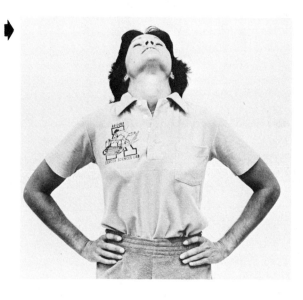

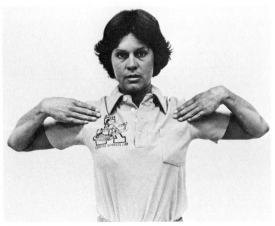

Chest and Shoulder Stretch. Standing erect, arms bent in front of chest at shoulder height, with finger tips touching shoulders, pull the elbows back as far as possible, and return to the starting position. Then swing the arms outward and sideward, and return them to the original position.

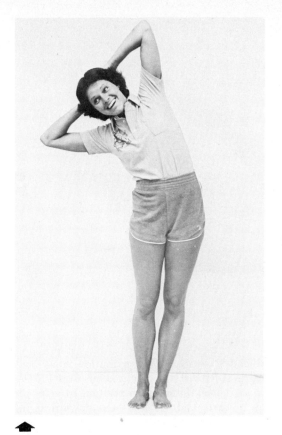

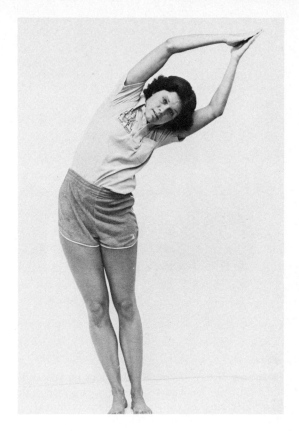

Trunk Rotation. Standing up straight, with feet placed together and hands behind the head, rotate the trunk as far as possible to the right and return, then to the left and return. Move at a moderate pace, and try to gradually increase the range of movement.

Side Body Bend. Standing up straight, with feet placed together and arms extended overhead, bend the trunk slowly to the left as far as it can go, and then return to the starting position. Repeat the same motion to the right. Again, try to increase the range of movement gradually.

Half-Knee Bend and Trunk Rotation. Standing up straight with feet together and hands on hips, bend the knees to a half-sit position, extend the arms out in front, and twist the trunk to the right. Return to the original position, and repeat this movement to the left.

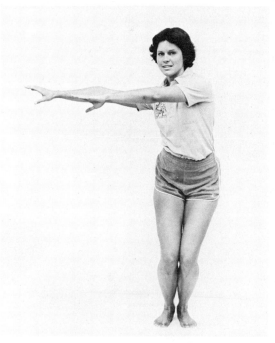

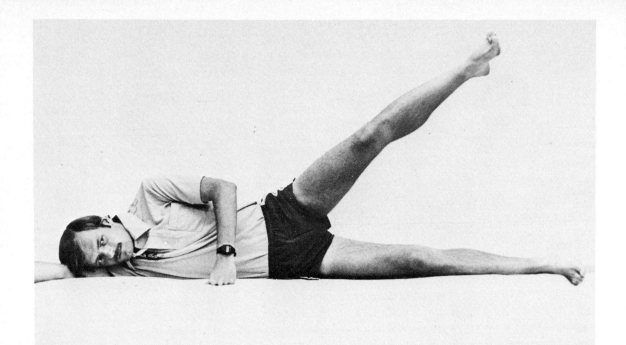

▲

Side Leg Raise. Lying on the floor on the right side with the head resting on the extended right arm, lift the leg upward to approximately a 45-degree angle. Hold in this position for three to five seconds then return to the starting position. Repeat on the opposite side.

Modified Push-Up. With a limited upper-body strength, start with the modified push-up. Lie flat on the stomach, hands in a position to push the trunk upward, and the legs bent upward at the knees. Keeping the back straight and in line with the buttocks, raise the trunk until the arms are fully extended at the elbow. Lower the body to a position where the chest just touches the floor, and then push back up to the fully extended position. This exercise is to be done with the arms only, so immobilize the rest of the body.

▼

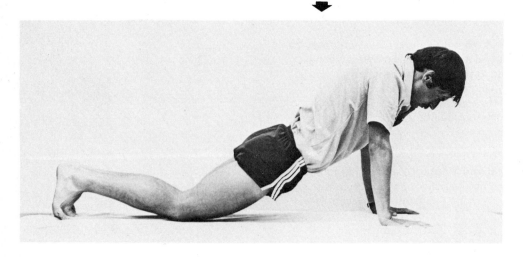

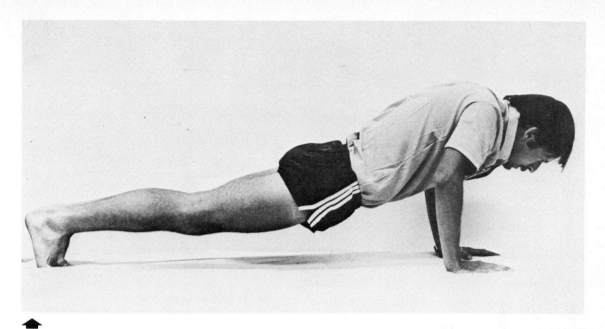

Full Push-Up. Once you have mastered thirty repetitions of the modified push-up, you have the strength to perform the full push-up. Perform this exercise exactly as you did the modified version, except now use the toes, and not the knees, as the point of support. This forces you to lift a greater percentage of your body weight.

Head and Shoulder Curl. Lie on the back with the legs fully extended in front. Place the hands behind either the head or neck. Now, slowly curl the head and shoulders up to about a 45-degree angle as illustrated in the figure. Hold this position for about five seconds, and then return to the starting position.

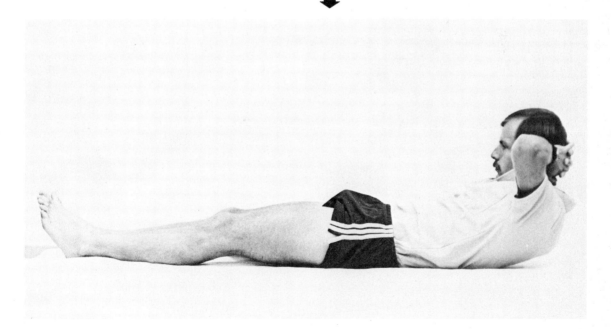

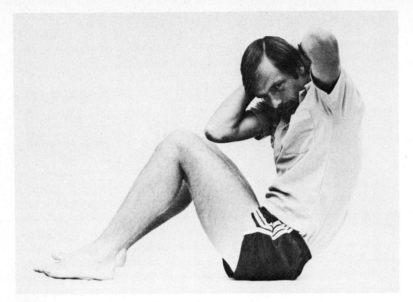

Full Sit-Up. Start in the same position as the head and shoulder curl, lying on the back, but this time bend the knees to a 90-degree angle. With the hands behind the head, curl the head, shoulders, and trunk slowly upward to a full sitting position and touch one of the knees with the opposite elbow. Return slowly to the starting position and repeat.

Start with ten repetitions and gradually build up to forty.

Trunk Lifter. Lying on the stomach with the hands behind the head and a partner holding the feet, slowly extend the trunk upward as far as possible and hold in this position for three to five seconds.

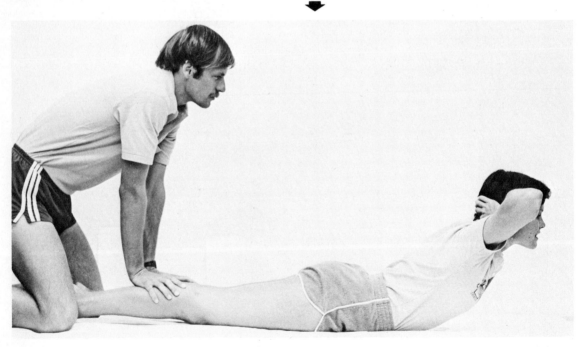

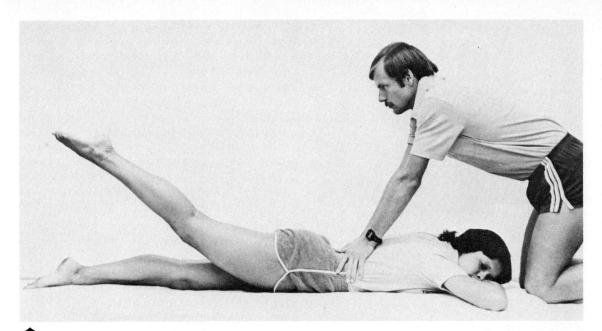

Leg Lifter. Lying on the stomach with a partner holding down the back, lift the right leg up as high as possible keeping the stomach and hips pressed flat against the floor. Hold in this position for three to five seconds, and then return to the original position. Repeat with the left leg.

Hip-Flexor Stretch. Lying on the back, bring the right knee to the chest, grab the leg below the knee, and pull the knee slowly toward the chest. Hold this stretched position for five seconds, and repeat with the opposite leg. Repeat for a total of five repetitions for each leg.

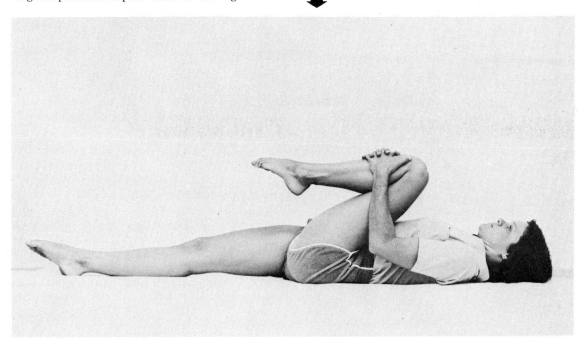

263

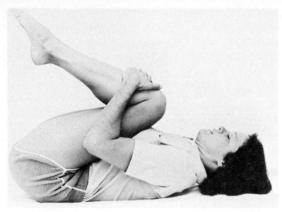

Lower-Back Stretch. Lying on the back, bring both knees to the chest, grab each leg below the knee, and pull both knees slowly toward the shoulder. Hold this stretched position for five seconds, and repeat for a total of five repetitions.

Upper-Trunk Stretch. Lying on the stomach, push the upper body off the mat to a position where the arms are fully extended. Concentrate on keeping the pelvis or hips flat on the floor. Hold in this stretched position for five seconds, and repeat for a total of five repetitions.

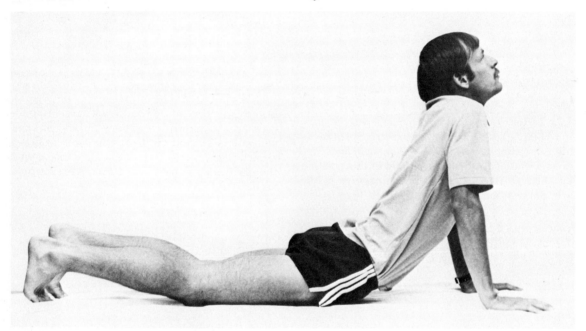

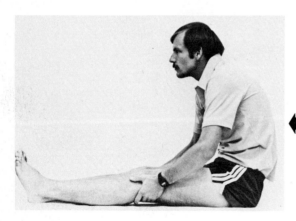

Hamstring Stretch. Sitting on the floor with the legs extended out in front, force the knees flat against the floor, grab behind the knees, and slowly pull the head down toward the knees. Do not bounce or bob, but move slowly. Hold in this stretched position for five seconds, and repeat for a total of five repetitions.

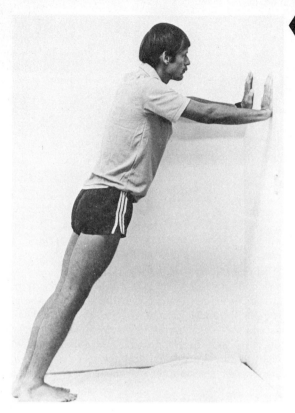

Lower-Leg and Heel Stretch. Standing approximately three feet from a wall, extend the arms out, touching the wall, and gradually let the body lean forward toward the wall, keeping the feet planted firmly on the ground. You will feel the stretch in the lower leg and heel area. Hold in the stretched position for five seconds, and repeat for a total of five repetitions.

Back Arch. Kneeling on the hands and knees, with the knees three to four inches apart directly under the hips, and the arms directly under the shoulders, drop the head forward, contract the stomach and buttocks muscles, and arch the lower back. Hold in this position for three to five seconds, and then relax, repeating for a total of five repetitions.

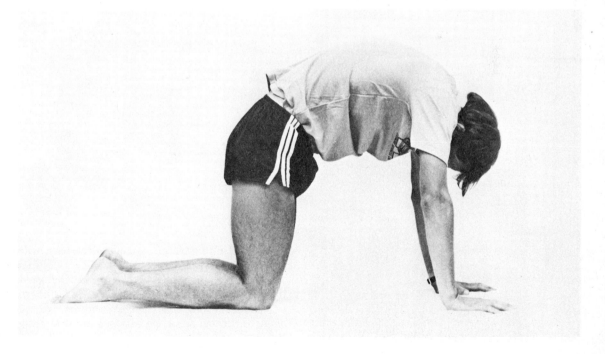

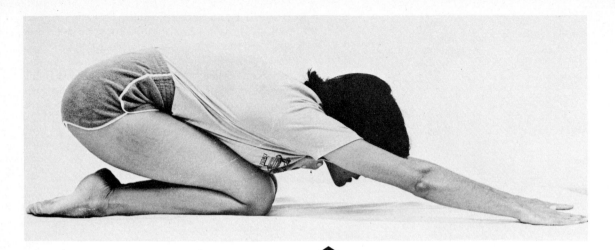

Bar Hang. Locate a bar or some other suitable object that is just slightly taller than the extended reach. Use a stool or jump up and grab the bar, and then hang from the bar for twenty to thirty seconds. Repeat for a total of two repetitions.

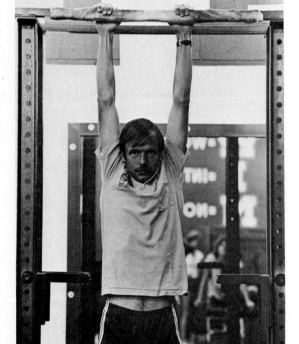

Abdominal Stretch. Starting in the kneeling position identical to that explained for the back arch, swing the trunk forward over the shoulders, bend the elbows and lower the chest to the floor. Then extend the arms forward, lower the head, and raise the buttocks as high as possible by arching the back. Hold in this position for five seconds, then relax, and repeat for a total of five repetitions.

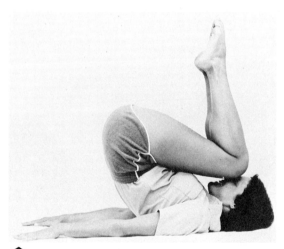

Back and Hip Stretch. Lying on the back with the arms extended to the sides, tilt the hips upward and bring the knees up and toward the head, keeping the arms and back pressed firmly against the floor. Hold in this stretched position for five seconds, and then relax, repeating a total of three times.

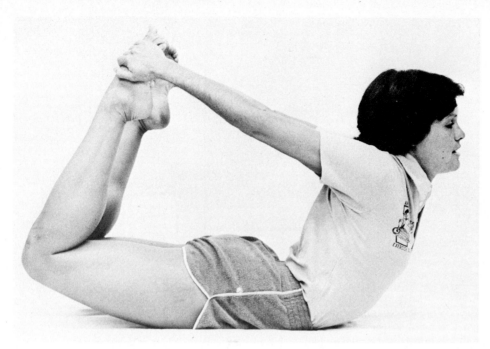

Lower-Trunk Stretch. Lying flat on the stomach, reach back and grab the ankles, arch the back and pull the head up slowly as high as possible. Hold in this position for five seconds, then relax, and repeat for a total of three repetitions.

Upper-Back Stretch. Lying flat on the back with the arms extended along the side of the body, raise the legs up and over the head and, keeping the knees locked in an extended position, attempt to touch the floor behind the head. Keep the back and arms flat on the floor. Hold in this position for five seconds, then relax, and repeat for a total of three repetitions.

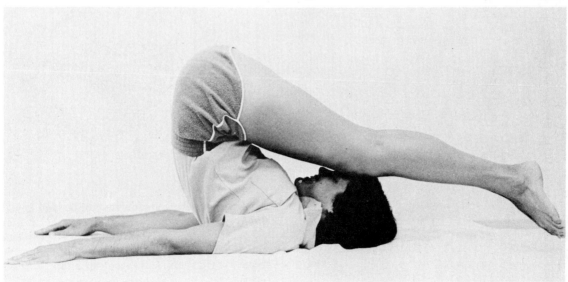

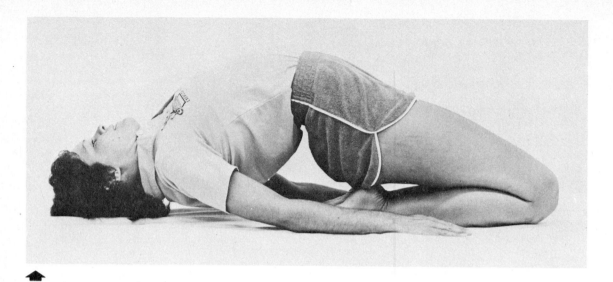

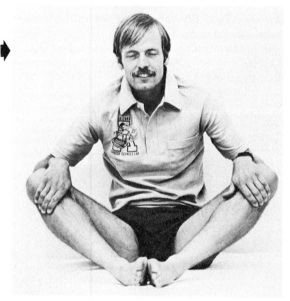

Kneeling Back Bend. Kneeling with both knees and ankles on the floor, very slowly lean backward, attempting to touch the head to the floor. This should be attempted only after having developed above-average flexibility. Repeat for a total of three repetitions.

Sitting Groin Stretch. Sitting with the soles of the feet touching and the knees pointing outward, slowly push down on the knees, attempting to gradually, over time, push them to the floor. Hold in the stretched position for five seconds, then relax, and repeat for a total of three repetitions.

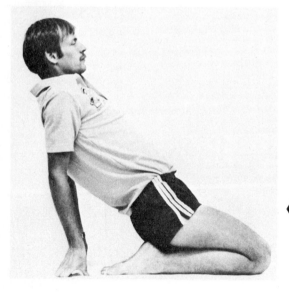

Toe Pointer. Kneeling on the ankles and knees, slowly sit back on the heels with the ankles stretched backward. Gradually raise the knees from the floor. Hold in a stretched position for five seconds, then relax, and repeat for a total of three repetitions.

268

C

Field Tests for Assessing Physical Fitness

INTRODUCTION

An extensive physical fitness assessment of athletes and the fitness-conscious public is available through elaborate testing facilities in human performance laboratories at most major universities and colleges, in some hospitals and research institutes, and even in several high schools. Unfortunately, however, these laboratory facilities cannot meet the volume of tests requested by coaches, athletes, and the general population. As a result, field tests of the various components of physical fitness and athletic performance must be relied on. A field test is a simple test, which requires minimum equipment and facilities but which provides an accurate estimate of a particular component. This appendix includes one, or more, field tests for each of the basic components discussed in Section B, Fundamentals of Physical Training, of this book.

STRENGTH

Strength can be easily assessed by the one-repetition maximum test (1-RM). The basic muscle or muscle group to be tested is selected and the individual is given a series of trials to determine the greatest weight that he or she can lift just once for that particular lift. If the individual is an inexperienced weight lifter, this test is conducted largely through trial and error. Start with a weight that the individual can lift comfortably, then keep adding

weight until he or she can lift the weight correctly just one time. If this weight can be lifted more than once, more weight should be added until a true 1-RM is reached. While 1-RM's can be obtained for any basic weight-training exercise, test batteries usually select three or four exercises that represent the body's major muscle groups. Table C–1 gives a series of values for selected strength exercises for both males and females on the basis of body weight. While the strength requirements will differ for each sport or activity, and even by position within each sport, these values represent optimal values for the average athlete who is training mainly for general fitness. Specific standards for each sport have yet to be developed.

Additional strength tests are available using dynamometers, cable tensiometers, and elaborate force transducers and recorders. These tests, however, require expensive equipment and do not cause any substantial improvement in measurement accuracy. Refer to a recent text in measurement and evaluation (e.g., Baumgartner and Jackson, 1975) for additional information on these laboratory-types of tests.

POWER

Power is the application of strength through distance per unit of time. Power can be assessed very accurately in the laboratory, using expensive force transducers and recorders. Several field tests have

Table C–1   *Optimal Strength Values for Various Body Weights (Based on the 1-RM test)*

Body Weight lb	Bench Press Male	Bench Press Female	Standing Press Male	Standing Press Female	Curl Male	Curl Female	Leg Press Male	Leg Press Female
80	80	56	53	37	40	28	160	112
100	100	70	67	47	50	35	200	140
120	120	84	80	56	60	42	240	168
140	140	98	93	65	70	49	280	196
160	160	112	107	75	80	56	320	224
180	180	126	120	84	90	63	360	252
200	200	140	133	93	100	70	400	280
220	220	154	147	103	110	77	440	308
240	240	168	160	112	120	84	480	336

been proposed but lack objective validation. The sitting shotput and medicine ball throw have been used to estimate upper-body power, while the standing long jump and vertical jump have been used to estimate lower-body power. Unfortunately, standards for these tests have not been established.

The Margaria-Kalamen leg-power test (Mathews and Fox, 1971) represents a more objective measure of lower-body power. The subject begins by standing six meters in front of a series of steps. On command, he runs as quickly as possible up the stairs, stepping on every third step. A microswitch embedded in a rubber mat is placed on the third step and activates a timer when the subject hits this step. A second microswitch is placed on the ninth step, which stops the timer when hit (Figure C–1). The elapsed time represents the time required to move the body weight the vertical distance between the third and ninth steps. Power is then calculated by the formula,

$$\text{Power (kg} \times \text{meters/sec)} = \frac{\text{Body weight (kg)} \times \text{vertical distance (meters)}}{\text{elapsed time (sec)}}$$

Standards for power on the basis of the Margaria-Kalamen leg-power test have not yet been calculated. Costill et al. (1968) tested a group of college football players using the original version of this test.

MUSCULAR ENDURANCE

Muscular endurance has been measured in a number of different ways, including the greatest number of sit-ups that can be performed in a fixed period of time (usually thirty seconds or one minute) or the maximum number of push-ups, pull-ups, or bar dips that can be performed continuously in an indefinite time period. Many of these tests penalize the participant who has long legs, short arms, or a heavy body weight. To eliminate this bias, a concept has evolved that uses a fixed percentage of the individual's body weight as the resistance. The individual lifts this weight as many times as possible, until reaching the point of fatigue or exhaustion. Firm guidelines have yet to be established for the percentages of the individual's body weight in relation to the muscle groups tested. In fact, it is debatable whether the weight used in the test should be a fixed percentage of the individual's body weight or a fixed percentage of the individual's 1-RM or absolute strength. For example, if the endurance test for the bench press movement were conducted using 50 percent of the individual's body weight as the resistance, a 180-pound man would be asked to lift 90 pounds as many times as he could. A strong man of this body weight would be able to lift this 90-pound weight twenty, or more, times, while a relatively weak man who weighed 180 pounds might not be able to lift the 90-pound weight even one time, i.e., the designated weight exceeds his 1-RM. In this case, the test for muscular endurance would be highly dependent on strength. To isolate muscular endurance as a pure component, so that the test is not so dependent on the individual's strength, it is advocated that the test battery be established on the basis of the individual's strength and not his body weight.

In accordance with these recommendations, it is

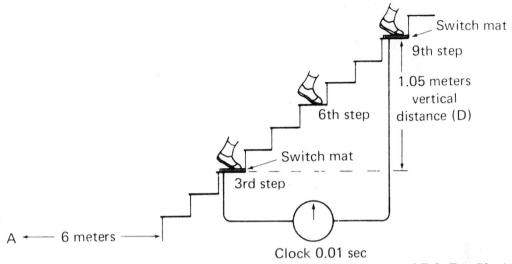

Figure C–1 The Margaria-Kalamen leg-power test. (From D. K. Mathews and E. L. Fox, *Physiological Basis of Physical Education and Athletics*. Philadelphia: W. C. Saunders Co., 1971. Reproduced by permission of the publisher.)

suggested that a fixed percentage of 70 percent of the maximum strength be used to test muscle endurance. This percentage would be the same for all movements tested. Since this is a relatively new concept, norms or standards have yet to be established, but they could be easily established for each specific population to be tested. On the basis of limited test data, the recreational athlete or health-seeking exerciser should be able to perform twelve to fifteen repetitions, and the competitive athlete, twenty to twenty-five repetitions at 70 percent of his or her maximum strength for each of the movements tested.

SPEED

Speed can be estimated simply by measuring the time it takes to cover a set distance. This can be accomplished for the individual body segments, such as for the arm or leg, by using an elaborate system of microswitches and an electronic timer. The limb is placed on the first microswitch, and when the movement starts, the microswitch contact is broken, starting the timer. When the limb has traveled a set distance, the clock is stopped when the limb makes contact with a second microswitch. Total body speed can be measured by timing the

athlete over a set distance from twenty to one hundred yards. Again, norms or standards have not been established and would vary considerably by sex, age, body size, and sport. It is suggested that each sport or activity, and position within each sport, have its own standards for optimal performance. Many coaches have already done this for football (forty-yard-dash time) and baseball (ninety-foot-dash or circle-the-bases time).

In order to differentiate speed into its two components, acceleration and peak velocity, the reader should refer to Chapter 5, where this was discussed at some length.

AGILITY

The concept of agility is difficult to precisely define operationally, even though there is general agreement among most coaches, athletes, and researchers as to what is meant by the term *agility*. Agility, typically, refers to the ability to move and change body position or directions rapidly, without losing balance or sacrificing speed. Agility is exemplified by the shifty halfback on a broken field run in football, or the supple gymnast, performing a complex, free-exercise routine. Unfortunately, there are no universally accepted tests of agility, although many test batteries exist, which use various shuttle run tests to estimate the agility component. While shuttle run tests have some merit, they are largely tests of speed and are far removed from assessing what is traditionally thought of in the athletic world as agility. This is an area where new tests or test batteries are needed. Refer to a standard measurement and evaluation text for examples of existing tests of agility (Baumgartner and Jackson, 1975).

FLEXIBILITY

Probably the most accurate tests of flexibility presently available are those that assess the actual range of motion of the various joints. While this is easily accomplished by instruments such as the Leighton Flexometer and the electrogoniometer (illustrated in Chapter 5), these pieces of equipment are not readily available. Simple field tests include

the sit-and-reach test (see Figure 5–2) and the back-hyperextension test (Figure C–2).

In the sit-and-reach test, the individual sits with the legs extended directly in front of him or her and the back of the knees pressed against the floor. The feet are placed against a stool to which a yardstick is attached, with the fourteen-inch mark placed at the point where the foot contacts the stool. The individual places the index fingers of both hands together and reaches forward slowly, as far as possible. The distance reached is noted on the yardstick and recorded. The knees must be kept in contact with the floor, and bouncing is to be discouraged. Standards for an athletic population are presented in Table C–2. Obviously, this test will be influenced by the length of the arms and legs of the individual, in addition to his or her flexibility.

The back hyperextension test is performed with the individual in the prone position, lying on the floor. With the individual's feet being held in place, the individual arches the back and lifts the chest

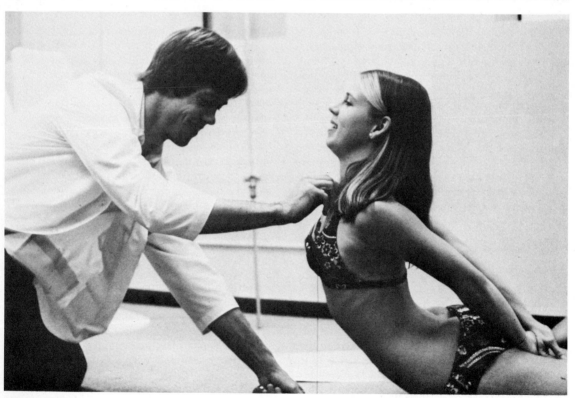

Figure C–2 Back hyperextension test.

Table C–2   *Standards for the Sit-and-Reach, and the Back-Hyperextension Flexibility Tests*

	Sit-and-Reach	Back Hyperextension
Excellent	22 inches or greater	56 or greater
Good	20–21 inches	46–55
Average	14–18 inches	36–45
Fair	12–13 inches	26–35
Poor	11 inches or less	25 or less

From Health Improvement Program, *National Athletic Health Institute, Inglewood, Calif. Reproduced by permission.*

and chin as far off the floor as possible (Figure C–2). The distance between the floor and the sternal notch is measured. Then, the individual sits on the floor with his or her back and buttocks against a wall, and the distance between the floor and sternal notch is measured again. The flexibility score is determined by the following equation:

Back hyperextension =
$$\frac{\text{hyperextension height}}{\text{seated sternal height}} \times 100$$

Dividing the hyperextension height attained by the seated sternal height provides an estimate of the angle of flexibility, and partially negates the advantage of having a long trunk. Standards for the back hyperextension test are presented in Table C–2.

CARDIOVASCULAR ENDURANCE CAPACITY

Aerobic or cardiovascular endurance capacity can be estimated on the basis of an endurance-run test. The Balke 1.5-mile run is suggested for general use by older adolescents and adults. For children and young adolescents, a shorter test of approximately 1.0 mile would be more appropriate. Running for a fixed distance has a distinct administrative advantage over a test that is based on the distance covered in a fixed time. With a fixed difference, each individual ends the test at the same place and scoring is accomplished simply by taking the time needed to complete that distance. Hundreds of individuals can be tested simultaneously when a fixed distance is used. Table C–3 lists the various 1.5-mile run times and the estimated equivalent $\dot{V}O_2$ max. Previous studies have shown from moderate to high

correlations, i.e., approximately $r = 0.60$ to $r = 0.90$, between running performance tests and $\dot{V}O_2$ max.

Table C–3   *Estimated $\dot{V}O_2$ max for 1.5 Mile Endurance-Run Time* [*][†]

Time min:sec	Estimated $\dot{V}O_2$ max ml/kg × min
7:30 and under	75
7:31– 8:00	72
8:01– 8:30	67
8:31– 9:00	62
9:01– 9:30	58
9:31–10:00	55
10:01–10:30	52
10:31–11:00	49
11:01–11:30	46
11:31–12:00	44
12:01–12:30	41
12:31–13:00	39
13:01–13:30	37
13:31–14:00	36
14:01–14:30	34
14:31–15:00	33
15:01–15:30	31
15:31–16:00	30
16:01–16:30	28
16:31–17:00	27
17:01–17:30	26
17:31–18:00	25

[*]*Adapted from K. H. Cooper, "A Means of Assessing Maximal Oxygen Intake," J. Amer. Med. Assoc. 203 (1968): 201–204.*
[†]*Refer to Table C–4 for a rating of the estimated $\dot{V}O_2$ max.*

Table C–4 *Range of Maximal Oxygen Uptake Values with Age* *

Age Group (yr)	Maximal Oxygen Uptake, ml/kg •min				
	Low	*Fair*	*Average*	*Good*	*High*
10–19	below 38	38–46	47–56	57–66	above 66
20–29	below 33	33–42	43–52	53–62	above 62
30–39	below 30	30–38	39–48	49–58	above 58
40–49	below 26	26–35	36–44	45–54	above 54
50–59	below 24	24–33	34–41	42–50	above 50
60–69	below 22	22–30	31–38	39–46	above 46
70–79	below 20	20–27	28–35	36–42	above 42

*Since females are generally 20 percent lower on the average compared to males, normal values for females can be obtained by shifting over one category to the right, e.g., the "fair" category for males would be considered "good" for females.

The 1.5-mile test can be run on either a track or on a 1.5-mile nonrepeating course. The latter may be preferred to assure that each individual covers a full 1.5 mile and does not stop a lap or two short. This test should be given only to those who are in condition or have been conditioned to run the distance. Pretraining is essential and will help resolve problems of pacing frequently encountered in endurance-running tests. Those over twenty-five to thirty years of age should not be encouraged to take this test until they have had a stress electrocardiogram (see Chapter 15) and been diagnosed as normal, in addition to having a routine physical examination.

BODY COMPOSITION

The individual's body composition can be most accurately estimated by the underwater weighing technique. While it is usually a laboratory technique, underwater weighing can be used as a field test also (see Figure 7–7). For the purposes of this book, it is assumed that the residual volume will not be assessable for measurement. It is possible in college-age individuals or younger to use an assumed constant residual volume without sacrificing too much accuracy. Estimated residual volumes by age and sex are listed in Table C–5.

A scale is attached to the diving board or is hung from some other form of support, approximately eighteen to twenty-four inches from the edge of the pool, at a point where the water is at least three feet

deep. The scale should be accurately calibrated prior to use, by hanging known weights from it and noting the readings. Since the residual lung volume is measured in liters, weight must also be expressed in metric units, i.e., kilograms (weight in pounds divided by 2.205). The individual to be assessed sits on a chair, a weight, or some other type of seat suspended from the scale, or simply hangs from a rope or chain attached to the scale. The underwater weight of the individual is determined by having him or her totally submerge, exhaling as he or she goes under water. The highest weight attained at

Table C–5 *Estimated Residual Lung Volumes by Sex and Age*

Age yr	Estimated Residual Volume (liters)
Females	
6–10	0.60
11–15	0.80
16–20	1.00
21–25	1.20
26–30	1.40
Males	
6–10	0.90
11–15	1.10
16–20	1.30
21–25	1.50
26–30	1.70

the conclusion of his maximal exhalation represents the person's gross underwater weight. A minimum of five to ten trials should be given each individual, since it takes practice and experience before an accurate weight can be obtained. The average of the two or three heaviest trials is selected as the representative gross weight for that individual. The weight of the seat, chain, or other supporting material must then be subtracted from the gross weight in order to obtain the individual's actual, or net, weight underwater. Body density is then calculated as follows:

$$\text{Density} = \frac{\text{Body weight}}{\text{Body volume}}$$

Body Volume =

$$\frac{[\text{Weight (kg)} - \text{net underwater weight (kg)}]}{\text{density of water}}$$

$$- \text{ estimated residual volume}$$

Since most pools are heated to approximately 76–78°F, a constant density of water of 0.997 will be used.

$$\text{Relative fat (\%)} = [(495/\text{density}) - 450]$$

$$\text{Fat weight} = \text{Weight} \times \text{Relative fat}/100$$

$$\text{Lean weight} = \text{Weight} - \text{Fat weight}$$

As an example of these calculations, a male eighteen years of age weighs 180 pounds and has a net underwater weight of 8 pounds. His estimated residual volume from Table C–5 would be 1.30 liters. His body composition would be calculated as follows:

$$\text{Weight} = 180 \text{ lb} = 81.6 \text{ kg}$$

$$\text{Net underwater weight} = 8 \text{ lb} = 3.6 \text{ kg}$$

Volume =
$$\frac{(81.6 - 3.6)}{0.997} - 1.3 = 78.2 - 1.3 = 76.9$$

$$\text{Density} = \frac{81.6}{76.9} = 1.061$$

Relative fat (%) =
$$[(495/1.061) - 450] = 466.5 - 450 = 16.5\%$$

$$\text{Fat weight} = 16.5\% \times 180 \text{ lb}/100 = 29.7 \text{ lb}$$

$$\text{Lean weight} = 180 \text{ lb} - 29.7 = 150.3 \text{ lb}$$

Anthropometric measurements can also be used to estimate the various components of body composition, i.e., body density, relative or absolute fat, and lean body weight. Skinfold thicknesses, body diameters or breadths, and body circumferences or girths have been used in the past with reasonable accuracy to estimate body composition. Table C–6 lists a series of equations derived by various authors for different ages and both sexes. When estimating body composition, select an equation representative of the population to be tested.

The anatomical landmarks for the various sites are illustrated in Figures C–3 and C–4 and described as follows:

Chest. Diagonal fold directly above the axilla.

Scapula. Inferior angle of the scapula with the fold running parallel to the axillary border.

Triceps. Midway between the acromion and olecranon processes on the posterior aspect of the

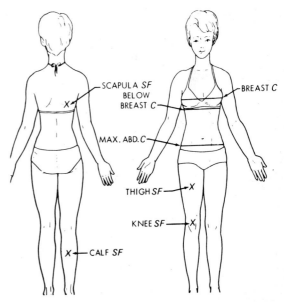

Figure C–3 Skinfold measurement sites. (From Albert R. Behnke and Jack H. Wilmore, *Evaluation and Regulation of Body Build and Composition,* © 1974, p. 28. Reprinted by permission of Prentice-Hall, Inc., Englewood Cliffs, New Jersey.)

Table C–6 *Equations Based on Sex and Age for Determining Body Composition*

Age (yr)	Equation	Study
Females		
9–12	Density = 1.079 − (0.043 × log of scapula skinfold*)	Parízková (1961)
13–16	Density = 1.102 − (0.058 × log of scapula skinfold*)	Parízková (1961)
17–35	Lean weight (kg) = 8.63 + [0.68 × weight (kg)] − [0.16 × scapula skinfold] − [0.10 × triceps skinfold] − [0.05 × thigh skinfold]	Wilmore and Behnke (1970)
18–55	Density = 1.214 − (0.0406 × log of triceps, thigh and suprailiac skinfold*) − (0.00016 × age)	Jackson, et al. (1980)
Males		
9–12	Density = 1.094 − (0.054 × log of scapula skinfold*)	Parízková (1961)
13–16	Density = 1.131 − (0.083 × log of triceps skinfold*)	Parízková (1961)
17–35	Lean weight (kg) = 10.26 + [0.793 × weight (kg)] − [0.368 × abdominal skinfold]	Wilmore and Behnke (1969)
36–67	Lean weight (kg) = 6.14 + [0.84 × weight (kg)] − [0.63 × midaxillary skinfold]	Lewis et al. (1975)
18–61	Density = 1.1886 − (0.0305 × log of chest, abdomen and thigh skinfold*) − (0.00027 × age)	Jackson and Pollock (1978)

*Take the log of the skinfold or the sum of the three skinfolds from a table of logarithms and multiply it by the designated constant.

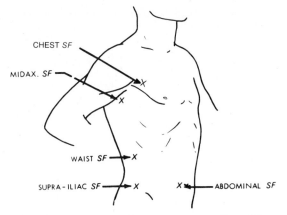

Figure C–4 Skinfold measurement sites. (From Albert R. Behnke and Jack H. Wilmore, *Evaluation and Regulation of Body Build and Composition,* © 1974, p. 28. Reprinted by permission of Prentice-Hall, Inc., Englewood Cliffs, New Jersey.)

arm, the arm held vertically, with the fold running parallel to the length of the arm.

Midaxillary. Vertical fold on the midaxillary line approximately at the level of the fifth rib.

Abdominal. Horizontal fold adjacent to the umbilicus.

Suprailiac. Vertical fold on the crest of the ilium at the midaxillary line.

Thigh. Vertical fold on the anterior aspect of the thigh midway between the hip and knee joints.

A special caliper* is used to assess the fat that lies directly beneath the skin. The skin-fold is grasped firmly by the thumb and index finger, and the caliper is placed on the exact site one-half to one inch from the thumb and finger (Figure C–5).

Once one of the body composition parameters is assessed, the remaining parameters can be estimated by using the relationships defined earlier. As an example of this, if lean weight were estimated from selected measurements, fat weight would be the difference between the total body weight and lean weight, and relative fat would be calculated by the ratio of fat weight to total weight multiplied by 100 to convert from decimal to percentage.

*The Harpenden caliper (No. 3496) is recommended. Quinton Instruments, 2121 Terry Ave., Seattle, Wash. 98121.

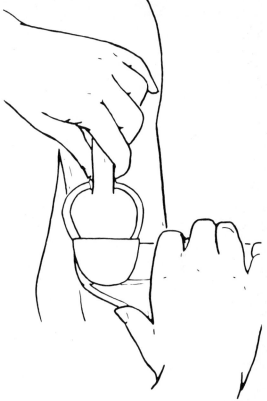

Figure C–5 Technique for obtaining the triceps skinfold thickness. (From Albert R. Behnke and Jack H. Wilmore, *Evaluation and Regulation of Body Build and Composition,* © 1974, p. 28. Reprinted by permission of Prentice-Hall, Inc., Englewood Cliffs, New Jersey.)

REFERENCES

Baumgartner, T. A., and Jackson, A. S. *Measurement for Evaluation in Physical Education.* Boston: Houghton Mifflin Co., 1975.

Behnke, A. R., and Wilmore, J. H. *Evaluation and Regulation of Body Build and Composition.* Englewood Cliffs, N. J.: Prentice-Hall, 1974.

Costill, D. L.; Hoffman, W. M.; Kehoe, F.; Miller, S. J.; and Meyers, W. C. "Maximum Anaerobic Power among College Football Players." *J. Sports Med. Physical Fitness* 8 (1968): 103–106.

Jackson, A. S., and Pollock, M. L. "Generalized Equations for Predicting Body Density of Men." *Br. J. Nutr.* 40 (1978): 497–504.

Jackson, A. S.; Pollock, M. L.; and Ward, A.

"Generalized Equations for Predicting Body Density in Women." *Med. Sci. Sports Exercise* 12 (1980): 175–182.

Lewis, S.; Haskell, W. L.; Klein, H.; Halpern, J.; and Wood, P. O. "Prediction of Body Composition in Habitually Active Middle-aged Men." *J. Appl. Physiol.* 39 (1975): 221–225.

Mathews, D. K., and Fox, E. L. *The Physiological Basis of Physical Education and Athletics.* Philadelphia: W. B. Saunders Co., 1971.

Parízková, J. "Total Body Fat and Skinfold Thickness in Children." *Metabolism* 10 (1961): 794–807.

Wilmore, J. H., and Behnke, A. R. "An Anthropometric Estimation of Body Density and Lean Body Weight in Young Men." *J. Appl. Physiol.* 27 (1969): 25–31.

Wilmore, J. H., and Behnke, A. R. "An Anthropometric Estimation of Body Density and Lean Body Weight in Young Women." *Amer. J. Clin. Nutr.* 23 (1970): 267–274.

Glossary of Terms

Acceleration: rate of change in velocity.

Acclimatization: adaptation to a particular environmental stress.

Acid-base balance: the proper balance of H and OH ions in the blood.

Acidosis: the situation in which the acid-base balance shifts to the acid side, due either to increased levels of unbuffered acids in the blood or to a reduction in the blood bicarbonates.

Actin: thin protein filament that acts with the protein filament myosin to allow muscle contraction.

Action potential: The change in the electrical potential across the cell or tissue membrane.

Acute: referring to something immediate or of short duration, e.g., a treadmill run to exhaustion would be an acute bout of exercise.

Adipose tissue: connective tissue in which fat is stored.

Adolescence: developmental period of time between the onset of puberty and the attainment of full physiological maturity.

ADP: adenosine diphosphate. A high energy phosphate compound from which ATP is synthesized.

Adrenal glands: endocrine glands located directly above each kidney, composed of the medulla (the hormones epinephrine and norepinephrine) and the cortex (cortical hormones).

Adrenaline: see epinephrine.

Adrenocorticotrophic hormone (ATCH): a pituitary hormone responsible for controlling the hormones released by the adrenal cortex.

Aerobic: in the presence of air or oxygen.

Aerobic power: synonomous with the terms maximal oxygen uptake, maximal oxygen consumption, and cardiovascular endurance capacity.

Afferent nerve: sensory nerve that carries impulses from the sensory receptors, e.g., skin, eyes, ears, to the central nervous system.

Agility: the ability to change directions rapidly while maintaining total body balance and awareness of body position.

Aldosterone: hormone from the adrenal cortex responsible for sodium retention.

Alkaline reserve: the amount of bicarbonate in the blood available for buffering acids.

Alkalosis: the situation in which the acid-base balance shifts to the alkaline, or basic, side.

Alveolar air: that air present in the alveoli which is involved in the exchange of gases with the blood in the pulmonary capillaries.

Alveoli: small air sacs, located at the termination of the pulmonary tree, in which the exchange of respiratory gases takes place with the blood in the adjacent capillaries.

Amino acids: the basic building blocks of protein.

Amphetamine: prescription drug that stimulates the central nervous system.

Anabolic steroid: a prescription drug that has the anabolic or growth-stimulating characteristics of the male androgen, testosterone. Frequently taken by athletes to increase body size and muscle bulk.

Anabolism: the building up of body tissue.

Anaerobic: in the absence of oxygen.

Anaerobic threshold: that point where the metabolic demands of exercise cannot be met totally by available aerobic sources and at which an increase in anaerobic metabolism occurs, as reflected by an increase in the blood lactate.

Androgen: male sex hormone from the testes, and, in limited amounts, from the adrenal cortex.

Anemia: inadequate number of red blood cells, or low hemoglobin levels, limiting oxygen transport.

Angina pectoris: chest pain associated with a lack of blood to the heart.

Angstrom: unit of measure equal to 10^{-8} cm.

Anorexia: inadequate appetite, which, if chronic, e.g., anorexia nervosa, can lead to eventual death.

Anoxia: inadequate oxygen in the blood or tissues.

Anthropometry: the study of body measurements.

Antidiuretic hormone: hormone from the posterior pituitary gland, which promotes water retention through its action on the kidney.

Arteriole: a small artery that regulates the flow of blood from the arteries to the capillaries.

Arteriosclerosis: loss of elasticity of the arteries, or hardening of the arteries. The precursor to various diseases of the cardiovascular system, e.g., stroke and coronary artery disease.

Artery: a vessel which transports blood away from the heart.

Aspartates: potassium and magnesium salts of aspartic acid.

Athlete's heart: an enlarged heart, typically found in endurance athletes, due, primarily, to hypertrophy of the left ventricle. It is no longer considered to be a pathological or diseased condition, as it once was.

ATP: adenosine triphosphate. A high-energy compound from which the body derives its energy.

Atrium: one of the chambers of the heart. The right atrium receives blood from the systemic circulation, and the left atrium receives blood from the pulmonary circulation.

Atrophy: loss of size, or mass, of body tissue, e.g., muscle atrophy with disuse.

Autonomic nervous system: that portion of the nervous system that controls involuntary activity, e.g., smooth muscle and the myocardium, and includes both sympathetic and parasympathetic nerves.

Axis cylinder: the central core of the axon of the nerve fiber.

Axon: the fiber-like extension of the nerve cell, which transmits the nerve impulse away from the cell body.

Balance: the ability to have complete control of the body as it is moved through space.

Basal metabolic rate (BMR): the rate of body metabolism under the most optimal conditions of quiet, rest, and relaxation. The lowest rate of metabolism compatible with life.

Blood pressure: the force that blood exerts against the walls of the blood vessels or heart.

Body density: the density of the body is equal to the body weight divided by the body volume.

Bronchiole: small terminal branch of the bronchus.

Bronchus: the subdivision of the trachea, as it splits into two branches.

Buffer: a substance in the blood that combines with either acids or bases to maintain a constant acid-base, or pH, balance.

Calorie: a unit of heat energy defined as the amount of heat required to raise the temperature of one kilogram of water 1°C, from 15 to 16°C.

Calorimeter: a device for measuring the heat production of the body or of specific chemical reactions.

Capillaries: the smallest vessels in the vascular system which connect the arterioles and venules, where all exchanges of gases or materials between the circulatory system and the tissues or lungs take place.

Carbohydrate: a food substance that includes various sugars and starches and is found in the body in the form of glucose and glycogen.

Cardiac: relating to the heart, e.g., cardiac muscle and cardiac output.

Cardiac muscle: the myocardium, or muscle, of the heart.

Cardiac output: output, or volume, of blood pumped by the heart per minute. The product of heart rate and stroke volume.

Cardiovascular endurance capacity: the term used to define overall body endurance, or stamina. See aerobic power or maximal oxygen uptake.

Catabolism: the tearing down, or destruction, of body tissue.

Catalyst: a chemical substance that initiates or accelerates a chemical action without being altered as a result of the action.

Central nervous system: that division of the nervous system that includes the brain and spinal cord.

Cerebellum: the hindbrain, responsible for the smooth coordination of body movements.

Cerebral cortex: the portion of the brain that contains the primary and supplementary motor areas which control all movement patterns of a voluntary nature.

Cerebrum: the large forebrain.

Cholesterol: a lipid or fatty substance essential for life and found in various tissues and fluids. Elevated levels in the blood have been associated with an increased risk of cardiovascular disease.

Chronic: referring to something of an extended or long-term nature, e.g., physical training program of six months' duration.

Cinematography: the use of films to analyze movement.

Circuit training: selected exercises or activities performed in sequence, as rapidly as possible.

Collagen: a protein substance found in bones, cartilage, and white fibrous tissues.

Concentric contraction: a muscular contraction in which shortening of the muscle occurs.

Conditioned reflex: a nervous reflex pattern that is learned.

Conduction: transfer of heat or cold through direct contact with an object or medium.

Connective tissue: specialized tissue, such as ligaments and tendons, that connects various body structures.

Convection: the transfer of heat or cold from a body to a moving liquid or gas.

Coordination: the act of movement in an organized, controlled, and precise manner.

Coronary arteries: those arteries that supply the heart muscle or myocardium.

Cortex: refers to the outer layer, e.g., cerebral cortex is the outer layer of the brain.

Cortisol: a hormone from the adrenal cortex.

Creatine phosphate: an energy-rich compound, which plays a critical role in providing energy for muscular contraction.

Dead space: the volume of the various parts of the respiratory system in which no gas exchange occurs.

Dehydration: loss of body fluids.

Dendrite: the projection of the nerve cell that transmits impulses toward the cell body.

Diaphragm: the major muscle of respiration, which separates the thorax from the abdomen.

Diastole: the relaxation phase of each cardiac cycle, immediately following the contraction, or systole, of the heart.

Diastolic pressure: the lowest pressure of the arterial blood against the walls of the vessels or heart resulting from the diastole of the heart.

Diuretic: a substance that increases kidney function leading to a loss of body fluids through frequent urination.

Dynamometer: a device for measuring muscular strength.

Dyspnea: labored breathing.

Eccentric contraction: lengthening of the muscle under tension, as when lowering a heavy object.

Ectomorphy: one of three categories of the somatotype in which the body is rated for the degree of linearity.

Edema: filled with fluid.

Effective blood volume: that volume of blood available to supply the exercising muscles.

Efferent nerve: also referred to as a motor nerve or motoneuron. Conducts impulses from the central nervous system to the various end organs, such as muscle.

Electrocardiogram (ECG): a recording of the electrical activity of the heart.

Electrocardiograph: an instrument that picks up and produces a record of the electrical activity of the heart.

Electromyogram (EMG): a recording of the elec-measure joint angles and changes in joint angles.

Electrolyte: any solution that conducts electricity by means of its ions.

Electromyogram (EMG): A recording of the electrical activity of a muscle or a group of muscles.

Endocrine gland: a ductless gland that produces and/or releases hormones directly into the blood stream.

Endomorphy: one of three categories of the somatotype in which the body is rated for corpulence or obesity.

Endurance: the ability to resist fatigue. Includes

muscular endurance, which is a local or specific endurance, and cardiovascular endurance, which is a more general, total body endurance.

Enzyme: an organic catalyst that speeds the velocity of specific chemical reactions.

Epinephrine: one of the hormones of the adrenal medulla. Also referred to as adrenaline.

Epiphysis: that part of the long bone that ossifies separately before uniting with the main shaft, or diaphysis, of the bone.

Ergogenic aid: substance or phenomenon that elevates or improves physical performance.

Ergograph: an instrument or device used for recording muscular work.

Ergometer: a device for exercising the subject in a manner in which the physical work performed can be measured, e.g., bicycle ergometer.

Estrogen: female sex hormone.

Evaporation: the loss of heat through the conversion of the water in sweat to a vapor.

Exercise prescription: individualizing the exercise program on the basis of the duration, frequency, intensity, and mode of exercise.

External respiration: the process of bringing air into the lungs and the resulting exchange of gas between the alveoli and the capillary blood.

Fartlek training: speed play, where the athlete varies his or her pace at will from fast sprints to slow jogging; normally performed in the country, using hills.

Fascia: connective tissue surrounding and connecting muscle.

Fast-twitch muscle fiber: one of several types of muscle fibers that have low oxidative capacity, high glycolytic capacity, and are associated with speed or power activities.

Fat: a food substance that is composed of gylcerol and fatty acids.

Fatigue: inability to continue work, due to any one or a combination of factors.

Fatty acid: along with glycerol, the product of the breakdown of fats.

Fat weight: absolute amount of body fat. Fat weight plus lean body weight equals total body weight.

Flexibility: the range of movement of a specific joint or a group of joints, influenced by the associated bones and boney structures, muscles, tendons, and ligaments.

Glucagon: a hormone from the pancreas that acts to increase blood glucose, or sugar, levels.

Glucose: a simple sugar which is transported in the blood and metabolized in the tissues.

Glycerol: a substance that combines with fatty acids to form fat.

Glycogen: the storage form of carbohydrates in the body, found predominantly in the muscles and liver.

Glycogen loading: manipulating exercise and diet to optimize the total amount of glycogen stored in the body.

Glycogenolysis: the metabolic breakdown of glycogen.

Glycolysis: breakdown of glycogen to lactic acid.

Golgi tendon organ: a proprioceptor located in series with muscle tendons.

Gonads: endocrine glands responsible for reproduction; the testes in males and ovaries in females.

Growth hormone (GH): a pituitary hormone responsible for contolling tissue growth. Also referred to as somatotrophic hormone.

Heat cramp: severe cramping of the skeletal muscles, due to excessive dehydration and the associated salt loss.

Heat exhaustion: a disorder due to an excessive heat load on the body, characterized by breathlessness, extreme tiredness, dizziness, and rapid pulse, and usually associated with a decrease in sweat production.

Heat stroke: the most serious heat disorder, characterized by a body temperature above 105°F, cessation of sweating, and total confusion or unconsciousness, which can lead to death.

Hematocrit: the relative contribution, or percentage, of the blood cells to the total blood volume.

Hemoconcentration: used in reference to an apparent increase in red blood cell number due to a plasma volume reduction, i.e., there is a relative, but not an absolute, increase.

Hemoglobin: iron pigment of the red blood cell that has a high affinity for oxygen.

Hormone: a chemical substance produced or released by one of the endocrine glands, which is transported by the blood to a specific target organ.

Hyperemia: an excessive amount of blood in a part of the body.

Hyperglycemia: elevated levels of glucose, or sugar, in the blood.

Hyperplasia: increase in size, due to an increased number of cells.

Hypertension: abnormally high blood pressure, usually defined in adults as a systolic pressure in excess of 140 mmHg and/or diastolic pressure in excess of 90 mmHg.

Hyperthermia: overheating.

Hypertrophy: increase in the size, or mass, of an organ or body tissue.

Hyperventilation: breathing rate and/or tidal volume increased above levels necessary for normal function.

Hypoglycemia: abnormally low blood glucose, or sugar, levels.

Hypotension: an abnormally low blood pressure.

Hypothalamus: that region of the brain involved in controlling or releasing many of the hormones of the pituitary gland.

Hypoxia: a lack of oxygen in the blood or tissues.

Inhibition: negative nervous control to restrict, or limit, the amount of force generated.

Innervation ratio: the ratio of the number of muscle fibers per motoneuron.

Insulin: a hormone produced by the pancreas that assists in the control of the blood sugar, or glucose, levels.

Internal respiration: the exchange of gases between the blood and tissues.

Interval training: training program that alternates bouts of heavy or very heavy work with periods of rest or light work.

In vitro: functioning outside of, or detached from, the body.

In vivo: functioning within the body.

Ion: an electrically charged atom or group of atoms.

Ischemia: a temporary deficiency of blood to a specific area of the body.

Isokinetic contraction: contraction in which the muscle generates force against a variable resistance where the speed of movement is maintained constant.

Isometric contraction: contraction in which the muscle generates force, but there is no observable movement, e.g., pushing against a building.

Isotonic contraction: contraction in which the muscle generates force against a constant resistance and movement results, either shortening (concentric) or lengthening (eccentric).

Kinesthesis: a sense, or awareness, of body position.

Lactic acid: the end product of glycolysis, or anaerobic metabolism.

Latent period: period of time between the stimulus and the response to that stimulus.

Lean body weight: determined by subtracting the fat weight from the total body weight. That weight of the body which is not fat, e.g., bone, muscle, skin, organ weights, etc.

Ligament: connective tissue that binds bone to bone, to maintain the integrity of a joint.

Lipid: fat, or fat-like, substance.

Manometer: an instrument for measuring pressure.

Maximal oxygen consumption: see maximal oxygen uptake.

Maximal oxygen intake: see maximal oxygen uptake.

Maximal oxygen uptake ($\dot{V}O_2$ max): the best physiological index of total body endurance. Also referred to as aerobic power, maximal oxygen intake, maximal oxygen consumption, and cardiovascular endurance capacity.

Menstruation: the periodic cycle in the uterus associated with preparation of the uterus to receive a fertilized egg.

Mental practice: mental rehearsal of the athletic event or sport.

Mesomorphy: one of three categories of the somatotype in which the body is rated for the degree of muscularity.

Metabolism: the sum total of the energy-producing and -absorbing processes in the body, i.e., the energy used by the body.

Micron: unit of measure equal to 0.001 mm.

Mitochondria: energy-producing bodies within the cell.

Motor area, or motor cortex: that area of the cerebral cortex which controls voluntary muscle movement.

Motor end plate: where the efferent or motor nerve attaches to the muscle fiber.

Motor nerve, or motoneuron: motor, or efferent, nerve which transmits impulses to muscles.

Motor unit: the motor nerve and the group of muscle fibers it supplies.

Muscle fiber: the structural unit of muscle. A single cell with multiple nuclei composed of a number of smaller units called myofibrils.

Muscle spindle: a sensory receptor located in the muscle itself, which senses changes in muscle tension.

Myelin sheath: the inner covering of the medullated nerve fiber.

Myocardium: the muscle of the heart.

Myofibril: the small elements which comprise the muscle fiber, composed of the proteins actin and myosin.

Myoneural junction: the junction between the muscle fiber and its nerve.

Myosin: a muscle protein that acts with actin, another muscle protein, to allow the muscle to contract.

Neurilemma: the outermost covering of a nerve fiber.

Neuron: the nerve cell; the basic structural unit of the nervous system. Conducts nervous impulses to and from various parts of the body.

Nitrogen narcosis: "rapture of the deep." A condition which is caused by breathing air underwater at depths where the partial pressure of nitrogen increases until it has a narcotic-like effect on the central nervous system, leading to distortions in judgment and sometimes to serious injury or death.

Norepinephrine: a hormone produced by the adrenal medulla and, also, a chemical transmitter substance at peripheral sympathetic nerve endings.

Obesity: an excessive amount of body fat. The state of being overfat.

One-repetition maximum (1-RM): the greatest amount of weight that can be lifted just one time.

Ossification: process of calcification or hardening of the bone during the growth process.

Overload: stressing the body or parts of the body to levels above that normally experienced.

Oxygen debt: the quantity of oxygen above normal resting levels used in the period of recovery from any specific exercise or muscular activity.

Oxygen poisoning: caused by breathing concentrations of oxygen for long periods of time during deep dives, resulting in visual distortion, confusion, rapid and shallow breathing, and convulsions.

Pacinian corpuscle: a proprioceptor located in muscle and tendon sheaths adjacent to joints.

Pancreas: an endocrine gland that produces both the hormones insulin and glucagon, which control blood glucose, or sugar, levels.

Parasympathetic nervous system: a major subdivision of the autonomic nervous system whose fibers arise from the midbrain, medulla, or sacral region of the spinal cord.

Parathormone: hormone produced by the parathyroid glands, which assists in controlling calcium and phosphorus levels.

Parathyroids: endocrine glands that are located on or embedded in the thyroid glands and that produce parathormone.

Pericardium: the fibrous sac that encapsulates the heart.

Periosteum: the fibrous membrane that surrounds bone.

Peripheral nervous system: that part of the nervous system that lies outside the central nervous system, i.e., spinal cord and brain.

pH: a system for expressing the degree of acidity or alkalinity of a solution, in which a value of 7.0 is neutral, greater than 7.0 alkaline, and less than 7.0, acidic.

Plasma: the liquid fraction of the whole blood.

Ponderal index: defined as height divided by the cube root of weight.

Power: the product of force and velocity. This is probably far more important than absolute strength alone.

Precapillary sphincter: small band of smooth muscle controlling the flow of blood to the true capillaries.

Progressive overload: gradually increasing the training stimulus in a systematic manner.

Progressive resistance exercise (PRE): the resistance used in training is progressively increased systematically as the body adapts to the training stimulus.

Proprioceptor: a sensory receptor sensitive to pressure, stretch, tension, pain, etc.

Protein: a food substance formed from amino acids.

Pulse: periodic expansion of the artery, resulting from the systole of the heart.

Pulse pressure: the mathematical difference between the systolic and diastolic pressures.

Radiation: the transfer of heat through electromagnetic waves.

Reaction time: the period of time between the presentation of a stimulus and the subsequent reaction to that stimulus.

Reciprocal inhibition: the inhibition of the antagonist muscles, which allows the agonists to move.

Reflex: an automatic, involuntary, unlearned response to a given stimulus.

Relative body fat: the ratio of fat weight to total body weight, expressed as a percentage.

Relative humidity: a ratio expressing the degree of moisture in the surrounding air.

Repetition running: similar to interval training but with long work intervals and long periods of recovery.

Residual volume: that volume of air remaining in the lung following a maximal expiration. Vital capacity plus residual volume equal total lung capacity.

Respiration: the exchange of gases at both the level of the lung and tissue.

Respiratory exchange ratio (R or RER): the ratio of carbon dioxide expired to oxygen consumed, at the level of the lungs.

Respiratory quotient (RQ): the ratio of the carbon dioxide produced in the tissues to the oxygen consumed by the tissues.

Ruffini receptor: a proprioceptor located in the joint capsule.

Sarcolemma: the membrane surrounding the muscle fiber.

Sarcomere: the functional contractile unit of muscle, which is a part of the myofibril.

Sarcoplasm: the fluid portion of the muscle fiber, or the muscle protoplasm.

Sarcoplasmic reticulum: network of tubules and vesicles within muscle fibers, which are necessary to allow excitation of the muscle fibers.

Sensory nerve: afferent or sensory nerves transmit impulses from the sensory organs to the central nervous system.

Skeletal muscle: muscle controlling skeletal movement that is normally under voluntary control.

Slow-twitch muscle fiber: one of several types of muscle fibers that have high oxidative capacity, low glycolytic capacity, and are associated with endurance type activities.

Smooth muscle: involuntary muscle, such as that which lines blood vessels and the gastrointestinal tract.

Somatic nervous system: the voluntary nervous system, including both cranial and spinal nerves.

Somatogram: a chart on which somatotypes are plotted.

Somatotrophic hormone: a hormone released by the pituitary gland that influences growth. Also referred to as STH, or growth hormone (GH).

Somatotype: the characterization of the body physique in an objective and systematic manner.

Sphygmomanometer: an instrument used to measure arterial blood pressure.

Spirometer: an instrument used to measure the various lung volumes and dynamic lung function.

Strength: the ability of a muscle to exert force.

Stroke volume: the volume of blood pumped per contraction of the ventricle.

Sympathetic nervous system: a major division of the autonomic nervous system.

Synapse: the junction between two neurons.

Systole: the contraction phase of the cardiac cycle.

Systolic pressure: the greatest pressure in the vessels or heart during a cardiac cycle, resulting from the systole.

Tendon: connective tissue that attaches muscle to bone.

Testosterone: the predominant male androgen.

Thyroid gland: an endocrine gland located at the base of the neck, which produces several hormones regulating total body metabolism.

Thyroid-stimulating hormone: a pituitary hormone which controls the thyroid gland's release of thyroxin.

Thyroxin: a hormone produced by the thyroid gland, which assists in the control of total body metabolism.

Tidal volume: the amount of air inspired or expired during a normal breathing cycle.

Tonus: that quality of a muscle which gives it firmness in the absence of a voluntary contraction.

Total lung capacity: the sum of the vital capacity and the residual volume.

Valsalva maneuver: increased intraabdominal

and intrathoracic pressure created by holding the breath and attempting to compress the contents of the abdominal and thoracic cavities.

Vasopressin hormone: a pituitary hormone which controls blood vessel diameter.

Vein: a vessel that transports blood back to the heart.

Velocity: speed, or the rate, of movement.

Ventilation: movement of air into and out of the lungs.

Ventricle: a chamber of the heart that expels, or pumps, blood into the lungs (right ventricle) or into the systemic circulation (left ventricle).

Venule: a small vein that provides the link between capillaries and veins.

Vestibular receptor: a proprioceptor located in the ear.

Viscosity: that quality of a fluid that describes its flow characteristics. Water has a low viscosity, while honey has a high viscosity.

Vital capacity: the greatest volume of air that can be expired following the deepest possible inspiration.

Work: the product of force and distance.

Index